D1453861

Concepts of
ONCOLOGY NURSING

PRENTICE-HALL, INC.   *Englewood Cliffs, New Jersey 07632*

Concepts of
ONCOLOGY NURSING

DONNA L. VREDEVOE, Ph.D.
Professor
Teaching in Graduate Nursing Oncology Program and Nursing Research
School of Nursing, UCLA

ANAYIS DERDIARIAN, R.N., M.N.
LINDA PATTI SARNA, R.N., M.N.
MAIRE FRIEL, R.N., M.N.
Assistant Clinical Professors
Teaching in Graduate Nursing Oncology Program
School of Nursing, UCLA

JOSEPHINE A. GATAN SHIPLACOFF, R.N., M.N.
Clinical Research Nurse Coordinator
Division of Surgical Oncology
Department of Surgery, UCLA

with contribution by
CAROL A. BRAINERD, R.N., M.N.
Oncology Program Director
Visiting Nurses Association of Pasadena and San Gabriel Valley
Pasadena, California

Library of Congress Cataloging in Publication Data

Main entry under title:

Concepts of oncology nursing.

   Includes bibliographies and index.
   1. Cancer—Nursing. I. Vredevoe, Donna L.
[DNLM: 1. Neoplasms—Nursing. WY 156 C745]
RC266.C66   610.73'698   80-27886
ISBN 0-13-166587-1   AACR1

Editorial/production supervision and
  interior design by Ros Herion
Cover design by Frederick Charles, Ltd.
Manufacturing buyer: John Hall

Printed in the United States of America

10 9 8 7 6 5 4 3 2

Prentice-Hall International, Inc., *London*
Prentice-Hall of Australia Pty. Limited, *Sydney*
Prentice-Hall of Canada, Ltd., *Toronto*
Prentice-Hall of India Private Limited, *New Delhi*
Prentice-Hall of Japan, Inc., *Tokyo*
Prentice-Hall of Southeast Asia Pte. Ltd., *Singapore*
Whitehall Books Limited, *Wellington, New Zealand*

Contents

CHAPTER THREE
Psychosocial Variables in Cancer Management:
Considerations for Nursing Practice *36*
by Anayis Derdiarian

CHAPTER FOUR
Concepts in the Nursing Care of Patients
Undergoing Cancer Assessment *51*
by Linda Patti Sarna

CHAPTER FIVE
Concepts in the Nursing Management of Patients
Receiving Cancer Chemotherapy and Immunotherapy *81*
by Linda Patti Sarna

Preface

This book is intended as a textbook for nursing students, primarily in graduate courses that include content on care of oncology patients. The list of topics could not be exhaustive, but it reflects considerable thought by each author in selecting those concepts and topics that are of greatest relevance to patient care.

The book begins with an introduction to cancer as a disease. It progresses to an examination of basic physiological, psychological, and sociological variables that are of concern in assessing and intervening with cancer patients. The next chapters explore the clinical variables that relate to cure and care of oncology patients. While the medical bases of the disease and its sequellae are explored, the main emphasis is on nursing aspects of cancer care. After this examination of nursing care of the cancer patient, the subject shifts to prevention of the disease, its secondary consequences, and side effects. This area of prevention emerges as one that involves patient education as a primary intervention tool. The knowledge of the predisposing factors in the etiology of cancer is transferred to the patient to allow the patient to discriminate danger signals of cancer. Rehabilitation is a most important aspect in the cancer process. The patient with the disease arrested, slowed, or eliminated faces the readjustment to his or her milieu. Here nursing plays an important role in facilitating the adjustment of the patient, in minimizing new problems, and in educating the patient and family as to how to cope with a return to a home and/or career environment. These situations, concepts, and ideas all generate countless researchable ideas. The next two chapters develop the role of the researcher and some approaches to clinical research in nursing oncology. The last chapter presents nursing models that are relevant to clinical assessment and research.

Donna L. Vredevoe
Anayis Derdiarian
Linda Patti Sarna
Maire Friel
Josephine A. Gatan Shiplacoff

Concepts of
ONCOLOGY NURSING

chapter one

DONNA L. VREDEVOE, Ph.D.
Professor
Teaching in Graduate Nursing
Oncology Program and Nursing Research
School of Nursing, UCLA

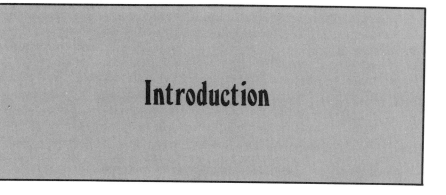

Introduction

When cancer occurs, varying degrees and types of changes occur in those affected. There are physiological changes ranging from subtle immunological alterations to disruption of functions of infected organs. Patients tend to focus on those physiological alterations that produce pain, discomfort, loss of function, disfigurement, or change in appearance. However, many profound changes in cell metabolism preceded these overt manifestations of malignancy. Patients who are diagnosed while asymptomatic or early symptomatic often anticipate and fear consequences of more serious forms of the malignancy. If patients could be certain that the probability of return to their normal health status was high and that treatment could be accomplished without major side effects, they likely would handle cancer much as an encounter with an infectious disease such as influenza. However, cancer, as a collection of a wide variety of malignant processes, offers too many permutations of possible consequences to the human mind. Somehow the human mind cannot always ignore the more hopeless of the consequences and focus on the more hopeful of the consequences. Hence fear, anxiety, feelings of loss of control, depression, and other psychological reactions begin to set in.

The nurse deals more with the reality of the disease. Entering into the care of a cancer patient the nurse will study the medical diagnosis and predicted consequences and work with the patient to help him* see what is really there now in regard to the disease process and what could come as a result of continuation of the disease process in treatment. The nurse helps the patient understand and cope with cancer. The nurse works with the patient and family to reestablish a pattern of normalcy after the disruption of the diagnosis of cancer. In some patients total cures are possible. In others the probability of death is very high. In the vast middle range are most of the cancer patients—somewhere between cure and death, caught up in the struggle by health care givers to bring them to as close to a cure or stability of disease as possible. Cancer treatment can range from risky and painful procedures to minor surgery with only follow-up exams. Again the range of possibilities in treatments is broad. Few diseases pose as many possible choices as to types of treatments. In this complex environment of multiple types of cancers, of known and unknown varying etiologies, with wide ranges of possible treatments, the nurse is the interpreter, care giver, teacher, and support for the patient.

Cancer is also a very visible disease. It affects one out of four to five Americans. It is present in people of all races, ethnic groups, social strata, occupations, and ages. While epidemiological and basic research studies are helping to identify conditions and substances that predispose subjects to develop cancer, the direct etiological agent of most cancers has not been identified. Vast sums of money have been spent in search of clues for cancer. More recently funds are being directed at utilizing existing knowledge for prevention of cancer.

This book is intended as a guide to the nurse and other care givers who are concerned with cancer patients. It is developed so as to present the fundamentals of the disease process and the psychological and sociological sequellae first. Then clinical applications are developed. Next, prevention and rehabilitation are considered. Finally the role of the researcher and ways to develop new knowledge are explored so that the cycle of creation of new knowledge for application of care of cancer patients is completed.

Since patient teaching is very important in care of cancer patients, many topics relating to cancer care are introduced with references to basic findings. It is hoped that the reader will search further

---

*In deference to both sexes, the pronouns "him" and "her" are used interchangeably throughout the book to describe a patient (except in discussions about cancer of sexual organs).

for the basic and current information relating to patient needs for information.

It is hoped, further, that the reader will be able to gain from this book a conceptual approach to problems in care of cancer patients. The process of moving from a discussion of basic systems in cancer to nursing care management to the development of new ideas through research is the theme developed here. By understanding the process developed in this book, readers can adjust this approach to topics that are not covered here in depth, but that are relevant to cancer care.

chapter
two

DONNA L. VREDEVOE, Ph.D.
Professor
Teaching in Graduate Nursing
Oncology Program and Nursing Research
School of Nursing, UCLA

Physiological variables related to cancer

INTRODUCTION

Many variables relate to the etiology, development, and treatment of cancer. This chapter is intended to introduce the reader to the broad spectrum of physiological variables involved in cancer. Psychological and sociological variables will be considered in Chapter 3. The reader should be aware, however, that all three types of variables—physiological, psychological, and sociological—tend to interact in cancer. Moreover, since there are so many physiological variables, not all can be presented here and described. Because a number of excellent review articles and books have been devoted to descriptions of some of the variables, this chapter has many references to direct the reader either to information on the original work on the variables or to subsequent studies or reviews on the subject.

In normal tissue, growth feedback mechanisms control cell multiplication so that tissues do not exceed their size capacity. In cancer the growth is uncontrolled to the extent that the cancerous cell eventually invades sites far distant from the point of origin and causes the tumor mass to disrupt normal cell funtions. In the early phase of tumor growth, tumor cells grow exponentially. As the tumor increases in size, the time it takes the tumor mass to double in volume increases. This is described as a Gompertzian function [13]. Three mechanisms have been proposed to explain the prolonged doubling time as the tumor mass increases: (1) The time from one cell mitosis to the next increases to thereby increase the cell cycle time; (2) the number of cells participating in cell division in the tumor decreases; and (3) there is an increase in cell loss from the tumor as it ages [13, 87].

Dividing cells, both normal and cancerous, go through the following series of phases: (1) the mitotic (M) phase; (2) the gap 1 (G_1) phase, which is a resting phase during which DNA synthesis for other than repair purposes is absent while RNA and protein synthesis continue; (3) the DNA synthetic (S) phase during which DNA synthesis occurs; and (4) the gap 2 (G_2) phase, another resting stage during which DNA synthesis ceases although RNA and protein synthesis continues [13,48]. The cell cycle is then completed as G_2 leads to the M phase. There is also another resting stage termed G_0. This G_0 stage is used to describe a stationary state for normal cells that are not in an active cycle but are capable of going into an active cycle after stimulation or release from inhibition [48].

Cancer cells can be in any of these stages. If the cells are in G_0 or in a prolonged G_1 they may be partially or completely insensitive to some chemotherapeutic agents. It is important to remember that a tumor mass contains both cancerous and normal cells. Normal cells in tumor masses could be fibroblasts, endothelial cells, lymphocytes, polymorphonuclear cells, mononuclear phagocytes, and so forth. The most important cell in the process of cancerous growth is the tumor stem cell [11]. This is the cell capable of extensive proliferation. In spontaneous animal tumors there are fewer tumor stem cells than in long-transplanted tumors in which almost all of the cells are stem cells. The growth potential of a tumor cell cannot be determined by morphology. The number of stem cells in an experimental animal tumor can be determined by transplantation assays or by in vitro cultivation of the tumor [48].

The transition to the neoplastic state is not necessarily an abrupt one. Accumulating evidence suggests that neoplastic development occurs in stages [6] and that a number of as yet undefined cellular events must occur before cancer cells result.

METASTASIS

In most cancers, excluding cancers of the skin, some metastasis, often micrometastasis, has occurred by the time the disease is diagnosed clinically [91,97,99]. This is not to say that metastasis has occurred in all patients at diagnosis. However, the transfer of cancer cells from the site of origin to distant sites in the body—that is, the process of metastasis—is so much a part of cancer that it can be regarded as a natural stage of the disease. The clinician must constantly be aware of the possibility of metastatic growth and treat the patient accordingly.

Animal models developed for studies of metastases [27] have provided experimental evidence for the concepts of this process. Although the actual mechanism of tumor invasion is unclear, the process has been described. Clearly there are factors related to the host and to the tumor that affect the rate of metastatic growth.

Metastases can occur by four major routes: (1) direct invasion in which tumor fragments invade nearby normal tissues; (2) via the lymphatic system; (3) via the hematogenous compartments of the circulatory system; and (4) by seeding of a body cavity [27,20,28, 101]. Tumors appear to gain advantages by: (1) entering the circulatory system, usually at vulnerable spots such as thin-walled venules in lymphatic channels; (2) having a well-established blood supply within the tumor and surrounding it, enabling entry of tumor cells into the circulatory system; (3) forming circulating emboli of tumor cells [60]; and (4) vascularizing micrometastases [30].

It has been hypothesized that the type of cell that metastasizes is one with unique properties. Fidler has summarized the evidence for this view: " . . . the metastatic lesion represents the end point of several destructive events that only a few cells can survive. . ." [27]. He provides evidence that, within a tumor, there is a subpopulation of cells that possess the unique potential to metastasize and that these cells do so by overcoming host defenses [27]. If this is so, special efforts would be necessary to direct chemotherapeutic effects to these cells in particular.

The observation of Higginson [47] that 60% to 90% of human cancers may have been caused by environmental factors led to great interest in chemical carcinogenesis. Haenszel and colleagues [36,37] demonstrated that epidemiological studies that linked cancer and geographical location could not be explained by genetics of the people in those geographical locations. Thus, the hypothesis that environmental factors played a role in carcinogenesis was strengthened.

Eighteen chemicals or groups of chemicals, including four industrial processes, are thought to be directly or indirectly involved in occurrence of cancer in humans [75]. The four industrial processes are: (1) manufacture of auramine with a target organ of the bladder; (2) underground hematite mining with a target organ of lung and a main route of exposure via inhalation; (3) nickel refining with target organs of the nasal cavity and lung and main route of exposure via inhalation; and (4) manufacture of isopropyl alcohol by the strong-acid process with a target organ of the paranasal sinuses. In these industries the exact carcinogen is unknown and the results cannot be generalized to all situations involving these processes [75,94].

The 14 chemicals or groups of chemicals with associated neoplasms are as follows [75, with specific references in that paper]:

1. 4-aminobiphenyl: bladder cancer
2. Arsenic and certain arsenic compounds: skin cancer, lung cancer in smelter workers inhaling arsenic trioxide, blood dyscrasias, and liver tumors
3. Asbestos: mesotheliomas and lung cancers, gastrointestinal tract cancers, cancer of larynx
4. Benzene: leukemia
5. Benzidine: bladder cancer
6. Chlornaphazine: bladder cancer
7. Bis (chloromethyl) ether (BCME) and technical grade chloromethyl methyl ether (CMME): oat cell carcinoma, lung cancer
8. Chromium and certain chromium compounds: lung cancer
9. Diethylstilbestrol: clear cell carcinoma of the vagina by in utero exposure
10. Melphalan: acute leukemia
11. Mustard gas: respiratory tract cancer
12. 2-naphthylamine: bladder cancer
13. Soots, tars, and certain mineral oils: cancer of skin, lung, bladder, and gastrointestinal tract

14. Vinyl chloride: angiosarcomas of liver and tumors of the brain, lung, and hemolymphopoietic system

In addition to these there are eighteen other chemicals, or groups of chemicals, that are probably carcinogenic for humans. This group includes cyclophosphamide [75]. The reader is urged to consult reference [75] for complete documentation of these associations between chemicals and cancer.

The evaluation of the carcinogenic risk to humans of these chemicals or processes was based on epidemiological or case studies. For several chemicals there was experimental evidence of carcinogenicity that led to the prediction of an association between exposure to the chemical and development of cancer. There are more than 200 other chemicals for which there is some evidence of natural carcinogenicity from at least one species of experimental animals [94, 45]. Suspected carcinogens also occur in some foods [67,77], for example, the aflatoxins. Food additives, herbicides, and pesticides have been evaluated for carcinogenicity and, where evidence supports a role in carcinogenesis, have been regulated [71,49,98]. The list of possible substances involved in carcinogenesis grows daily. It is important to note that natural as well as manufactured substances [67, 75] can be potential carcinogens.

The implications of chemical carcinogenesis for nursing are many. Patient teaching to avoid exposure or reexposure is of great importance. As industries move more and more to adapting protective measures for employees exposed to carcinogenesis, it is important to understand factors in motivation to use protective equipment. Since some of the exposure is through drugs used in medical treatment (for example, melphalan and cyclophosphamide [75]) patients should be alert to the carcinogenic side effects when they consent to use the drugs and as they participate in monitoring their treatment.

In 1964 strong evidence was presented that a high proportion of all human lung cancers is associated with cigarette smoking [85]. This observation has led to warnings in advertising about the potentially harmful effects of smoking, and to promotion of smoking-cessation programs, patient education about the need to avoid smoking, and the search for new types of nonhazardous cigarettes.

Efforts are being made to develop ways of predicting carcinogenicity of chemicals. Chemical carcinogens are thought to have one or both of the following characteristics:

1. Activity only after metabolism to ultimate carcinogens, the derivatives that initiate oncogenesis. The known exceptions are carcinogens that are alkylating or acylating agents per se.
2. Strong electrophilic reactants. Ultimate carcinogens contain relatively electron-deficient atoms that seek to react with nucleophilic sites—that is, atoms that have easily shared electrons. Nucleophilic sites are relatively abundant in DNA, in RNA, and in proteins [66].

There is evidence that tumor induction by chemical carcinogens is a two-stage process. Studies on induction of skin cancers in experimental animals demonstrated that local administration of low doses of a known chemical carcinogen did not result in induction of tumors [8,9,95]. This stage was termed *initiation*. Initiation is considered to be essentially irreversible. The second stage, *promotion*, may follow during the next months. The promotion stage is reversible. Promotion requires repeated doses of a promoter [66]. The classical promoter agent in mouse studies is croton oil used in the induction of skin tumors. Basically then, carcinogens are better able to produce cancers if agents that enhance their action are present after contact with the carcinogen.

The same type of two-stage tumor development was seen in tumors of the bladder [12,46], liver [70,4], lung [4], mammary gland [3], and thyroid [39] in laboratory animal systems. Thus the complexity of the induction of tumors by chemical carcinogens can be addressed in patient education so as to reassure people that a one-time exposure to a potential carcinogen does not necessarily mean that they will get cancer.

Several steps are being taken in prevention of initiation of cancer by chemical carcinogens. Mutation systems in vitro are being used to screen potential carcinogens. The most commonly used system is that of Ames and his associates [1,63], in which *Salmonella typhmurium* acts as a tester strain. Other assays utilize other bacteria, fungi, plants, insects, and mammalian cells [44,72,89]. The tests are relatively accurate in predicting carcinogenic activity of test chemicals for experimental animals and humans, but there are still problems of false-negatives and false-positives. Thus these tests cannot yet be regarded as specific for determining action of potential carcinogens in humans. While the in vitro transformation and mutation assays are exciting developments, in vivo animal carcinogenicity assays have not been replaced.

Environmental studies are being directed at early recognition of hazardous materials, reduction of pollution, and emphasis on education. Clinical evaluation and follow-up of workers exposed to hazardous materials have been initiated. The vigorous attempts to follow workers exposed to asbestos have resulted in earlier case finding and treatment.

Efforts are also directed at prevention of promotion of initiated cells. The administration of certain retinoids can reduce the incidence of some types of cancers. The incidence of cancer of the skin, lungs, bladder, and breast in experimental animals has been reduced by the administration of retinoids after administration of the chemical carcinogen [86]. The retinoids are able apparently to prevent the promoting influence.

The obvious preventive measure most pertinent to nursing is patient education about ways to avoid initial exposure or to lessen the risk of cancer from a previous exposure. Patient screening for early warning signals of cancer is important when clinical carcinogens are used in industry.

The mechanism of chemical carcinogenesis is still not understood. Most carcinogens are mutagens, either directly or after metabolism. Among the mechanisms proposed for chemical carcinogenesis are: (1) direct transformation due to mutation of genetic material; (2) change of essential control mechanisms of the genome; (3) activation of endogenous oncogenic virus carried on the cell genome; (4) immunosuppression which favors proliferation of cancer cells that would normally be suppressed by immune systems; or (5) a combination of these mechanisms [69].

―――――――――――――― VIRUSES AND CANCER ――――――――――――――

While strong evidence for viral etiology of animal tumors exists [35], the evidence for viral etiology of human cancers is less convincing. Three groups of viruses have been associated with cancers in humans and animals: (1) DNA herpesviruses; (2) the "C-type" RNA viruses; and (3) the "B-type" RNA mammary tumor viruses [58]. The designation "C-type" and "B-type" are morphological classification categories for oncogenic viruses or viruses related to cancer. Human cancers and their suspected viral etiological agents are

1. Burkitt's lymphoma and the DNA Epstein Barr virus (EBV) [103, 56]
2. Acute leukemia and an RNA C-type leukemia virus [31,25]

3. Mammary carcinoma and an RNA B-type virus [24,5,64]
4. Cervical carcinoma and the DNA herpes simplex virus type 2 [73]

Evidence for the association of EBV and Burkitt's lymphoma perhaps is the strongest. The EBV virus is a human virus known to be the etiological agent of infectious mononucleosis, a lymphoproliferative disease. EBV is oncogenic in subhuman primates. In seroepidemiological studies, Burkitt's lymphoma and nasopharyngeal carcinoma are associated with elevated EBV antibody titers [21,22,102]. The viral nucleic acid has been shown by biochemical studies to be present in Burkitt's lymphoma biopsies and in epithelial tumor cells of nasopharyngeal carcinomas. Indeed, based on this knowledge, a scheme of EBV-induced pathogenesis has been proposed for experimental testing [103]. There have been proposals that a preventive vaccine for Burkitt's lymphoma be developed [54]. This is based on the success of a vaccine for Marek's disease, a herpes virus-induced lymphoma in chickens [7]. However, preliminary work to determine whether there is more than one type of EBV and the possible natural sources of subclinical disease or disease produced by related viruses that cross-immunize to EBV must be completed first.

The case for the association of acute leukemia in humans and an RNA virus is most tenuous. It is based largely on inferences from work in animals that clearly associated RNA viruses with leukemias [35]. However, even in the animal studies the exact role of the viruses in production of leukemia remains to be elucidated.

Evidence for a viral cause of mammary carcinoma is weak and rests on two observations: (1) of biochemical and immunological cross-reactions of human breast cancer with murine mammary tumor virus (MTV); and (2) of the presence of virus particles, similar to those associated with MTV, in human milk and in an occasional tissue culture line of human breast cancer tissues [90].

Herpes simplex virus (HSV) was first isolated from primary lesions of three cases of acute vulvovaginitis in 1946 [83]. Convalescent sera of the three patients showed neutralizing antibody. The HSV cytological features in vaginal and cervical Pap smears were supported by virus isolation and neutralizing antibody in convalescent sera in studies in 1963 [88].

Evidence associating HSV with cervical carcinoma came from a screening of Pap smears for cervical anaplasia and detectable genital herpes virus [68]. These and other studies led to seroepidemiological studies that confirmed the association between HSV-2. However, direct evidence that HSV-2 is the etiological agent of cervical carcinoma is lacking. Two variables that discriminate between women with cervical cancer and the control group are the initiation of sexual activity at an early age and exposure to multiple sexual partners [76]. Metaplastic changes normally occur in cervical epithelium during puberty and during the first pregnancy. It has been hypothesized that infection by HSV-2 during a period of normal cervical metaplasia is an event leading to the development of cancer [74]. While there is an association between neutralizing antibody to HSV-2 of cervical carcinoma it has not been shown that the virus is the etiological agent of cancer [74].

There is also preliminary epidemiological evidence for a viral etiology of Hodgkin's disease [84,96]. Further, there is evidence for an association of Herpes simplex virus, type I and oral carcinoma [80]. In the case of most cancers, viral etiology has been considered at some time in the past or present.

Even if viral etiology were conclusively shown, one would have to consider whether the virus was transmitted horizontally—that is, from one person to another person in the environment—or vertically—that is, by the viral genome that is transmitted from generation to generation or by introduction of the virus via the placenta or nursing milk. Immunization against horizontally transmitted viruses would be successful if the immunization suppressed virus genetic expression and hence controlled tumor development. Other considerations in immunization would be: (1) whether the incidence of the type of cancer was sufficiently high to warrant immunization; (2) whether previous natural exposure to the virus has occurred; and (3) whether factors other than virus are involved in the etiology of the cancer and what effects viral immunization would have on the other factors.

PHYSICAL CARCINOGENESIS

Irritation and trauma are known to be involved in carcinogenesis. Tumors arise in experimental animals when materials such as cellophane, nylon, bakelite, or polystyrene are implanted. Whether this is due to a chemical carcinogen in the materials, irritation, induction of oncogenic viruses, or other factors is not known.

One of the most important physical carcinogens is irradiation. Sunlight is known to increase the risk of skin cancer. A condition known as xeroderma pigmentosum is an autosomal recessive disease in which there is a defect in the mechanism for repair of ultraviolet-induced damage to DNA. Patients with this condition are particularly prone to skin cancers induced by sunlight [48]. The incidences of human squamous cell carcinoma, basal cell carcinoma, and melanoma have been shown to be related to direct exposure to sunlight [48]. In the case of squamous and basal cell carcinomas the exposure of the site of primary tumor origin seems to be a factor in development of cancer. However, particularly in melanoma there is some evidence for influence of genetic and viral factors [14].

The most important type of radiation injury in oncogenesis is that induced by ionizing radiation. A major source other than natural radiation is medical radiation used in diagnostic procedures. There is evidence in some conditions that radiation is associated with an increase in cancer. X-ray therapy for ankylosing spondylitis was associated with an increase in leukemia in the treated group [18]. Radiation therapy for so-called "enlarged thymus" in the 1930s was associated with an increased incidence of thyroid cancer and leukemia years later [41]. Atomic bomb survivors showed an increased incidence of leukemia [59]. Radium watch dial paint resulted in an increased rate of bone and other cancers in those workers who ingested small amounts of the material in licking their brushes to make a fine point. The list of associations between exposure to ionizing radiation and radionuclides is a long one. The greatest risk from radiation seems to be the development of leukemia [48].

Many factors are involved in estimation of risk of developing cancer as a result of exposure to radiation. Tumor induction would depend on many factors such as the type of tissue; the hormonal state, age, and immunological status of the host; as well as genetic factors and the dose, route, rate and type of irradiation.

The exact mechanism of radiation-induced carcinogenesis is unknown. It is known that radiation damages DNA and causes mutations and chromosomal structural alteration. In one mouse system radiation has been shown to cause the activation of an oncogenic virus [52,53].

FETAL ANTIGENS IN CANCER

It is known that embryonic genes may be activated in human cancers. Expression of the embryonic genes is detected by their protein products termed *oncodevelopmental proteins*. Examples of these proteins are human chorionic gonadotrophin (HCG), alpha-fetoprotein, carcino-embryonic antigen (CEA) and Regan isoenzyme (placental alkaline phosphatase) [29]. While it was originally thought that these proteins were restricted to certain tumors, it is now known that they are on more types of tumors than expected and that minimal amounts of some of the proteins are found in noncancerous people.

No single oncodevelopmental substance has been found in all tumors.

Efforts are being made to use these proteins in cancer diagnosis and in understanding events in oncogenesis. A radioimunoassay for CEA is useful in early detection and management of some types of cancer, particularly colonic cancer. Gold and Freedman [32,33] showed that a CEA-like substance is released from cells of colonic carcinoma, but not from normal colon. Subsequent work has shown that CEA is associated with nonmalignant conditions as well [100]. Indeed, a glycoprotein has been isolated from the colonic lavages of healthy people that is immunologically equivalent to CEA from tumor tissue [81]. Hence cautious interpretations of the presence of this marker must be made if it is to be used in diagnosis and clinical tracking of the cancer.

HORMONES AND RISK OF CANCER

It has been suggested that risk of breast cancer is inversely related to urine estriol ratio, which reflects estrogen metabolism [17,57]. Epidemiological studies indicated that the estriol ratio and breast cancer rates are inversely correlated [23,61,62]. For example, young primiparas, who have a low rate of breast cancer, have a high estriol ratio [15]. On the other hand, case-control studies failed to support the relationship of estrogen metabolism, as measured by the estriol ratio, and incidence of breast cancer [16]. These studies indicate that there may be a relationship between estrogen metabolism and breast cancer, but that a great deal more work needs to be done to define the nature of the relationship. This is only one example of research into the hormonal status of the host as it relates to incidence of cancer. Hormonal status is an important area which will be the focus of much future research in cancer.

HORMONES IN TREATMENT OF CANCER

Information regarding the presence of estrogen receptors on breast cancer tissue is of considerable interest in selecting therapy for breast cancer patients. A significant percentage of these patients have hormone-dependent tumors that respond to hormonal manipulation such as additive hormonal therapy, or hormonal withdrawal through such procedures as oophorectomy, adrenalectomy, or hypophysectomy. Estrogen target tissues such as the uterus and certain mammary tumors have receptor macromolecules that have an affinity for binding with estrogen (specifically, estradiol-17 beta) [50]. A great deal of effort has been directed at determining whether identification of these receptors on breast cancers diagnosed will be useful in predicting prognosis and response to hormonal therapies. It is now clear that if estrogen receptors are not present on the breast cancer tissue, the chances of tumor regression in response to endocrine therapy are minimal. If the tumor tissue contains the estrogen receptors, approximately 55% of the cases will respond to endocrine therapy [65].

The concentration of estrogen receptors has been found to be the same in the primary tumor and its axillary node metastases [43]. Thus it appears that there is no detectable cell selection or modification during cell division and migration to the nodes. Benign tumors or noncarcinomatous breast tissue rarely contain estrogen receptors. Thus if a biopsy is found to contain estrogen receptors this is a characteristic of the cancer cells. There are then two types of breast carcinomas from a biochemical point of view: (1) those that contain specific estrogen receptors (termed estradiol-17 beta receptors by biochemists) and thus are like the target organs for estrogens such as the uterus, and (2) those that contain no specific receptors for estrogen and may bind estradiol-17 beta in only a nonspecific way such as skeletal muscles [38]. There does not appear to be a correlation between the clinical stage of the patient and the quantity of estrogen receptors present [65].

Great care must be exercised in handling biopsy specimens for determination of estrogen receptors since the receptors are labile at room temperature. In explaining the nature of the test to patients, it should be emphasized that presence of estrogen receptors does not necessarily mean a favorable response to endocrine therapy. In recent years the percentage of primary tumors shown to contain the receptors has risen from approximately 50% to 70–80% as a result of increased sensitivity to detection methods for the receptors. However, only about 55% of those who have tumors with estrogen receptors will respond to endocrine therapy and then with variable long-term success [65].

HYPERTHERMIA AS AN ADJUNCT TO THERAPEUTIC PROTOCOLS

Hyperthermia is the induction of temperatures that exceed normal body temperature. Temperatures of 40° to 45°C would be considered moderate hyperthermia in humans. Experimental evidence has been accumulating over a number of years to indicate that malignant cells may be more sensitive to heat than normal cells and that hyperthermia may potentiate the effects of irradiation and chemotherapy in the treatment of cancer. The time sequence of administration of the various modalities is important. Although the molecular basis for the potentiating effect of hyperthermia is not well understood, there are indications that DNA damage [10] and stimulation of the immune system may be factors [79]. However, these effects are dependent on the mode of administration and duration of the hyperthermia [40].

Hyperthermia has been induced by whole-body heating, localized heating, microwaves, ultrasound, pyrogenic toxins, and bacteria. The pros and cons of these types of heat administration have been reviewed [40]. The most promising techniques are those that involve focusing of delivery as is possible with microwaves and ultrasound. These techniques are under study by several groups. Many technical improvements are needed such as ways of monitoring temperatures in normal and malignant tissue and analyses of optimal conditions for use of hyperthermia alone or in combination with X-irradiation or chemotherapy. There is mounting evidence that whole body hyperthermia may be hazardous to the host [79]. Thus this is a type of adjunct to therapy that requires more research.

IMMUNE SYSTEMS

The cancer cell is an invader in the community of normal cells in the body. Key to the elimination of the cancer cells by immune mechanisms is recognition of them as foreign cells with surface determinants different from those of the normal tissue. These surface determinants have been termed *tumor specific antigens*. Clear evidence that tumor cells carry on their surface specific foreign antigens that can be recognized by the host came from experimental mouse tumors in inbred animals. Resistance to subsequent challenge with the same type of tumor was shown in mice in which intradermal tumors had grown for a while and then regressed to confer immunity on the host. Many other experiments confirmed that experimental tumors could induce immunity to subsequent rechallenge in hosts. Two types of tumor-specific antigens occur: (1) physically or chemically induced antigens; and (2) virus-induced antigens. In addition there are embryonic reversion antigens that represent reversions of antigenic specificities from adult to embryonic forms and are therefore not truly tumor specific. Such antigens were discussed previously.

The "foreignness" of a tumor cell is an important concept in tumor immunology. The immune system recognizes foreign substances, termed *antigens,* and responds in different ways. At this point a general overview of the immune response system will be made.

Perhaps best known is the humoral immune response in which an antibody immunoglobulin is produced in response to antigen. The antibody is specific in that it reacts only with that antigen or antigens very similar to it. This is the concept of specificity of the immune response. It used to be thought that antibodies for all of the specific antigens in the universe were shaped by the specific binding to the antigen. This template theory of antibody formation was one of several that provided alternative ways of viewing the immune response mechanism. After years of work it became apparent that the true explanation was that during development of an individual certain lymphocytes grew receptors for antigens on their surfaces. These receptors would then be available to bind with the specific antigen were it to be introduced into the body. When the antigen enters the body it binds to that small fraction of lymphocytes, termed *antigen binding cells,* which bears receptors to it. The antigen-binding cells divide and mature to secrete specific antibodies by a process termed *clonal selection.* Thus the specificity of the immune response rests with the interaction of antigen with the correct antigen-binding cells bearing the matching receptors.

Two classes of cells play predominant roles in the immune response. Lymphocytes have the property of specific response as just described. Macrophages play a nonspecific role in the immune response. There are two major classes of lymphocytes that have specific functions in the immune response (see Fig. 2.1). The thymus is the source of one class of lymphocytes termed *T cells.* The main function of the thymus is to produce and disseminate immunologically competent T lymphocytes. These T cells reside in the periarterial lymphatic sheath of the spleen and in the interfollicular and deep cortical areas of the lymph nodes. T cells have specific surface receptors, not related to immune functions, which can be used to identify them. By means of these markers, the T cells can be tracked to the peripheral blood, thoracic duct, and tissue sites. It is estimated that $65 \pm 15\%$ of peripheral blood lymphocytes are T cells [55]. Upon appropriate antigenic stimulation the small T lymphocytes can undergo blast transformation and proliferation to give rise to progeny. These activated lymphocytes play a direct role in cell-mediate immune responses such as the graft-versus-host reaction, delayed hypersensitivity, and resistance to microbial infections.

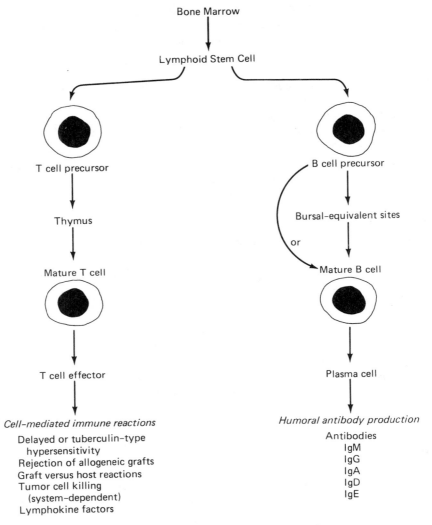

FIGURE 2.1 Origin and function of T and B lymphocytes.

These types of immune responses are termed *cell-mediated* as distinguished from the *humoral* responses mediated by immunoglobulins.

In addition to being effector cells (for example, T "killer" cells) in cell-mediated immunity, T cells also function as regulator "helper" cells in immunoglobulin production in the humoral immune mechanisms. They may also function as "suppressor" cells in inhibiting immune responses. Memory in the T cell system is thought to reside in long-lived T cells.

The counterpart lymphocyte system in the humoral immune response is the B lymphocyte system. These cells originate from the bone marrow in mammals or bursa in fowl. Stem cells develop into B cells, which are precursor cells for a variety of types of immunoglobulins. B lymphocytes home to the peripheral lymphoid organs where they predominate in the follicles and medullary cords. Fewer B than T cells circulate in peripheral blood. B cells carry specific receptors. When B cells contact antigen they undergo differentiation to eventually become plasma cells. It is the plasma cell that secretes large quantities of specific immunoglobulins [78,55,42,92].

Macrophages are also involved in the immune system. The macrophages develop from differentiation of bone monocytes which in turn develop from stem cells in the bone marrow. Macrophages may live several months. Macrophages play several important roles in the immune response. They phagocytose and process antigen for immune responses. Phagocytosis can release internal antigens of the microbial and other more complex antigens. There are, however, some antigens, termed *thymus-independent antigens,* that apparently stimulate lymphocytes directly. Another macrophage function is production of factors that regulate the B cell response. Macrophages can also act directly in certain cell-mediated immune responses and in tumor destruction [2]. Macrophages also have the ability to produce some components of *complement,* a component of lytic immune responses.

KINETICS OF ANTIBODY PRODUCTION

When an antigen enters the body there is a latent period of 4–24 hours before antibody-forming cells begin to appear [55]. During the next two weeks or longer, depending on the nature of release of the antigen, antibodies in the serum rise exponentially as the number of antibody forming cells increases. A complex feedback inhibition mechanism possibly regulated by T cells, macrophages, and the circulating antibodies themselves operates to depress the immune responses with time. This initial response to antigen is termed the *primary response.* If the same antigen is reintroduced, a more rapid antibody response occurs termed the *secondary response.* Different types of immunoglobulins are produced depending upon the phase of the immune response. Initially an immunoglobulin termed IgM is produced to be followed by IgG and later IgA. The primary response is primarily IgM, which is comparatively high molecular weight molecules

(19S). The secondary response is primarily IgG, a lower-weight immunoglobulin (7S) that constitutes more than 85% of total circulating antibody molecules. IgA may be either a circulating globulin or a globulin secreted on the surface of some organs. For example, it is found in milk, colostrum, tears, intestinal fluids, bronchial fluids, bronchial secretions, and saliva. It appears to play a role in protection of mucosal surfaces from microbial invasion [78]. The kinetics of IgM to IgG to IgA production are thought to be the result of antigen inducing B lymphocytes to switch from one type of globulin production to another.

Another immunoglobulin, IgE, has a profound ability to bind to tissues. This is the globulin that is produced in response to sensitization with allergens such as pollens and foods that induce the so-called *atopic hypersensitivities.* The antibody has also been termed *reagin.* It sensitizes mast cells in tissue or basophils in peripheral blood so that, when response to antigen occurs, the mast or basophils release biologically active materials upon contact with antigen that mediate the profound effects of atopic hypersensitivities such as sneezing, rhinitis, tearing, and skin rashes. The substances producing these effects are histamine, heparin, bradykinin, slow-reacting substance, serotonin, and acetylcholine [78]. Many factors are involved in atopic allergies and this topic cannot be dealt with in depth here.

Protein malnutrition has been associated with deficiencies in both humoral and cellular immunity. However, T cell-mediated immunological functions were increased by either protein or protein-calorie malnutrition of laboratory animals of various species [34]. The reasons for these contradicting findings are under study. Furthermore, a diet deficient in zinc resulted in depression of many aspects of immune functioning [77]. Since a well-functioning immunological system is important to general health and, very likely, to cancer prevention, these findings point to the need for special attention to nutritional studies on human subjects both with and without cancer. Fortunately, this is an active area of research.

─────────────── TUMOR IMMUNOLOGY ───────────────

There are several observations in human cancers that indicate that immune responses may be involved in rejection of tumors [19]:

1. Spontaneous remissions of pathologically proven cancers have occurred [26]. The highest incidence is seen in neuroblastoma, hypernephroma, choriocarcinoma, and malignant melanoma.

While there is no direct evidence of immune responses by the host to the tumor, the likelihood of an immune response is strong.

2. Tumor tissue may become infiltrated with lymphocytes, suggesting an immune response.

3. There is a higher incidence of cancer in patients with immunologic deficiencies either occurring as a result of a natural pathologic process or induced by immunosuppressive drugs.

4. Autopsies of persons for deaths unrelated to cancer reveal in some instances evidence of beginning cancers.

5. Some cancer patients appear to have decreased cell-mediated immune responses which are related to an increased growth rate of the cancer as compared to cancer patients with normal cell-mediated immune responses.

6. In a few cancers success of chemotherapy cannot be accounted for by direct cytotoxicity of the drug for the neoplastic cells. It is likely that residual cells are removed by immune responses.

If one accepts that tumors may possess tumor-specific antigens that could be recognized by the host and lead to an immune response, then one must ask how tumors escape immunological rejection. Mechanisms for escape of tumors are particularly important to understand since these mechanisms of escape might be those which could be overcome and thus result in therapy of the cancer. It has been postulated that an "immune surveillance" system operates to screen out emerging tumor cells. When this system is functioning well clones of tumor cells, which some theorists postulate may arise frequently in normal people, are cut off before they can reach clinically detectable size. The existence of such a system is based on inferences drawn from some of the evidence just presented that immunosuppression increases the incidence of cancer.

How then do tumors escape such a surveillance mechanism and grow in what should be a normally hostile immune response environment that recognizes the foreign tumor specific antigens? Several mechanisms have been proposed:

1. Immunological unresponsiveness, either induced by extraneous factors such as drugs or irradiation, or the result of a disease process or congenital immunodeficiency could create an environment freed of some of the immunological restraints found in normal individuals.

2. Specific immunological tolerance to cancer cell antigens may have occurred. Tolerance is a specific failure of the immune response to a known antigen [78]. It is specific to that antigen and

immune responses to other antigens are not affected. Tolerance could be predicted by the clonal selection theory if the contact with antigen occurred before or during maturation of the immune response system—that is, in fetal or early postnatal life when immunological stem cells could not yet recognize the invading antigen as foreign and hence could not develop cell receptors for it. By this theory, the body would develop immunological stem cells only with receptors to foreign antigens, and any antigen in the environment during fetal or very early postnatal life would be seen as self and hence could never be recognized by the immune system. This would be tolerance induced during embryonic or neonatal life. There is evidence that introduction of an antigen to a newborn experimental mouse induces tolerance to the antigen so that upon second contact with that antigen at an age when an immune response would be expected, the tolerant animal does not respond. Tolerance can also be induced in adult animals if an antigen is presented during an appropriate regimen of irradiation or antimetabolic drugs.

There is, however, no direct evidence that cancer patients are tolerant to autologous tumor cells. It seems more likely that, if tolerance plays a role in oncogenesis, it is at the level of tolerance to viral agents that might directly transform cells or create an environment for transformation of normal to neoplastic cells.

3. Tumor growth potential may so exceed the ability of the immune response to recognize antigen and contain it that tumors grow to the destruction of the host.

4. Tumors may be able to modulate their surface antigens through immunologically based genetic selection so that those antigens that produce minimal immune responses in the host survive. Such modifications of antigens have been seen in experimental systems.

5. Blocking immune factors may occur to favor the growth of the tumor. Immunological enhancement of tumor growth was noted many years ago. As originally observed by Kaliss [51] the growth of a strain-specific murine tumor in a genetically nonidentical mouse recipient (allogenic) would fail to be rejected in the foreign recipient if the recipient had been pretreated with antiserum to the tumor (passive enhancement) or had been immunized previously with antigenic material of the tumor genotype (active enhancement). Thus the allogenic tumor which would normally be rejected grew in the host bearing certain types of humoral antibodies. This system was extended to one in which the tumor and recipient were genetically identical (syngeneic) and the tumor was chemically or virally induced. The mechanism of

this enhancement is complex. It is thought that antibody inter-feres with immune responsiveness either by competing with potentially reactive lymphocytes for antigen, by exerting a central feedback-inhibiting control, or by a combination of these mechanisms [93].

--------------------- IMMUNOTHERAPY ---------------------

Immunotherapy is based on the assumption that tumors bear anti-gens that are distinctly foreign to the host and that, if introduced in an appropriate way into an immunologically responsive environment, could induce an immune response capable of destroying the tumor. The idea of redesigning the immunological environment of a host so that it becomes more responsive to antigens is an old one. Almost 400 years ago Jenner noted that milkmaids who contracted cowpox de-veloped resistance to smallpox. Although concepts of cross-immunity were unknown then, the observation that introduction of one antigen could induce resistance to another was fundamental. Many other observations were made of cross-immunity or nonspecific stimulation of the immune response with microbial and even chemical antigens. These observations stimulated a great deal of research into the phenomenon of cross-immunity and the nature of nonspecific stimulation of immune mechanisms. However, application of this knowledge to therapy of cancer was not made until there was clear-cut evidence that cancer cells did indeed bear antigens slightly different from those of the host.

Immunotherapy is a term used to encompass a variety of ap-proaches. *Active immunization* involves antigens thought to be tumor specific or antigens that are nonspecific and hence would stimulate immune responses to a variety of antigens including the real target, the tumor-specific antigen. *Passive immunization* involves the transfer of immunoglobulins that are tumor specific and that would induce a transient immunity in the recipient. *Adoptive im-munization* involves the transfer of immune lymphoid cells or subcellular fractions that confer an immunity mediated by the transferred materials themselves [93].

Active nonspecific immunotherapy is based on the observation that certain microbial substances, synthetic replicas, or chemicals can nonspecifically stimulate immunity to a wide variety of antigens such as viruses, bacteria, and fungi. Examples of materials used to induce this type of therapy are bacillus Calmette-Guérin (BCG) used to im-munize against tuberculosis, fractions of BCG such as methanol extractable residue (MER), glucan, *Corynebacterium parvum,* polynucleotides, and bacterial endotoxins. Clinical trials using BCG in stimulation of immune responses to a variety of tumors are numerous. Several observations regarding the requirements for successful therapy are apparent.

1. The tumor size must not be excessive. The definition of *excessive* varies from one clinical situation to another. In general, local tumors that have been excised are more vulnerable to immunotherapy with BCG than are tumors that have metastasized. BCG immunotherapy is particularly effective in treatment of subcutaneous melanoma nodules if the patient is immunologically competent. In this situation freeze-dried BCG is administered by scarification, intradermal injection, or even more easily by a multiple puncture tine technique.
2. The host must be immunologically able to react to tumor specific antigens and other antigens. This is frequently determined by sensitizing the recipient to a chemical such as 2,4 dinitrochlorobenzene (DNCB), which will sensitize 95% of normal people. A small amount of the chemical is placed on the skin to sensitize the individual. In 14 days a delayed hypersensitivity response can be elicited by readministration of a smaller amount of the chemical. A delayed hypersensitivity reaction characterized by erythema and a slight induration at the site of the second dose of DNCB is evidence that the host's immune response is intact.
3. Live BCG often preserved in lyophilized or freeze-dried form appears to be better than nonliving BCG in producing therapy. This is not unexpected since live vaccines are usually more effective than vaccines of dead organisms in microbial immunizations.
4. There must be an opportunity for contact between BCG and tumor cells. Intralesional injection of BCG is effective for cutaneous nodules. Systemic administration has been used for postsurgical therapy or leukemias in a few experimental trials.

BCG stimulates the reticuloendothelial system which is a scavenger system of the body. There are increases in "activated" macrophages which can nonspecifically destroy the neoplastic cells. The presence of these activated macrophages may facilitate the presentation of tumor-specific antigens to lymphocytes which then produce the cell-mediated or humoral responses that destroy the tumor.

This is the good news about BCG therapy. The bad news is that there may be side effects that range from minimal to severe. Serous discharges may result at the site of BCG inoculations. Fevers may result from both local and systemic complications. Repeated intralesional injections of BCG may produce severe hypersensitivity reactions and even anaphylaxis. If live BCG is being used, a persistent BCG infection may result in immunosuppressed patients. Erythema nodosum, uveitis, pancytopenia, hepatic dysfunction, hepatosplenomegaly, and jaundice may also result. However, clinical trials of BCG therapy have contributed a great deal to our understanding of how and why such adverse reactions develop. Administration of BCG by the multiple puncture tine technique or scarification is usually well tolerated. Adverse side effects can be readily controlled. The nurse should be particularly alert to side effects and ways to control them. A search of clinical trial data on the technique being used will give clues as to side effects and ways to minimize them.

One cannot discuss BCG immunotherapy without mentioning the serious potential of enhancement of the tumor. Such a hazard is real when large doses of BCG are administered. The conditions for induction of enhancement are complex and vary from protocol to protocol. Since this topic cannot be covered in depth here the reader should be alert to the possibility and seek additional information on the possibility of enhancement depending upon the protocol being used. Careful monitoring of the immune response(s) should be carried out to determine if any types of immunosuppression are occurring that could eventually lead to enhancement of tumor growth.

BCG is frequently used in combination with agents that could induce active immunization to specific tumor cell antigens. For example, it is used with tumor-cell vaccines and extracts. *Corynebacterium parvum* has been substituted for BCG as the nonspecific stimulant in some protocols. In experimental animal systems other avirulent bacteria and products are being tested for their ability to induce nonspecific immunotherapy.

Passive immunotherapy with antiserum is an old idea that is fraught with many problems. The protection is transient in that immunoglobulin molecules are transfused into the cancer patient from someone who has recovered from a similar cancer or from an animal that is specifically immunized to tumor antigens. When antisera from animals are transfused into people (heterologous antisera) there is the problem that the foreign globulins are recognized and reacted to by the host resulting in sensitization to further injections of this antiserum and to more rapid elimination of the transfused immunoglobulins. There are also problems with specificity of the immunoglobulin transferred to the cancer patient. Frequently antisera to normal tissue components contaminate the antisera. A

creative approach to the problem is emerging in that the heterologous antisera, in purified form, are being used simply as carriers
of therapeutic agents. These immunologic couriers can deliver
the therapeutic agent to its target with far more specificity than
can the therapeutic agent on its own.

Adoptive immunotherapy with viable cells is virtually impossible in humans who are not extremely similar in histocompatibility
antigens. Thus, attention has been directed at transferring those
components of an immune cell that may be able to perpetuate immunity in the recipient. There has been a great deal of interest in
"immune" RNA extracted from lymphoid cells of even other species
of animals that had been sensitized with tumor-specific antigens. The
immune RNA has been shown to be able to confer specific immunological reactivity on nonimmune lymphoid cells of the recipient
by a complex series of events. The RNA extracts are not immuno-
genic in themselves and thus do not create the problem of sensitization to the passively administered material.

An alternative approach in adoptive immunotherapy is sensitization in vitro of the recipient's own cells. Here the autologous lymphocytes are incubated in vitro with tumor antigens. The results with
this type of therapy are not yet exciting. It remains largely an experimental approach.

Immunotherapy is an intriguing approach to therapy of cancer.
Success of this approach varies widely depending on factors such as
the stage of the cancer, the protocol for administration, the experience of the clinicians involved, and the recognition of side effects at
an early stage. Immunotherapy is most useful as an adjunct to
chemo- and radiotherapy. The need for good nursing care of the
patient undergoing immunotherapy is apparent. Patients need to
understand the new approach. They must be alert to reporting side
effects and must understand both the care of the lesions resulting
from local immunotherapy, and the experimental nature of the
procedures.

BONE MARROW TRANSPLANTATION

Bone marrow transplants are used in an attempt to replace malignant
bone marrow stem cells, found in acute myelogenous leukemia, with
the bone marrow stem cells from a normal donor, free of malignant
disease. Bone marrow transplants have also been used for patients
with aplastic anemia and severe immunodeficiency diseases. In order
to replace the diseased bone marrow with healthy stem cells, total

body irradiation, cytotoxic drugs, and/or antilymphocytic globulins are used with the goal of destroying as many as possible of the malignant cells and creating "living space" for transplanted cells. This is necessary, first, to abort the progress of the cancer and, second, to prevent graft-versus-host disease. In graft-versus-host disease the surviving immunologically competent cells in the host react against any foreign components of the transplanted bone marrow to destroy it as the body would any foreign antigen [82].

An effort is also made to minimize the possibility of graft-versus-host disease by matching the transplantation antigens of the donor and the recipient as closely as possible. Two types of matching tests are used, identified as HLA and MLC. The former is a test utilizing antibodies to identify the HLA antigens (human leukocyte antigens) on the surface of the human lymphocytes. The latter is a test in which mixtures of donor and recipient cultured lymphocytes (mixed lymphocyte cultures) are tested for the ability of either donor or recipient cells to react by blastogenesis to the antigens of the other cell (donor or recipient) depending on the design of the test. With identical twins these tests would indicate matching lymphocyte antigens and lack of reactivity between the donor and recipient test lymphocytes. While every attempt is made to make matches between bone marrow cells from related or unrelated donors and recipient as similar as possible, there is always the possibility of graft-versus-host disease to the unmatched antigens. Hence, efforts are made to monitor the onset and progression of graft-versus-host disease if it intervenes. If the transplant is successful the donor stem cells mature in the recipient's bone marrow to replace the functions of the diseased stem cells.

Extensive irradiation of the recipient in preparation for the bone marrow infusion of donor cells creates a critical stage for the patient. Extensive precautions must be taken to minimize the chance of infection during the stages when the recipient has little or no immune response capacity. As the engrafted bone marrow cells home to the bone marrow of the recipient, the recipient begins to regain immunological competency by means of the donor stem cells which then have the potential to differentiate into immunologically competent cells by means discussed previously.

Bone marrow transplantation presents a challenge to nursing. Tissue matching, irradiation, and monitoring of the patient can go only so far in ensuring patient survival. The constant day-to-day attention to the environment of the patient, education of the patient and the family as to the critical nature of the treatment, and support of the patient and family are constant challenges.

THE CHALLENGES

There are many challenges ahead in understanding the biology of cancer and its treatment. As information regarding possible etiological agents and risk factors in oncogenesis accumulates, prevention becomes a reality. The complexity of the treatment of cancer indicates a need to educate patients about the events that lie ahead for them in their treatment and rehabilitation. For terminal patients there is a need to develop humane protocols for reducing pain and complications. The interaction of the physiological, psychological, sociological, and cultural factors in cancer care poses one of the greatest challenges to the clinician and researcher. There has been a thrust to develop valid, reliable, and sensitive diagnostic techniques for early cancer. It is inevitable that even the best of such tools will be fraught with false positive and false negatives leading to anxiety, fear, guilt, and recrimination in some instances. As these many facets of cancer research and therapy develop, the care of the patient will be most critical. Important in this care will be interpretation to the patient by the nurse of the physiological changes that occur because of the cancer and its treatment. This chapter has highlighted the present status of the many interacting fields. It is meant to stimulate the nurse oncology clinician to ask questions, to probe for answers, and to create new approaches.

REFERENCES

[1] AMES, B.N.; McCANN, J.; and YAMASAKI, E. Methods for Detecting Carcinogens and Mutagens with the Salmonella/Mammalian—Microsone Mutagenicity Test. *Mutation Research,* 31:347-364, 1975.

[2] ADAMS, D.O., and SNYDERMAN, R. Do Macrophages Destroy Nascent Tumors? *Journal of the National Cancer Institute,* 62:1341-1345, 1979.

[3] ARMUTH, V., and BERENBLUM, I. Promotion of Mammary Carcinogenesis and Leukemogenic Action by Phorbol in Virgin Female Wistar Rats. *Cancer Research,* 34:2704-2707, 1974.

[4] ARMUTH, V., and BERENBLUM, I. Systemic Promoting Actions of Phorbol in Liver and Lung Carcinogenesis in AKR Mice. *Cancer Research,* 32:2259-2262, 1972.

[5] AXEL, R.; SCHLOM, J.; and SPIEGELMAN, S. Presence in Human Breast Cancer of RNA Holologous to Mouse Mammary Tumour Virus RNA. *Nature,* 235:32-36, 1972.

[6] BARRETT, J.C. A Preneoplastic Stage in the Spontaneous Neoplastic Transformation of Syrian Hamster Embryo Cells in Culture. *Cancer Research,* 40:91-94, 1980.

[7]   BIGGS, P.M.; PAYNE, L.N.; MILNE, B.S.; CHURCHILL, A.E.; CHUBB, R.C.; POWELL, D.G.; and HARRIS, A.H. Field Trials with an Attenuated Cell Associated Vaccine for Marek's Disease. *Veterinary Record,* 87:704–709, 1970.

[8]   BOUTWELL, R.K. Some Biological Aspects of Skin Carcinogenesis. *Progress in Experimental Tumor Research,* 4:207–250, 1964.

[9]   BOUTWELL, R.K. The Function and Mechanism of Promoters of Carcinogenesis. *CRC Critical Reviews in Toxicology,* 2:419–443, 1974.

[10] BRONK, B.V. Thermal Potentiation of Mammalian Cell Killing: Clues for Understanding and Potential for Tumor Therapy. *Advances in Radiation Research,* 6:267–324, 1976.

[11] BRUCE, W.R., and LIN, H. An Empirical Cellular Approach to the Improvement of Cancer Chemotherapy. *Cancer Research,* 29:2308, 1969.

[12] BRYAN, G.T., and SPRINGBERG, P.D. Role of the Vehicle in the Genesis of Bladder Carcinomas in Mice by the Pettet Implantation Technic. *Cancer Research,* 26:105–109, 1966.

[13] CARTER, S.K.; BABOWSKI, M.T.; and HELLMANN, K. *Chemotherapy of Cancer,* pp. 9–19. New York: John Wiley, 1977.

[14] CHALMERS, A.H.; LAVIN, M.; ATISOONTORNKUL, S.; MANSBRIDGE, J.; and KIDSON, C. Resistance of Human Melanoma Cells to Ultraviolet Radiation. *Cancer Research,* 36:1930–1934, 1976.

[15] COLE, P.; BROWN, J.B.; and MacMAHON, B. Oestrogen Profiles of Parous and Nulliparous Women. *Lancet,* 2:596–598, 1976.

[16] COLE, P.; CRAMER, D.; YEN, S.; PAFFENBARGER, R.; MacMAHON, B.; and BROWN, J. Estrogen Profiles of Premenopausal Women with Breast Cancer. *Cancer Research,* 38:745–748, 1978.

[17] COLE, P., and MacMAHON, B. Oestrogen Fractions during Early Reproductive Life in the Aetiology of Breast Cancer. *Lancet,* 1:604–606, 1969.

[18] COURT-BROWN, W.M., and DOLL, R. Leukemia and Aplastic Anemia in Patients Irradiated for Ankylosing Spondylitis. London: Medical Research Council, Special Report Series No. 295, 1957.

[19] CURRIE, G.A. *Cancer and the Immune Response.* Baltimore: Williams and Wilkins, 1974.

[20] del REGATO, J.A. Pathways of Metastatic Spread of Malignant Tumors. *Seminars in Oncology,* 4:33–38, 1977.

[21] de SCHRYVER, A.; FRIBERG, S., JR.; KLEIN, G.; HENLE, W.; HENLE, G.; dé-THÉ, G.; CLIFFORD, P.; and HO, H.C. Epstein-Barr Virus-Associated Antibody Patterns in Carcinoma of the Post-Nasal Space. *Clinical and Experimental Immunology,* 5:443–459, 1969.

[22] de SCHRYVER, A.; KLEIN, G.; HENLE, G.; HENLE, W.; CAMERON, H.M.; SANTESSON, L.; and CLIFFORD, P. EB-Virus Associated Serology in Malignant Disease: Antibody Levels to Viral Capsid Antigens (VCA), Membrane Antigens (MA) and Early Antigens (EA) in Patients with Various Neoplastic Conditions. *International Journal of Cancer,* 9:353–365, 1972.

[23] DICKINSON, L.E.; MacMAHON, B.; COLE, P.; and BROWN, J.B. Estrogen Profiles of Oriental and Caucasian Women in Hawaii. *New England Journal of Medicine*, 291:1211–1213, 1974.

[24] DINOCHOWSKI, L. The Viral Factor in the Genesis of Breast Cancer: Present Evidence. *Triangle*, 12:37–47, 1972.

[25] DOLL, R. The Epidemiology of Leukemia. Seventh Annual Guest Lecture, Leukemia Research Fund, 61 Great Armond Street, London, W.C., 1N3JJ, 1971.

[26] EVERSON, T.C., and COLE, W.H. Spontaneous Regression of Cancer. Philadelphia: Saunders, 1966.

[27] FIDLER, I.J. Tumor Heterogenicity and the Biology of Cancer Invasion and Metastasis. *Cancer Research*, 38:2651–2660, 1978.

[28] FISHER, E.R., and FISHER, B. Recent Observations on the Concept of Metastasis. *Archives of Pathology*, 83:321–324, 1967.

[29] FISHMAN, W.H. Activation of Developmental Genes in Neoplastic Transformation. *Cancer Research*, 36:3423–3428, 1976.

[30] FOLKMAN, J. Tumor Angiogenesis. In *Cancer: A Comprehensive Treatise*, ed. F.F. Baker, Vol. 3, pp. 355–388. New York: Plenum Press, 1975.

[31] GALLAGHER, R.E., and GALLO, R.C. Type C RNA Tumor Virus Isolated from Cultured Human Acute Myelogenous Leukemia Cells. *Science*, 187:350–353, 1975.

[32] GOLD, P., and FREEDMAN, S.O. Demonstration of Tumor-Specific Antigens in Human Colonic Carcinomata by Immunological Tolerance and Absorption Techniques. *Journal of Experimental Medicine*, 121:439–462, 1965.

[33] GOLD, P., and FREEMAN, S.O. Specific Carcinoembryonic Antigens of the Human Digestive System. *Journal of Experimental Medicine*, 122:467–481, 1965.

[34] GOOD, R.A., and FERNANDES, G. Nutrition, Immunity and Cancer— A Review. Part I: Influence of Protein or Protein-Calorie Malnutrition and Zinc Deficiency on Immunity. *Clinical Bulletin*, 9:3–12, 1979.

[35] GROSS, L. Viral Etiology of Cancer and Leukemia: A Look into the Past, Present and Future—G.H.A. Clowes Memorial Lecture. *Cancer Research*, 38:485–493, 1978.

[36] HAENSZEL, W. Migrant Studies. In *Persons at High Risk of Cancer. An Approach to Cancer Etiology and Control*, ed. J.F. Fraumeni, Jr., pp. 361–371. New York: Academic Press, 1975.

[37] HAENSZEL, W., and KURIHARA, M. Studies of Japanese Migrants. I. Mortality from Cancer and Other Diseases among Japanese in the United States. *Journal of the National Cancer Institute*, 40:43–68, 1968.

[38] HÄHNEL, R., and VIVIAN, A.B. Biochemical and Clinical Experience with the Estimation of Estrogen Receptors in Human Breast Carcinoma. In *Estrogen Receptors in Human Breast Cancer*, ed. W.L. McGuire, P.P. Carbone, and E.P. Vollmer, pp. 205–345. New York: Raven Press, 1975.

[39] HALL, W.H., and BIELSCHOWSKY, F. The Development of Malig-

nancy in Experimental Induced Adenomata of the Thyroid. *British Journal of Cancer,* 3:534–541, 1949.

[40] HAR-KEDAR, I., and BLEEHEN, N.M. Experimental and Clinical Aspects of Hyperthermia Applied to the Treatment of Cancer with Special Reference to the Role of Ultrasonic and Microwave Heating. *Advances in Radiation Research,* 6:229–266, 1976.

[41] HEMPELMANN, L.H. Risk of Thyroid Neoplasms after Irradiation in Childhood. *Science,* 160:159, 1969.

[42] HERSCOWITZ, H. B. Immunophysiology: Cell Function and Cellular Interactions. In *Immunology II,* ed. J.A. Bellanti, pp. 151–202. Philadelphia: Saunders, 1978.

[43] HEUSON, J.C.; LeCLERCQ, G.; LONGEVAL, E.; DEBOEL, M.C.; MATTHEIEM, W.H.; and HEIMANN, R. Estrogen Receptors: Prognostic Significance in Breast Cancer. In *Estrogen Receptors in Human Breast Cancer,* ed. W.L. McGuire, P.P. Carbone, and E.P. Vollmer, pp. 57–72. New York: Raven Press, 1975.

[44] HOLLAENDER, A., ed. *Chemical Mutagens: Principles and Methods for Their Detection,* Vols. 1–3. New York: Plenum Press, 1971–1973.

[45] HEIDELBERGER, C. Chemical Carcinogenesis. *Annual Review of Biochemistry,* 44:79–121, 1975.

[46] HICKS, R.M.; WAKEFIELD, St. J.; and CHOWANICE, J. Evaluation of a New Model to Detect Bladder Carcinogens or Co-Carcinogens; Results Obtained with Saccharin, Cyclamate and Cyclophosphamide. *Chemico-Biological Interactions,* 11:225–233, 1975.

[47] HIGGINSON, J. Present Trends in Cancer Epidemiology. *Canadian Cancer Conference,* 8:40–75, 1969.

[48] HILL, H.Z., and LIN, H. Carcinogenesis and Tumor Growth. In *Clinical Oncology,* ed. J. Horton and G.J. Hill, II, pp. 1–33. Philadelphia: Saunders, 1977.

[49] IARC Monographs on the Evaluation of the Carcinogenic Risk of Chemicals to Man, Vol. 15, *Serne Fumigants, The Herbicides 2, 4-D and 2, 4, 5-T, Chlorinated Dibenzodioxins and Miscellaneous Industrial Chemicals.* Lyon, France: International Agency for Research on Cancer, 1977.

[50] JENSEN, E.V.; BLOCK, G.E.; SMITH, S.; KYSER, K.; and DeSOMBRE, E.R. Estrogen Receptors and Breast Cancer Response to Adrenalectomy. *National Cancer Institute Monographs,* 34:55–79, 1971.

[51] KALISS, N. Immunological Enhancement of Tumor Homografts in Mice: A Review. *Cancer Research,* 18:992, 1958.

[52] KAPLAN, H.S. On the Etiology and Pathogenesis of the Leukemias: A Review. *Cancer Research,* 14:535, 1954.

[53] KAPLAN, H.S. The Role of Radiation on Experimental Leukemogenesis. *National Cancer Institute Monograph,* 14:207, 1963.

[54] KLEIN, E.; KLEIN, G.; and LEVINE, P.H. Immunological Control of Human Lymphoma: Discussion. *Cancer Research,* 36:724–727, 1976.

[55] KONGSHAVN, P.A.L.; HAWKINS, D.; and SHUSTER, J. The Biology of the Immune Response. In *Clinical Immunology,* ed. S.O. Freedman and P. Gold, pp. 1–64. New York: Harper & Row, 1976.

[56] KUFE, D.; HEHLMANN, R.; and SPIEGELMAN, S. RNA Related to That of a Murine Leukemia Virus in Burkitt's Tumors and Nasopharyngeal Carcinomas. *Proceedings of the National Academy of Sciences U.S.*, 70:5–9, 1973.

[57] LEMON, H.M.; WOTIZ, H.H.; PARSONS, L.; and MOZDEN, P.J. Reduced Estriol Excretion in Patients with Breast Cancer Prior to Endocrine Therapy. *Journal of the American Medical Association*, 196:1128–1136, 1966.

[58] LEVINE, P.H. Approaches to Immunological Control of Virus–Associated Tumors in Man: Introductory Remarks. *Cancer Research*, 36:565–569, 1976.

[59] LEWIS, E.B. Leukemia and Ionizing Radiation. *Science*, 125:965, 1957.

[60] LIOTTA, L.A.; KLEINERMAN, J.; and SAIDEL, G.M. The Significance of Hematogenous Tumor Cell Clumps in the Metastatic Process. *Cancer Research*, 36:889–894, 1976.

[61] MacMAHON, B.; COLE, P.; BROWN, J.B.; AOKI, K.; LIN, T.M.; MORGAN, R.W.; and WOO, N. Oestrogen Profiles of Asian and North American Women. *Lancet*, 2:900–902, 1971.

[62] MacMAHON, B.; COLE, P.; BROWN, J.B.; AOKI, K.; LIN, T.M.; MORGAN, R.W.; and WOO, N. Urine Oestrogen Profiles of Asian and North American Women. *International Journal of Cancer*, 14:161–167, 1974.

[63] McCANN, J., and AMES, B.N. Detection of Carcinogens as Mutagens in the *Salmonella* Microsome Test: Assay of 300 Chemicals. Discussion. *Proceedings of the National Academy of Sciences*, 73:950–954, 1976.

[64] McGRATH, C.M.; GRANT, P.M.; SOULE, H.D.; GLANCY, T.; and RICH, M.A. Replication of Oncornavirus-like Particle in Human Breast Carcinoma Cell Line, MCF-7. *Nature*, 252:247–250, 1974.

[65] McGUIRE, W.L.; CARBONE, P.P.; SEARS, M.E.; and ESCHER, G.C. Estrogen Receptors in Human Breast Cancer: An Overview. In *Estrogen Receptors in Human Breast Cancer*, ed. W.L. McGuire, P.P. Carbone, and E.P. Vollmer, pp. 1–7. New York: Raven Press, 1975.

[66] MILLER, E.C. Some Current Perspectives on Chemical Carcinogenesis in Humans and Experimental Animals: Presidential Address. *Cancer Research*, 38:1479–1496, 1978.

[67] MILLER, J.A., and MILLER, E.C. Carcinogens Occurring Naturally in Foods. *Federal Proceedings*, 35:1316–1321, 1975.

[68] NAIB, Z.M.; NAHMIAS, A.J.; and JOSEY, W.E. Cytology and Histopathology of Cervical Herpes Simplex Infection. *Cancer*, 19:1026–1031, 1966.

[69] NEXO, B.A., and ULRICH, K. Activation of C-type Virus during Chemically Induced Leukemogenesis in Mice. *Cancer Research*, 38:729–735, 1978.

[70] PERAINO, C.; FRY, R.J.M.; and STAFFELDT, E. Reduction and Enhancement by Phenobarbital of Hepatocarcinogenesis Induced in the Rat by 2-Acetylaminofluorene. *Cancer Research*, 31:1506–1512, 1971.

[71] Public Law 85–929, The Delany Amendment, September 6, 1958.

[72] PURCHASE, I.F.H.; LONGSTAFF, E.; ASHBY, J.; STYLES, J.A.; ANDERSON, D.; LEFEVRE, P.A.; and WESTWOOD, F.R. Evaluation of Six Short-Term Tests for Detecting Organic Chemical Carcinogens and Recommendations for Their Use. *Nature*, 264:624–627, 1976.

[73] RAPP, F., and REED, C. Experimental Evidence for the Oncogenic Potential of Herpes Simplex Virus. *Cancer Research*, 36:800–806, 1976.

[74] RAWLS, W.E.; GARFIELD, C.H.; SETH, P.; and ADAM, E. Serological and Epidermiological Considerations of the Role of Herpes Simplex Virus Type 2 in Cervical Cancer. *Cancer Research*, 36:829–835, 1976.

[75] *Report of an IARC Working Group: An Evaluation of Chemicals and Industrial Processes Associated with Cancer in Humans Based on Human and Animal Data.* IARC Monographs Vol. 1-2. *Cancer Research*, 40:1–12, 1980.

[76] ROTKIN, I.D. A Comparison Review of Key Epidemiological Studies in Cervical Cancer Related to Current Searches for Transmissible Agents. *Cancer Research*, 33:1353–1367, 1973.

[77] SCHOLEN, L.H.; FERNANDES, G.; GAROFALO, J.A.; and GOOD, R.A. Nutrition, Immunity and Cancer—A Review: Part II. Zinc, Immune Functions and Cancer. *Clinical Bulletin*, 9:63–75, 1979.

[78] SELL, S. *Immunology, Immunopathology and Immunity.* New York: Harper & Row, 1972.

[79] SHAH, S.A. and DICKSON, J.A. Effect of Hyperthermia on the Immunocompetence of VX2 Tumor-bearing Rabbits. *Cancer Research*, 38:3523–3531, 1978.

[80] SHILLITOE, E.J., and SILVERMAN, S. Oral Cancer and Herpes Simplex Virus—A Review. *Oral Surgery*, 48:216–224, 1979.

[81] SHIVELY, J.E.; TODD, C.W.; GO, V.L.W.; and EGAN, M.L. Amino-terminal Sequence of a Carcinoembryonic Antigen-like Glycoprotein Isolated from the Colonic Lavages of Healthy Individuals. *Cancer Research*, 38:503–505, 1978.

[82] SKAMENE, E., and GOLD, P. Organ Transplantation. In *Clinical Immunology*, ed. S.O. Freedman and P. Gold, pp. 449–481. New York: Harper & Row, 1976.

[83] SLAVIN, H.B., and GAVETT, E. Primary Herpetic Vulvovaginitis. *Procedings of the Society for Experimental Biology and Medicine*, 63:343–345, 1946.

[84] SMITH, P.G., and PIKE, M.C. Current Epidemiological Evidence for Transmission of Hodgkin's Disease. *Cancer Research*, 36:660–662, 1976.

[85] *Smoking and Health.* Report of the Advisory Committee of the Surgeon General of the Public Health Service. Public Health Service Publication No. 1103, pp. 149–196, Washington, D.C.: U.S. Government Printing Office, 1964.

[86] SPORN, M.B.; DUNLOP, N.M.; NEWTON, D.L.; and SMITH, J.M. Prevention of Chemical Carcinogenesis by Vitamin A and its Synthetic Analogs (Retinoids). *Federal Proceedings*, 35:1332–1338, 1976.

[87]   STEEL, G.G.; ADAMS, K.; and BARRETT, J.C. Analysis of Cell Popu-
        lation Kinetics of Transplanted Tumors of Widely Differing Growth
        Rate. *British Journal of Cancer,* 20:784, 1966.

[88]   STERN, E., and LONGO, L.D. Identification of Herpes Simplex Virus
        in a Case Showing Cytological Features of Viral Vaginitis. *Acta Cyto-
        logica,* 7:295–299, 1963.

[89]   STOLTZ, D.R.; POIRIER, L.A.; IRVING, C.C.; STICH, H.F.; WEIS-
        BURGER, J.H.; and GRICE, H.C. Evaluation of Short-Term Tests for
        Carcinogenicity. *Toxicology and Applied Pharmacology,* 29:157–180,
        1974.

[90]   STUTMAN, O., and HERBERMAN, R.B. Immunological Control of
        Breast Cancer: Discussion. *Cancer Research,* 36:781–782, 1976.

[91]   SUGARBAKER, E.V.; COHEN, A.M.; and KETCHAM, A.S. Mecha-
        nisms and Prevention of Cancer Dissemination: An Overview. *Seminars
        in Oncology,* 4:19–32, 1977.

[92]   THALER, M.S.; KLAUSNER, R.D.; and COHEN, H.J. *Medical Im-
        munology,* pp. 113–138. Philadelphia: Lippincott, 1977.

[93]   THOMSON, D.M.P. Immunotherapy and Immunosuppression. In *Clini-
        cal Immunology,* ed. S.O. Freedman and P. Gold, pp. 532–573. New
        York: Harper & Row, 1976.

[94]   TOMATIS, L.; AGTHE, C.; BARTSCH, H.; HUFF, J.; MONTESANO,
        R.; SARACCI, R.; WALKER, E.; and WILBOURN, J. Evaluation of the
        Carcinogenicity of Chemicals: A Review of the Monograph Program of
        the International Agency for Research on Cancer (1971 to 1977). *Can-
        cer Research,* 38:877–885, 1978.

[95]   VAN DUUREN, B.L. Tumor-Promoting and Co-carcinogenic Agents in
        Chemical Carcinogenesis. In *Chemical Carcinogens,* ed. C.E. Searle, pp.
        24–51. American Chemical Society Monograph No. 173, Washington,
        D.C.: American Chemical Society, 1976.

[96]   VIANNA, N.J. Evidence for Infectious Component of Hodgkin's Disease
        and Related Considerations. *Cancer Research,* 36:663–666, 1976.

[97]   WEISS, L. A Pathobiologic Overview of Metastasis. *Seminars in On-
        cology,* 4:5–17, 1977.

[98]   WHO. *Fifth Report of the Joint FAO/WHO Expert Committee on Food
        Additives: Evaluation of Carcinogenic Hazard of Food Additives.* WHO
        Technical Report Series No. 220, 1961.

[99]   WILLIS, R.A. *The Spread of Tumors in the Human Body.* London:
        Butlerworths, 1972.

[100]   ZAMCHECK, N., and KUPCHIK, H.Z. The Interdependence of Clinical
        Investigations and Methodological Development in the Early Evolution
        of Assays for Carcinoembryonic Antigen. *Cancer Research,* 34:2131–
        2136, 1974.

[101]   ZEIDMAN, I. Metastasis: A Review of Recent Advances. *Cancer Re-
        search,* 17:157–162, 1957.

[102]   ZIEGLER, J.L.; BLUMING, A.Z.; FASS, L.; and MORROW, R.H.,
        JR. Relapse Patterns in Burkitt's Lymphoma. *Cancer Research,* 32:
        1267–1272, 1972.

[103] ZUR HAUSEN, H. Biochemical Approaches to Detection of Epstein-Barr Virus in Human Tumors. *Cancer Research*, 36:678–680, 1976.

ADDITIONAL READINGS

COLMAN, K., and PAUL, J. *An Introduction to Cancer Medicine.* New York: John Wiley, 1978.

KRUSE, L.; REESE, J.; and HART, L. *Cancer Pathophysiology, Etiology and Management.* St. Louis: C.V. Mosby, 1979.

PITOT, H. *Fundamentals of Oncology.* New York: Marcel Dekker, 1978.

SUSS, R.; KINZEL, V.; and SCRIBNER, J.D. *Cancer, Experiments and Concepts.* New York: Springer-Verlag, 1973.

chapter three

ANAYIS DERDIARIAN, R.N., M.N.
Assistant Clinical Professor
Teaching in the Graduate Nursing
Oncology Program
School of Nursing, UCLA

Psychosocial variables in cancer management: Considerations for nursing practice

INTRODUCTION

The intent of this chapter is not to discuss or apply the nursing process for the management of the psychosocial problems of the cancer patients. Although attempts have been made to develop methodologies to apply the nursing process to describe the psychosocial problems and the effectiveness of the nursing interventions in the solution of these problems, these attempts are essentially embryonic beginnings. Such attempts to refine the nursing process to more theoretical and scientific soundness, such as Newlin's work [7], deserve a comprehensive treatment that would be too cumbersome to fit in this chapter. Thus the nursing process in part or in whole will not be included in this chapter.

The intent of this chapter is to present a conceptual framework through which the psychosocial problems important for nursing's treatment can be viewed within a more focal context than the broad context of the patient's experiences from the time of diagnosis through the terminal stage. These problems will be discussed in terms of their specificity to the clinical stage in which they occur and their morphological differences along the clinical stages over time. Therefore the express intent is to propose a fresh view of those problems for more specific and effective methods of their management.

There are several implications in this chapter. First, it is to raise awareness about the difficulties of assessment and definition of the psychosocial problems, as they relate specifically to a particular stage of the clinical process of the cancer management. For such description, those problems need to be analyzed in terms of the physical and psychosocial determinants peculiar to the clinical stage. This would encourage the clinician to explore the biological and medical variables underlying the psychosocial problems such as grieving, hopelessness, feeling anxious, and the like. The second implication is to spare the clinician from the naive confidence that some theoretical understanding of such problems is adequate for their appropriate definitions in nursing diagnostic terms. In-depth understanding of the theories respective to those problems is necessary. For example, theoretical understanding of anxiety would culminate in problem definition as it specifically relates to the cancer patient at a specific clinical stage, such as prediagnosis, post-diagnosis, or during treatment. The third implication is to view nursing interventions as they relate to a particular stage with the same theoretical soundness and clinical specificity. Therefore it is essential for the reader to develop and update knowledge about problem definition and intervention by reviewing the literature on: (1) the theories related to nursing problems and interventions in the psychosocial realm; and (2) medical technology relative to specific stages. Thus the overall implication of this chapter is to provide a conceptual framework to be utilized in conjunction with the nursing process.

Despite brilliant medical and technological advances in the war against cancer, the diagnosis of cancer still produces terror in the hearts of those who have it. Perhaps the connotations that this diagnosis had centuries ago prevail today. Healy [4] has suggested that despite increased control of the disease and extention of survival time over the past quarter of a century, cancer continues to be shrouded by negative attitudes and defeatism. The most noted and mentioned attitudes and emotions are fear of death, fear of separation, fear of abandonment, fear of loneliness, fear of disability, fear of helplessness, fear of dependency, fear of pain, fear of disfigurement, and fear of extreme discomfort resulting from treatments. Past as well as current literature is abundant in descriptions of the various psychological and emotional reactions of the patient in adapting to the physical and life changes imposed by the diagnosis and treatment of cancer. Although each patient and family is unique in the way they will choose to react to the diagnosis and all that it implies for the future, it is being proposed here that many patients and families experience common reactions in adapting to the physical and psychosocial implications of cancer. Common as those reactions may be, however, they may differ in the way they present themselves as problems and thus demand different specific interventions depending on the clinical stage of the disease within which they occur. For example, although grief, anxiety, dependence, and hope, among other reactions, are commonly present during diagnosis determination, early treatment, chronic, preterminal, and terminal stages of the disease, the nature of problems of grieving, anxiety, dependence, and hopelessness is different and specific to each stage, and therefore these reactions require different management also specific to those stages. Implied here are two things: (1) Theoretical understanding of those phenomena is essential and yet not sufficient to identify those problems specifically and descriptively enough to formulate specific nursing diagnoses; and (2) such understanding must be coupled with adequate understanding of the respective stages of the clinical course of cancer. Further, it is being proposed that adaptive reactions such as grieving, anxiousness, hopelessness or hopefulness, and dependence are natural, usual reactions as long as: (1) they are not intense enough to interfere with the individual's health-attaining or health-promoting behavior; and (2) they are acceptable as natural or expected behavior given a specific situation. For example, denial in the face of the recent diagnosis is expected and acceptable as natural behavior and it becomes problematic if it is intense to the extent of preventing the person from seeking medical attention and/or it persists with the same intensity even after treatment.

Therefore, the challenge ahead is multidimensional. First, descriptions of those reactions the patients and the families experience need to be explored along the clinical course of the disease. Second, descriptions of the maladaptive reactions also need to be explored along the same course. Third, the determinants of the maladaptive reactions need to be identified. Fourth, interventive strategies specific to the natural adaptive as well as to the maladaptive (and therefore problematic) reactions need to be explored and identified. The challenge is indeed immense, and yet it must be faced if adequate understanding of the psychosocial problems or appropriate interventions is expected to exist.

The management of the psychosocial problems of cancer is complex and demands the collaboration of several other disciplines. The coordination of the teamwork of the physician, the nurse, the psychologist, the psychiatrist, the social worker, the clergyperson, the patient, and the family is of paramount importance. The coordination of the team's effort implies that the funneling of the efforts of individual team members to the patient is done through the nursing care. Thus the nurse is the central figure not only in orchestrating the teamwork but also in nursing systematically and in methodically generating observations with regard to problems and interventions. The nurse is naturally best situated in this strategic position on the team to deliver care and generate hypotheses and therefore knowledge about nursing care as well as about the care provided by other members of the interdisciplinary team.

THE FOUR STAGES OF CANCER

Systematization of practice and observation requires that the clinical context be considered in examining the reactions of the patients and of their families. Essentially, the clinical course of cancer needs to be divided into stages at critical points that distinguish one stage from the others. It is believed that each stage embodies psychosocial reactions intrinsic to the stage from the standpoint of the disease and treatment. Therefore, four stages are identified: (1) the stage of determination of diagnosis and treatment; (2) the stage of treatment; (3) the preterminal stage; and (4) the postterminal stage.

The Stage of Determination of Diagnosis and Treatment

The stage of determination of diagnosis and treatment encompasses the period of initial awareness of suspicious changes, the diagnostic work-up and consultation, as well as the actual determination of the diagnosis and the treatment. One of the most difficult and critical tasks of this stage is informing the patient of her disease. How this is done bears influence on the way the patient and the family will experience the postdiagnosis life. Although there are differing positions on whether or not to tell and when, what, and how much to tell, considerations regarding the individual patient, her diagnosis, and ability and readiness to absorb and withstand the sort of information must guide those decisions. It is generally accepted that whatever the decision, trust between the patient, the family, and the professionals is of critical value here. Trust is most likely to develop and be maintained if the truth, in whole or in part, is imparted coupled with empathy, concern, and an aura of confidence and willingness to support the patient and the family along the course of the disease and the treatment.

Linderman [6] has summarized the reactions of the patient following the shocking news about her disease into four stages. An initial natural (usual) reaction is one of grief, which is defined as "an emotion that is involved in the work of mourning, whereby a person seeks to disengage himself from the demanding relationship that has existed and to reinvest his emotional capital in new productive directions for the health and welfare of his future life" [5].

Engel [3] distinguishes various phases of the grief work. The first is shock and disbelief characterized by responses, at least in the case of the cancer patient, as, "It cannot be true," "They made a mistake," or, "It is just a tumor." It is believed that denial or disbelief is a mechanism in which the ego strength is preserved to save psychic energy necessary to complete successful grief work and as such it need be accepted as natural and functional. However, it must be distinguished from longstanding denial that interferes with the patient's or the family's acceptance of prescribed treatment. Understanding and skill are required in helping the patient and the family to accept reality.

The second phase is the beginning of awareness and acceptance of reality. Anger and depression set in gradually. Typically present are anxiety, insomnia, anorexia, depression, inability to concentrate, irritability, and feelings of loneliness. Among usual expressions are "Why me," "What did I do wrong," and the like. Often the patient or the family experience guilt related to their feelings or expressions of anger, and inability to concentrate. They need help in accepting such reactions as natural and surmountable and that, given time and assistance, control over their inner or external affairs is possible. Acceptance of reality may lead to resolution which is achieved through various forms. It is desirable, of course, that the patient feel an alliance with the therapeutic team and that a treatment plan be established in which the patient's and the family's voice is heard. The most functional outcome of this alliance is the success in keeping the patient and the family as active members of the therapeutic team waging war against the disease. The undesirable resolution may be one of defeatism that leads to refusal of or passive participation in the treatment with no or little hope for success.

Some of the particular apprehensions of this stage are those related to the diagnostic procedures and their outcomes. The determination of the extent of the disease then leads to the apprehension about the treatment even before this is determined. Treatments may include surgery, chemotherapy, radiotherapy, and/or immunotherapy. Thus the grief reactions to the initial diagnosis of cancer may be mixed with grief reactions to the possible loss of body part or function. Those reactions may be founded in the fear of adverse, debilitating, and disfiguring effects of chemotherapy, radiotherapy, or surgery which pose possible loss of self-esteem. Most authorities agree that truthfulness, openness, and realistic hopefulness on the part of the therapeutic team members help focus the patient's and the family's apprehensions on the realities about: (1) the extent of the disease; (2) the expected outcomes of the treatments; (3) the goals of each treatment and how these work; and (4) the mode of administration of each and whether pain or discomfort will be experienced and how much. Also, good communication in imparting those characteristics helps free the patient and the family from possible and potential misconceptions about any or all aspects of the disease and/or the treatments. Explanations need to be given after a careful analysis of the patient's concerns: (1) What is the patient verbalizing? (2) What, really, is the patient saying? (3) What does the patient want to know but is unable or unwilling to formulate as question(s)? When explanation is based on such assessment, it is more efficient and effective. Often such explanations need to be repeated to ensure the patient's and the family's understanding of the explanation to the extent that they are comfortable with the information. Often when diagnosis, treatment, and expected outcomes are discussed with the patient and the family for the first time, they may not be assimilated by the patient due to possible denial, extreme anxiety, or lack of understanding of the terminology used by the professional. The patient and the family need to feel welcome to ask questions or request further explanations. The nurse may assess the patient's or the family's need for an additional conference with the physician or any other member of the team. Most patients adjust more readily to certainty about the diagnosis or the treatment, than to the uncertainty that the team may cause inadvertently.

The third phase is that of acceptance and resolution. This stage is especially crucial because of the many resolutions the patient and the family must make in reorganizing and restructuring their lives. Decisions about the future in terms of accepting the treatment and all that it implies in the way of physical, financial, and psychosocial changes and adjustments need to be made. It is very important that the patient and the family are given honest and supportive communication during the process of the decision making. They may be under the illusion that death will never come or the inevitable adverse outcomes of the disease will be handled by some new miracle medical technique. Or, they may be locked in pessimism despite evidence of a more optimistic reality. They need be helped to make realistic and meaningful decisions. Care needs to be given to help reserve the family's emotional, psychological, physical, and financial energies for the times when the patient will need them most. Thus, resolutions regarding means of accepting the inevitable and choosing strategies for coping with it are partially made during this time.

The Stage of Treatment

The treatment stage is the intermediate stage that encompasses the events between the patient's initial reactions to the diagnosis and her reactions prior to the onset of the terminal period. This stage also pertains to the periodicity of illness, its relapses, remissions, progress, and periods of arrest.

The treatments for cancer are sometimes more loathsome to the patient than the disease itself. Each treatment modality has its peculiar physical, psychological, emotional, and social stresses. Often the patient is given combined treatment and thus is expected to cope with the various stresses of each modality. It is useful to look at some stresses peculiar to treatment modalities.

Surgical Treatment. Surgical treatment is particularly frightening. Mutilation of the body, loss of a body part or function, and altered body image are believed to affect the person's self-esteem and view of her future life. Uncertainty regarding the eradication of disease through removal of the body part adds to the ambivalence the patient experiences in anticipating the surgery. Preparation for the surgery must include the expectation of loss of the body part or function. Means of dealing with such loss need to be explained to the patient in terms of the care specific to this treatment—nursing, medical, physical, social, psychological, and spiritual—in meeting her needs. It is not unusual for the patient or the family to experience anticipatory grief with respect to any loss that they may see as impending. Therefore, anxiety, insomnia, anger, irritability, depression, and lack of concentration may well occur. They may continue, even intensify, after surgery, as the patient grieves the many losses ensuing from surgery.

Chemotherapeutic Treatment. In addition to the side effects of certain drugs, the patient's perceptions and interpretations regarding the treatment need to be assessed. Patients often regard chemotherapeutic treatment as indicative of advanced disease unmanageable by means of surgery or other treatment. This may be true, particularly if chemotherapy is adjuvant treatment to surgery or radiotherapy. Nausea and vomiting not only interfere with the nutritional status and therefore the well-being of the patient, but they reinforce the patient's withdrawal from physical and social activities through weakness, malaise, or effects of antiemetic medication. This not only may intensify the depression (if present) and its concomitant physical and emotional symptoms, but it may add to the feelings of helplessness. Other threats are those related to change of body image due to alopecia, lesions of oral cavity, skin disorders, mood changes associated with steroid treatment, and life-threatening infections. Some drugs have neurological effects, and some profound loss of cognitive functions. Each may be interpreted as signs of debilitation and further threat to life. Each needs careful assessment and intervention. Explanations regarding the treatments, the mode of their administration, the expected outcomes, and the objectives to be achieved need to be explained to the patient and the family prior to and during the treatment course.

Radiological Treatment. As in other treatment modalities, misconceptions about the reason for radiotherapy, the mode of treatment, and its effects are not uncommon. Careful explanation must be given about the objectives, outcomes, possible side effects, equipment to be used, and length of time of the treatments. Allowing the patient a visit to the radiotherapy facility at this time will enhance her understanding of the mode of the administration of the treatment and thus alleviate anxiety.

Reactions to Isolation During Chemotherapy and Immunotherapy. Although isolation technique is commonly exercised in treatment modalities for a variety of diseases, isolation of the cancer patient entails stricter measures. The room contains nothing more than is needed for the care of the patient, usually physically distant from the noise and the life of the ward. Those attending the patient are gowned, capped, masked, and shoed in sterile apparel. Visits to the caring persons are minimized to as few entries to the room as possible. Visits of the family usually are limited to only a few on a one-at-a-time basis. Physical contact with loved ones such as kissing and hugging are not permitted. Foods are sterilized prior to coming to the patient; these are usually always cooked. Many familiar objects such as photographs, favorite hobbies, or books are limited to few or none. Thus the environment is sterile in the biological, psychological, social, and emotional senses of the word.

In addition to the sensory deprivation experienced by a patient removed from her usual stimulations, there is the problem of sensory overload from new, often annoying stimulation. Several outcomes have been reported as manifestations of the patient's reactions: mental disorientation, hallucinations, emotional and physical extreme fatigue and insomnia, withdrawal, intensification of pain, and other similar behavior.

Other sources of psychosocial problems peculiar to this stage are: (1) remission; and (2) relapse. Lingering anxieties related to both need continuous attention and management. Ability to live with those anxieties and function at the optimal level demands more than the patient's stamina. It demands also, the stamina of the family, and indeed the stamina of the therapeutic team.

Remission. Being in remission, as much a triumph as it may be, is not free of problems. The truth is that neither the patient and the family, nor the caregivers, are free of doubt that recurrence of disease in metastatic or another primary form is possible. Therefore, whatever adjustments the patient and the family or the caregiver may make are made with constant awareness that they are subject to change. The possibility of recurrence and all of its ramifications tends to maintain the physical, psychological, and emotional dependence of the patient and the family on the therapeutic team for support. For many patients disease may not recur, but for many it will recur. For some patients and families, remission may mean total eradication of disease and unrealistic optimism. The underlying message for the patient, the family, and the therapeutic team must be one of realistic expectation. Both facts and wisdom are required to convey this to them throughout the period of remission. Insight into the reality of the situation should guide the approaches to physical and psychosocial rehabilitation.

Recurrence. Recurrence of the disease subjects the patient, the family, and the therapeutic team to profound psychic trauma. The grieving process begins all over again, possibly with more intensity, since the patient and the family may carry unresolved feelings from previous griefs. The trauma is experienced with equal devastation by the therapeutic team. The particular emotional reactions are feelings of defeat, deceit of the patient and the family, guilt related to both, loss of control, and feelings of powerlessness. The tendency to want to avoid the patient and the family results from those feelings. This is a critical time for open communication between the patient, the family, and the therapeutic team. Sharing of mutual feelings not only has a cathartic action on all concerned, but more importantly, renews feelings of being supported, cared for, and hope in the patient and the family. Exploration of alternatives in terms of treatment, new adjustments, and expectations with the patient and the family will help formulate realistic goals. Renewal of feelings to fight on may be more difficult to initiate and maintain than they were prior to the recurrence. The stresses then were relatively more bearable since cure was a possibility; now recurrence is more of a reality.

Recurrence may result in treatment with a positive outcome or slow progression into a chronic disease. Even when the disease is controlled there is always the possibility of further recurrence. The expectation of adaptation on the part of the patient and the family is that of coping with symptoms. The goal of rehabilitation is maximal functioning. Among the less-adaptive reactions are: physical and psychological dependence on the treatment, family, and the caregivers; anger; withdrawal; fear of abandonment; hopelessness; and lack of cooperation with rehabilitative efforts. Severe depression is one of the most difficult problems and is almost always prevalent in the first or subsequent recurrences of the disease. The most helpful messages the therapeutic team may convey are understanding and acceptance of the patient's and the family's feelings, willingness to try alternative approaches for interventions, and assurance that the patient and the family will not be abandoned. Clear view of realistic expectations of interventions and open communication with the patient and the family will help them make realistic decisions regarding cooperation with the interventions as well as regarding the future. Hope and despair ever vacillate during this stage.

The Preterminal Stage

No treatment other than palliative interventions is usually attempted once the diagnosis is made that the disease is terminal. The goal for treatment is maintenance of physical, psychological, emotional, and social functioning as much as is possible. The medical interventions are aimed at symptom control such as relief of pain, nutritional substitutes, and infection control. The patient's as well as the family's physical, psychological, emotional, and financial reserve is markedly depleted during this stage. The dominant fears of the patient are those of abandonment by the family or the caregivers, being a burden to the family or friends, and being left alone at the time of death. Hopes of the patient are for many simple things all related to physical and psychological comfort. Sarna found that being able to sleep, and to be free of pain, were things that patients with lung cancer hoped for in this stage [8].

Awareness of the impending death may exist on the part of the patient and the family, yet open communication between them may not exist. Each resorting to pretention of not knowing or not wanting to discuss may create an emotionally inhibiting atmosphere. Casey found that closed communication substitutes for open communication—while patient and family avoid open discussion of imminent death, each in their own way communicates covertly [1]. For example, the family or the caregivers may begin disengaging from the patient's care unintentionally, or the patient disengages from the family psychologically, socially, or emotionally. Or, a kind of game playing exists in which each pretends to accept the other's pretense which usually is not free of feelings of guilt and anger. The caregiver(s), the clergyperson, or a trusted friend may be very helpful in initiating open communication in which feelings are aired, shared, and hopefully resolved.

The Postterminal Stage

The funeral is a very important event. At the time the patient dies, many family members or loved ones experience a sense of relief along with grief. The sense of relief is usually out of feelings of deliverance of the patient from the agony of terminal illness, as well as feelings of their own deliverance from intense physical and emotional involvement with the patient and the patient's suffering. The first several weeks are lived with a kind of numbness. Much talk is carried about the deceased and the illness. Often family members feel depleted of physical and psychic energy and thus unable to support one another. Help of other family members, friends, and even members of the therapeutic team are needed.

During the following weeks feelings of guilt, ambivalence toward accepting death as the inevitable event, feelings of having failed, and even of anger toward the deceased are common. Often, with the death of the patient, the relationship of the caregivers and the family comes to a halt. Families do appreciate the presence of a caregiver, usually the nurse, at the funeral and during the grieving period. The work of resolution of feelings, acceptance of the death of the loved one, and reintegration work demands the support of others.

PROBLEMS IN MANAGEMENT OF PSYCHOSOCIAL PROBLEMS

Problems in Assessment

As we have noted, reactions common to one stage are also common to others if not to all stages of the clinical course of cancer. However, there may be differences in the intensity or longevity of re-actions, or differences specific to a situation which is specific to a stage. For example, reactions of grieving, anger, anxiety about the future, depression, sexual dysfunction, and fears of various kinds occur in all stages of the disease. The clinician is able to assess and determine whether those reactions are natural (usually seen), adapta-tional, or maladaptational. Obviously there are no well-established differential diagnostic indicators or procedures that, when considered and applied, may circumscribe the problem to a more specific area. The observer makes a gross assessment regarding the observed reac-tions, their nature, their possible determinants, and whether they are adaptive or maladaptive. The adaptiveness or maladaptiveness of the reactions can be distinguished in terms of the function of these reactions in the overall behavior of the patient toward achieving the goals of the interventions. Some relevant considerations are:

1. The particular stage of the clinical course of the disease
2. The medical diagnosis
3. The medical treatment
4. The entering behavior—previous knowledge and experience
5. The age, sex, role, education background, the family, and cul-tural background
6. The level of awareness and knowledge of the patient about the disease and the treatment
7. The meaning of the disease to the patient
8. The outcome expected of the treatment—both desirable (in-tended) and undesirable (unintended) outcomes
9. The outcome obtained by the treatment—both desirable (in-tended) and undesirable (unintended) outcomes
10. The meaning of the outcome of the treatment to the patient—both desirable (intended) and undesirable (unintended) outcomes

An additional difficulty in the assessment of psychosocial problems is the lack of reliable tools with which to identify and measure the problems. One way of dealing with this difficulty is to utilize theo-retical constructs respective to those reactions most prevalent in the adaptation of individuals to the diagnosis and treatment of cancer. This will take the observations and interpretation of reactions a step further away from intuitive observations and interpretations. Docu-mentation of such systemized observations will help develop re-searchable questions. The ideal is to develop valid and reliable tools, through methodological research, to describe and measure prob-lems related to those and other reactions. There are tools in the behavioral disciplines to measure some problems such as anxiety, powerlessness, and the like. But these are highly specific to the phenomena in healthy or nondiseased populations and therefore may have limited clinical usefulness. The efforts of nurses to develop tools more specific to clinical use in identifying psychosocial problems are increasing. One such effort resulted in the Dependence-Independence Observational Tool developed by Derdiarian, Clough, and Wittig [2].

Problems in Intervention

As we found with assessment, interventions in the psychosocial problems also lack support in knowledge. Unfortunately, interventions rely on empirical and often intuitive knowledge based on scant or topical understanding of their underlying theories. However, their theoretical underpinnings can be subjected to systematic and methodical practice. Their theoretical constructs can be defined in operational terms of interventive nursing practice, expected patient outcomes, and development of criteria for the evaluation of interventions. For example, teaching as a nursing intervention may be more effective in alleviating a specific degree of anxiety in some patients than in other patients. The question is, then, What level of anxiety is alleviated, in which patient population, as a result of which teaching content or method? Such analysis would link the theoretical relationships between anxiety and teaching to the determinants intrinsic to the clinical stage of the patient's disease and treatment. Documentation of this sort will in time yield researchable questions and thus generate knowledge respective to those interventions. Obviously, it is imperative that the nurse keep abreast of new developments of knowledge and technology. Although there are many interventive methods for each of a number of psychosocial problems, practice in cancer patient care reveals that there are some major interventive approaches in dealing with those problems. These are based on theories related to teaching, communication, crisis intervention, reality orientation, motivation, hope maintenance, and the like. The implementation of these or other interventions needs to be based on diagnoses that are as carefully assessed, well formulated, and precisely stated as possible.

Implications for Nursing

Nursing Practice. It is imperative that nursing practice be systematized, that is, that a theoretical framework be utilized to guide data collection, analysis, and interpretation in both assessment and implementation of interventions. Theoretical as well as technical knowledge must be updated and kept current. Furthering nursing's primary goals along with furthering the goals of other professionals with whom the nurse collaborates demarcates nursing's scope within the overall scope of interdisciplinary care of the cancer patient. Systematization of practice as described facilitates generation of knowledge on two levels: (1), knowledge related to nursing; and (2) knowledge related to other disciplines.

Nursing Education. Content and practice related to management of psychosocial problems of cancer patients and their families are integral to the training of the neophyte nurses. Proficient practice in this area of nursing requires specialized training on the graduate level or intense and comprehensive training on the continuing education level. Theoretical as well as practicum content should be given equal emphasis in such training.

Nursing Research. Systematization of nursing practice is the basis for generating testable hypotheses related to practice. Research can and ought to be integral to the training of the professional whether generic or postgraduate. Nursing can develop research both in the field of nursing and in collaboration with other disciplines.

CONCLUSION

Management of psychosocial problems subsequent to the diagnosis and treatment of cancer is a challenge that demands deliberate and well-coordinated interdisciplinary teamwork. The challenge comprises two major components of equal importance—assessment and intervention—each needing sophisticated skills in practice and scientific treatment. By nature, the nursing profession holds the most strategic position on the interdisciplinary team. The importance of this position to the patient lies in the nurse being the primary contact person all along the clinical course of the disease, giving the patient systematic and deliberate nursing care as she funnels into the patient's care the therapeutic efforts of each member of the team. The importance of this position to the team lies in the nurse providing the team with feedback and being an active participant in formulating diagnoses of psychosocial problems and interventions specific for their solutions. The importance of this position to the development of knowledge about the nature, extent, and source of psychological problems, as well as effectiveness of various interventions in all stages of the clinical disease, lies in the nurse's ability to develop skills and tools to systematize her or his observations.

REFERENCES

[1] CASEY, K. The Family of the Terminal Patient: An Exploration of Behavior and Feelings. *Conference on Cancer Nursing Research*, Los Angeles, 1979.

[2] CLOUGH, D., and DERDIARIAN, A. A Behavioral Checklist to Measure Dependence and Independence. *Nursing Research*, 28:55–58, 1980.

[3] ENGEL, G. Grief and Grieving. *American Journal of Nursing*, 61:93–98, 1974.

[4] HEALY, J., ED. *Ecology of Cancer Patient*, p. 184. Washington, D.C.: Interdisciplinary Communications Program, The Smithsonian Institute, 1970.

[5] JACKSON, E.N. *Understanding Grief*, p. 18. Nashville: Abingdon, 1957.

[6] LINDERMANN, E. Symptomatology and Management of Acute Grief. *American Journal of Psychiatry*, 101:104, 1944.

[7] NEWLIN, N. *Conference on Cancer Nursing Research*, Los Angeles, 1979.

[8] SARNA, L. An Investigation of the Hopes of Terminally Ill Cancer Patients. *Conference on Cancer Nursing Research*, Los Angeles, 1979.

ADDITIONAL READINGS

ABRAMS, R.D. The Patient With Cancer—His Changing Pattern of Communication. *The New England Journal of Medicine*, 274(6):317–322, 1966.

BAHNSON, C. Psychological and Emotional Issues in Cancer: The Psychotherapeutic Care of the Cancer Patient. *Seminars in Oncology*, 2:300–310, 1975.

FREIDENBERGS, I.; GORDON, W.; HIBBARD, M.R.; and DILLER, L. Assessment and Treatment of Psychosocial Problems of the Cancer Patient, a Case Study. *Cancer Nursing*, 3:111–119, 1980.

FRIEDMAN, B.D. Coping With Cancer: A Guide for Health Care Professionals. *Cancer Nursing*, 3:105–110, 1980.

HOLLAND, J.C.B. Coping with Cancer: A Challenge to the Behavioral Sciences. In *Cancer, The Behavioral Dimensions*, ed. J.W. Cullen, B.H. Fox, and R.N. Isom, pp. 263–267. New York: Raven Press, 1976.

KENNEDY, B.J.; PELLEGEN, A.; KENNEDY, S.; and HAVERNICK, N. Psychological Response of Patients Cured of Advanced Cancer. *Cancer*, 38(5): 2184–2191, 1976.

PAYNE, E.C., and KRANT, M.J. The Psychological Aspects of Advanced Cancer. *Journal of the American Medical Association*, 210:1238, 1969.

PECK, A., and BOLAND, J. Emotional Reaction to Radiation Treatment. *Cancer*, 40:180–184, 1977.

SHANDS, H.C. The Informational Impact of Cancer on the Structure of the Human Personality. *Annals of New York Academy of Science*, 125:883–889, 1966.

WEISMAN, A.D. *Coping with Cancer*. New York: McGraw-Hill Book Company, 1979.

chapter four

LINDA PATTI SARNA, R.N., M.N.
Assistant Clinical Professor
Teaching in Graduate Nursing
Oncology Program
School of Nursing, UCLA

Concepts in the nursing care of patients undergoing cancer assessment

INTRODUCTION

Understanding the principles of diagnosis and staging of malignant tumors and the relationship of those principles to therapeutic options facilitates the comprehensive nursing care of cancer patients. The physical, emotional and social dimensions of a patient's response to the diagnosis of cancer are important considerations in the selection of appropriate therapy. An appreciation of the events leading to a patient's initial presentation to the physician and the subsequent pathways of diagnosis and treatment also will direct nursing actions on the patient's behalf.

This chapter will focus on the basic concepts underlying the nursing care of patients faced with the prospect of cancer. It will provide a review of the essential principles involved in the screening, diagnosing, and staging of malignancy and will incorporate nursing implications for patient care. Nursing assessment parameters evaluating the impact of the diagnosis will be discussed. Further examination of current treatment options available to patients with cancer will be addressed. Nonapproved cancer therapy will also be discussed, particularly as it relates to the nurse-patient relationship.

Purpose and Function

The purpose of cancer screening is to detect abnormalities that may indicate a malignant process. Screening tests and procedures should be sensitive enough to detect early, subtle changes before overt symptoms occur. Theoretically, cancer screening would ensure accurate identification of potential malignancies with minimal risk to the patient. The availability of effective treatment promising reduced mortality and disability is implicit in attempts at cancer detection [17].

Screening is currently a controversial area in cancer health care. Malignancies that do not have effective treatment alternatives despite early detection and malignancies with effective treatment despite late detection would not benefit from screening procedures in terms of reduced mortality [17]. Screening efforts are designed to identify malignancies that can be effectively treated if diagnosed early. Optimally, cancer screening will provide information for the patient and the health team to guide further health care.

Early detection of cancer may have a significant impact on the prognosis of malignancy and the quality of the patient's life. Localized tumors may be more easily and effectively treated with curative intent than those tumors that have spread throughout the body.

Risks

The risks involved in any cancer screening program should be carefully evaluated in terms of the potential benefits it can offer. Screening may cause unnecessary anxiety due to equivocal results requiring further testing [3,17]. Unnecessary surgery, such as breast biopsies, may be performed when the patient has a benign lump and is symptom free [17]. There is also a potential risk of false reassurance after a patient has been told he is free of cancer in the specific sites evaluated. The patient may assume he is is totally healthy and ignore subsequent provocative signs and symptoms.

Of considerable concern in any medical procedure are the risks of morbidity. This is especially true in screening procedures aimed at the population at large. The risk of radiation-induced breast cancer from mammography is an example of a recent controversy regarding risks of screening [17].

New Recommendations

Recent evaluation by the American Cancer Society of the results of cancer screening procedures has resulted in recommendations for changes from previous guidelines [1]. (See Table 4.1.) Revised guidelines for screening for lung cancer, breast cancer, colon cancer, and cervical cancer indicate an attempt to reduce unnecessary cost and risk while continuing to provide benefits in cancer detection. The previous recommendation for annual chest X-ray for high-risk persons was changed due to the disappointing results in the evaluation of the impact of screening procedures (including sputum cytology) on morbidity and mortality. Prevention (for example, smoking cessation) may be the major variable in reducing mortality due to lung cancer. While recommended, the breast self-examination is controversial in terms of its high yield of false positives, its questionable impact on disease course, and the difficulties with compliance [17]. The American Cancer Society recommends changes in the frequency of Pap smears after two initial annual negative tests. In this case, high-risk women benefit from more frequent screening. Endometrial tissue samples for women at high risk for endometrial cancer (due to history of infertility, for example, or estrogen therapy) are recommended at menopause. Though stool-guiac testing has a small yield, its cost is minimal and it has minimal false positives or false negatives as well as an acceptable degree of patient compliance [24]. The impact of digital exams on cure and survival in colon cancer is unclear. But, the exam has low morbidity and cost and a high yield, making

TABLE 4.1
Guidelines for Cancer Screening [1]

Type of Cancer	Screening Recommendations
Breast	Breast self-examination every month for women over 20 years, physical examination of breast every 3 years for women 20–40 years,[a] (annually after 40 years), baseline mammogram at age 35–40, annual mammograms after 50 years
Colon and rectum	Sigmoidoscopy every 3–5 years for persons over 50 years (with two previous annual negative tests), stool-guiac slide test annually for persons over 50 years, digital rectal examination annually for persons over 40 years
Cervix	Papanicolaou smear every 3 years for women 20–65 years,[b] pelvic examination every 3 years for women 20–40 years, annually for women over 40 years
Lung	No current effective screening procedures

[a] After 40 years consult with physician annually.
[b] Every 3 years for sexually active women under 20 years.

it acceptable for cancer screening [24]. Health counseling, including assessment of risk factors and a physical examination for a cancer check are recommended every three years for persons over 20 and annually for persons over 40 years who are asymptomatic. The presence of symptoms should be an indication for immediate health assessment.

Accuracy

Screening procedures may be evaluated for their efficiency in terms of their ability to recognize normal as well as abnormal. The following labels are used in evaluation of a screening test's accuracy:

1. True positive—an abnormality suggestive of cancer is detected; cancer is truly there.
2. False positive—an abnormality is detected; there is no cancer.
3. True negative—there is no abnormality; there is no cancer.
4. False Negative—the cancer is present but not detected.

While no screening procedure can claim 100% accuracy, the error should be on the side of false positives rather than false negatives. Validity can be reflected in both the sensitivity and specificity of the test [27]. Assessment of the patient's understanding of the meaning and accuracy of the test results is an important nursing consideration. The patient's experience with ambiguous test results may influence his trust in future information from medical procedures.

Mass Screening

Mass screening involves surveying the entire population. Such efforts may be ineffective and costly [27]. By necessity, the procedures need to have significant validity, be easy to administer, be cost effective, and be relatively benign. Patient compliance may depend on the availability of the health care service and the positive reinforcement—verbal rewards by health team, social sanction, health insurance benefits—that they receive for undergoing the procedure.

Screening in High-Risk Groups

Screening of groups at high risk for cancer may be different in frequency and scope of cancer detection. Determination of patients at risk includes identification of predisposing pathologic conditions, environmental and occupational exposure to known carcinogens, per-

TABLE 4.2
Examples of Variables To Be Assessed in Identification
of High-Risk Groups for Cancer Screening [24]

Type of Malignancy	Risk Factors
Breast cancer	Breast cancer in sister or mother,[a] cancer in other breast, early menarche or late menopause, nulliparous or first pregnancy after 25 years, benign breast disease[b]
Colon cancer	Hereditary polyposis syndromes, family history of adeno-carcinoma or colonic cancer, ulcerative colitis, villous adenomas, diet rich in animal fat and cholesterol, previous colonic cancer
Lung cancer	Older men, smoking, miners of radioactive isotopes (uranium), exposure to heavy pollutants, industrial pollution (exposure to nickel, asbestos, chloro-methyl-methyl ether), previous history of lung cancer

[a] Especially if bilateral or premenopausal breast cancer.
[b] Especially if lobular histology.

sonal habits (for example, smoking), family history of cancer, past and current health history, and presence of precancerous lesions [7,15,26]. (See Table 4.2.) The person at "risk" has an unusual susceptibility to the development of cancer. Multiple variables may influence the cancer development directly or as precursors to a pathologic condition. Additional variables may influence the mortality to the specific disease [8,27,28]. Chapter 10 details nursing's preventive role in interrupting the links in cancer development. Nursing assessment of factors predisposing to malignancy may be an important screening function [32].

Patient education regarding cancer prevention and detection can begin in cancer screening [31,32]. The patient should be able to identify personal risk factors for oncogenesis. Patient education should include information regarding self detection measures (such as the breast self-examination) and cancer's warning signals [1,11, 22]. The patient should know when, where, and how to seek help if there is a change in health status.

Physical Examination in Cancer Screening

The physical examination of the patient during a diagnostic work-up will include the principles of inspection and palpation. Physical signs and symptoms may be due to direct effects of the tumor, metastases, or to indirect metabolic or immunologic results of cancer. The physical exam may reveal signs which have varying degrees of specificity and sensitivity for the diagnosis of cancer.

Physical examination of the patient is an important procedure in cancer detection in which nurses may play a greater role in the future [32]. Precancerous and cancerous lesions may be detected by inspection and palpation of accessible sites.

Occult Malignancies

Occult tumors may be uncovered with radiographic techniques, cytologic examinations of exfolliated cells, and laboratory tests examining chemical, hematological, hormonal and genetic abnormalities. No one test, at this point, is diagnostic for cancer [6]. These tests will be able to discriminate between normal and abnormal and may with varying degrees of accuracy suggest a malignant process. When suspicious results occur, further diagnostic testing is warranted.

Patient Concerns

Patient fears and concerns regarding cancer screening may involve emotional as well as physical parameters. The fear of the results may influence the patient's behavior throughout the procedure. Embarrassment and discomfort of a test—proctoscopy, for example—may be the major concern of the patient experiencing that procedure. A person's sense of vulnerability to cancer as well as his trust in the results obtained from a screening procedure can promote preventive health care behaviors. Health behaviors will also be influenced by the perceived benefits of the action in reducing susceptibility to disease and in preventing the consequences of illness [27]. (Specific elements of health behavior as they relate to prevention of cancer are dealt with in Chapter 9.)

Nursing Assessment in Cancer Screening

In cancer screening, a nursing assessment should include an evaluation of any pertinent signs and symptoms that might indicate a malignant process [32]. Recognition of recent changes in life-style and habits and assessment of personal appearance may also be very important in cancer screening. High-risk variables associated with cancer development should also be assessed [7,19]. The patient should also be made aware of these factors [20]. The nurse should assess the patient's cancer "set," which would include previous personal experiences with cancer patients and views related to cancer causation and cancer cure.

Patient education regarding cancer screening procedures involves relaying:

1. Purpose and importance of the procedure
2. How the results will relate to the patient's plan of health care
3. What activities occur during the procedure
4. Relative risks of procedure
5. Possible discomfort, side effects during the procedure
6. Environmental setting, equipment necessary
7. Length of time involved
8. Precautions after the procedure
9. Frequency necessary for repeating screening procedure
10. Financial cost
11. When and how notification will be received regarding results

Emotional support of the patient may be given by decreasing fear and anxiety associated with the procedure by providing the patient with understandable answers to his questions [3,13]. However, education may not be the most effective way to comfort the patient. Physical contact, diversion, relaxation techniques, and having an important friend accompany the patient may provide other ways of decreasing a patient's discomfort during the screening procedure. Environmental alterations such as the provision of privacy may also be within the nursing domain. The totality of the experience may dramatically influence the patient's future decisions to be involved in preventive health care. Many patients may have little stress associated with screening procedures.

Clinical considerations in the nursing care of patients undergoing screening tests may involve aiding or monitoring the performance of the test. Prevention or minimization of untoward side effects may require nursing action. Conscientious care of the specimen and test result may also be an important nursing function. The time interval before the notification of the results of the test will be important information for the patient.

CANCER DIAGNOSIS

Diagnostic Testing

Diagnostic testing may be necessary when screening procedures reveal positive or suspicious results. If the patient presents with suggestive signs and symptoms, diagnostic testing will begin immediately. The correct diagnosis of cancer is essential for appropriate treatment selection and determination of the potential prognosis. The diagnosis may also predict the propensity for the tumor to metastasize. The diagnosis may include the anatomic location, tissue of origin, cellular type, and degree of cellular dysplasia [5,6].

Diagnostic testing involves evaluation of clinical signs and symptoms directly or indirectly caused by cancer. It also may include histologic diagnosis as well as various laboratory examinations (for example, cytology), radiographic and endoscopic procedures.

Presentation of Malignancy

The symptoms and signs that may be the first indications of malignant disease are varied. (See Tables 4.3 and 4.4.) The dissemination through the media of information about signs and symptoms suspicious for cancer has helped to educate the public. This increased awareness of warning signals and the emphasis on the importance of early detection of cancer has made many people sensitive and responsive to subtle body changes. Sometimes it is the type of sign or symptom (for example, bleeding) rather than the degree of change that influences the patient to seek medical attention. The point at which a symptom becomes bothersome to the patient may be a more critical event in prompting the patient to receive medical care than the degree of visibility or abnormality. Some patients deny even gross signs of disease, diminishing the possibility of early diagnosis and cure [2]. In some cases, the signs and symptoms that are first presented may be evidence of metastatic lesions rather than the primary tumor.

Direct Effects. Signs and symptoms related to cancer growth and development may be characterized as local or distant effects of the tumor. Local effects of a tumor mass depend on its location as well as its size [6,30]. (See Table 4.3.)

Five major types of symptomatology may result from the direct presence of a malignant tumor: pain, obstruction, destruction, hemorrhage, and infection. Pain may result from the pressure and invasion of other anatomical structures. The pain will vary in type and degree depending upon the location and size of the tumor as well as a myriad of psychologic and physiologic variables influencing the perception of pain. It is also important to note that tumors may arise and obtain significant size before any pain is perceived.

Obstruction and destruction of normal anatomical structures by

TABLE 4.3
Presentation of Malignancy:
Direct Effects

Site	Signs and Symptoms[a]
Skin	Change in mole, rash, roughness, and ulceration
Lung	Cough, dyspnea, hemoptysis, and chest pain
Breast	Mass, change in texture, mobility, and nipple discharge
Colon	Change in bowel habits and abdominal pain
Cervix	Abnormal, persistent vaginal bleeding, and postcoital pain
Larynx	Persistent cough and hoarseness

[a] Suggestive but not specific to malignancy.

the tumor can cause mild to severe functional defects. These alterations may be significant to the patient because of the impact on his life activities. Symptoms related to obstruction and destruction will also vary in kind and degree according to the site of tumor.

Hemorrhage may also result as a direct effect of tumor growth and invasion into major vessels. Generalized bleeding may occur with bone marrow depression caused by primary or metastatic disease. Bleeding may be a profound initial symptom necessitating emergency treatment.

The tendency for bulky masses to become necrotic and bleed also sets up an ideal environment for an infectious process. Cancer's impact on the function of the bone marrow as well as the immune system may also increase a patient's vulnerability to infection. Obstruction will also contribute to factors predisposing to development of infection. Thus, the patient with a malignancy may first present with symptoms related to the infectious process caused by the presence of cancer.

Distant Effects. Cancer can also present with dramatic constitutional effects [10, 16, 30]. Body wasting, sudden weight loss, and anorexia are associated with many tumors. The generalized feelings of malaise and lassitude are also frequently reported by patients and may precede other more specific symptoms. Some patients may experience febrile episodes not directly related to an infectious process. The fever may come in cycles or patterns.

Distant effects can also be mediated by tumor metastases. A tumor may spread through direct extension and cause symptoms by encroaching upon adjacent anatomical structures. A tumor may also spread through the lymphatic system, often becoming evident in the nearest regional lymph nodes first. Implantation of the tumor throughout the body may be mediated through the circulatory system [3]. The physical signs and symptoms of these metastatic tumors will be similar to those described under direct effects.

Paraneoplastic syndromes are metabolic consequences of the cancerous state which may occur in up to 75% of patients with advanced stages of malignancy [16]. These syndromes are a constellation of signs and symptoms resulting from circulating products created by the tumor directly or indirectly. (See Table 4.4.) They do not have a direct relation to the size of the tumor or its interference with normal organ function. Ectopic hormone production is the most common class of these syndromes. Hormones may be produced by the nonendocrine tumors and found in unusual sites or in abnormal quantities. They may be produced in excess and result in abnormal endocrinologic effects. The tumor may induce a decrease in immune competence (with subsequent opportunistic infections) or acquired autoimmune conditions such as hemolytic anemia [4].

Other classes of paraneoplastic manifestations would include skin rashes (dermatomyositis, for example, or acanthosis nigricans),

TABLE 4.4
Examples of Paraneoplastic Syndromes

Tumor	Syndromes
Lung cancer	Hypercalcemia, Cushing's disease, peripheral neuropathy
Breast cancer	Hypercalcemia, cerebellar degeneration
Renal cell cancer	Anemia
Hodgkin's disease	Decreased cellular immunity, hemolytic anemia
Multiple myeloma	Decreased humoral immunity
Colon cancer	Melanotic pigmentation of the skin, acanthosis nigricans
All tumors	Cachexia, anorexia, fatigue

skeletal abnormalities (such as clubbing), renal abnormalities (such as nephrotic syndrome), neurologic changes (peripheral neuropathy or muscle weakness, for example), and hematologic changes including hypercoagulability or erythrocytosis.

Recognition of the propensity for some tumors to result in paraneoplastic syndromes is important in clinical screening efforts as well as in diagnostic testing. These signs and symptoms may be very difficult for the patient to relate to a cancerous process. Successful treatment of the primary tumor may result in long-term control of the signs and symptoms. Often in an acute presentation, and in patients with advanced disease, therapy is directed toward interrupting the pathophysiologic mechanism of the paraneoplastic syndrome as well as providing symptomatic relief for the patient.

Histologic Diagnosis

While other diagnostic tests (such as radiographic exams) may suggest malignancy, histologic testing can result in "proof" of malignancy. Histologic examination can determine the type of cancerous cell (for example, adenocarcinoma) and the degree of cellular aplasia (grading) [6]. Accurate histologic diagnosis of a tumor may be obtained only after an examination of suspect tissue [6,30]. This sample may be obtained in a variety of ways. Histologic confirmation of the tumor via frozen or permanent section may be obtained by tissue biopsy. Needle, incisional, or excisional biopsies may be performed to obtain tissues for diagnostic clarification. These may be done prior to or as part of a therapeutic procedure (for example, surgery). Biopsies may also be done to ascertain presence of metastatic lesions in other organ sites such as liver, lymph nodes, and bone. Other information influencing treatment decisions may be obtained via biopsy (for example, presence of estrogen receptors).

The major purpose of the biopsy is to detect and obtain a sample of malignant growth for examination. The risk of the procedure varies with the tumor location and type. Risks of any biopsy technique include tumor implantation as a result of the procedure, infection, and hemorrhage.

Diagnostic Cytology

In some cases, diagnosis of malignancy may be made with a cytologic examination. This involves collection and slide preparation of exfoliated cells without the tissue framework provided in a frozen or permanent section. The Pap smear is a familiar example of diagnostic cytology. Bronchial washings, fluid or tissue aspiration, and collections of sputum, urine, or spinal fluid are other methods of obtaining material for diagnostic cytology. This may be an excellent method for diagnosing asymptomatic cancer of some sites.

Determination of malignancy and the specific cell type varies depending upon the procedure and tumor involved. Differentiation of dysplasia from malignancy may be difficult in cytologic examination [6].

For any invasive diagnostic procedure, nursing assessment of the patient's understanding and concerns regarding the test is important. Comfort measures to reduce pain and anxiety are important nursing responsibilities in enabling the patient to endure the procedure. In some cases, as in sputum collections, the patient's involvement and cooperation will be essential in obtaining the specimen.

Laboratory Tests

Clinical laboratory tests are important adjuvants to histologic and cytologic examinations in the diagnosis of cancer [6,12,16,30]. (See Table 4.5.) The results of laboratory tests may be related to impaired physiologic functioning mediated by direct effects of the primary tumor or of tumors in metastatic sites. Distant effects of the

TABLE 4.5
Significant Laboratory Tests in Cancer Diagnosis and Staging

Test	Significance in Cancer Diagnosing/Staging
Chemistry	
Alkaline phosphatase	Increased in bony or liver metastases
Electrolytes	Reveals organ obstruction or malfunction as well as hormonal syndromes
Calcium	Increased with multiple myeloma, boney metastasis, ectopic parathyroid hormone or prostaglandin secretion
Calcitonin	Increased in medullary carcinoma of the thyroid
SGOT, SGPT	Increased in liver cancer
5HIAA (5-hydroxyl acetic acid)	Increased in carcinoid syndrome
Protein electrophoresis	Reveals abnormal proteins in myeloma, lymphoma, and chronic lymphatic leukemia

TABLE 4.5 (continued)

Test	Significance in Cancer Diagnosing/Staging
Alpha-fetoprotein	Increased in liver cancer and testicular malignancy
Glucocorticoids Parathyroid hormone ACTH (adrenocorticotropic hormone)	Increased in paraneoplastic syndromes
Carcinoembryonic antigen (CEA)	May increase with many types of cancer, particularly cancer of bowel
Serum or urine immunoelectrophoresis	Antigen-antibody test may reveal para-proteins in myeloma, lymphoma, and chronic lymphocitic leukemia
EB virus titer	Increased in Burkitt's lymphoma and nasopharyngeal carcinoma
Beta-HCG (human chorionic gonadotropin)	Increased in testicular malignancy
Uric acid	Increased in leukemia
Acid phosphatase	Increased in carcinoma of the prostate

Hematology

Hemoglobin/Hematocrit	Presence of anemia common in colorectal or gastrointestinal tumors; erythro-cytosis in renal cell cancer
Differential	Number and quality of leukocytes and lymphocytes altered in bone marrow disease
Platelet count	Decreased in bone marrow involvement of malignancy
Bone marrow aspiration	Evidence of primary and metastatic infiltration of bone marrow
Leukocyte alkaline phosphatase (stain)	Decreased in chronic myelogenous leukemia
Acid phophatase stain	Present in some T cell lymphomas and hairy cell leukemia (tartrate resistant)

Chromosomal analysis

Philadelphia chromosome	Often present in chronic myelogenous leukemia

Note: These test results may be altered due to other pathology.

tumors, as described in the section on paraneoplastic syndromes, may also be uncovered.

Tumor Markers

Tumor markers in the form of biochemical abnormalities or abnormal proteins revealed by radionuclide immunoassays may aid in the diagnosis and selection of treatment [16]. They may be also useful in following patients after treatment for signs of recurrence. Carcinoembryonic antigen (CEA) may be elevated in both malignant and benign conditions. It is most commonly associated with colorectal, breast, and pancreatic tumors, but also may be found in a variety of other cancers. CEA is not useful for screening alone, because it lacks specificity as well as sensitivity to the early stages of a malignant process. Alpha-fetoprotein and lactic dehydrogenase (LDH) are markers that may be helpful in both diagnosing and staging malignancy.

Radiographic Exams

Radiographic procedures may indicate the presence of the tumor or the deviation of normal anatomic landmarks that it may produce [4, 29]. These tests are rarely able to make an absolute diagnosis of cancer alone. They may be important in defining suspected tumor and planning therapy. Of special note are ultrasound examinations, which can provide noninvasive imaging of normal and abnormal structures. Computerized axial tomography can be very effective in the diagnosis of brain tumors. Occasionally, selective arteriography of brain, GI tract, pancreas, liver, and some retroperitoneal tumors can suggest a preoperative diagnosis of cancer [2].

Endoscopic Exams

Endoscopic examinations such as bronchoscopy, sigmoidoscopy, colonoscopy, gastroscopy, and esophagoscopy provide an opportunity for inspection in otherwise unobservable areas [6]. The procedure also facilitates the collection of biopsy and cytology specimens for the purpose of histologic diagnosis.

Nursing Assessment During the Diagnostic Phase

Patients entering the hospital for diagnostic testing may be experiencing a variety of symptoms related to the direct or indirect effects of malignancy. Weight loss, fatigue, and a general sense of malaise are frequent complaints of many with cancer. The gamut of physical symptomatic disturbances may be augmented by the often even more acute psychic stress that may accompany the threat of cancer. Some patients may have had a positive result from a screening test for cancer, but others may be undergoing diagnostic testing due to their presentation of signs and symptoms suspicious of cancer.

A careful systematic nursing assessment of the patient's wellbeing both physically and emotionally can aid in individualizing care. These initial experiences during diagnostic testing may well set the style for future communication and cooperation between the patient and nurse and members of the health team [33]. A key step in establishing trust and building this relationship is through an understanding of the patient's "story" or experience with cancer and his present illness.

Crucial elements of the nursing assessment and history that must be elicited in initial patient interviews during diagnostic testing are listed. (Refer to Chapter 13 for a guide to models of nursing assessment.)

1. What was the patient's life like before his illness (including job, family, social activities, nutrition, elimination, sleep pattern, sexual activity, personality)?
2. What was the patient's past experience with illness, including cancer?
3. How has this illness affected the patient's life?
4. What life changes due to the illness are most disturbing to the patient? How has the patient dealt with these?
5. What are the patient's major concerns at this time related to the possibility of a cancer diagnosis?
6. How has the patient coped with stressful situations?

In addition to the assessment of the impact of the illness on the patient's life, information that may be pertinent to the present hospital experience may also be relevant in determining patient needs.

1. Previous hospitalizations, experiences, fears and anxieties
2. Anticipated events, length of stay, and perceived reason for hospitalization
3. Past reactions to and present concerns regarding hospital activities and procedures
4. Presence and availability of significant others

Feelings of guilt plague many cancer patients throughout their illness with cancer. Some of these feelings are first manifest during diagnostic testing if the patient perceives that some action (or lack of action) may have contributed to his present state. Sometimes these feelings may be reinforced by family members or members of the health team.

This time can be particularly painful and lonely for the patient and the family. The social isolation that many with illness encounter can be even more poignant for those with the stigma of cancer. In addition to the fears of pain and death, the fear of cancer as a contagion can significantly affect social relationships.

Use of denial as a protective mechanism can be encountered at varying levels during this diagnostic phase [3,13]. Sometimes the denial of the existence or meaning of symptoms may have contributed to delay in seeking health care [2]. As a defense mechanism it can also minimize the emotional stress associated with the diagnostic process and enable the patient to endure painful testing. Rarely is it a long-term coping mechanism, but it is often present in varying degrees throughout the cancer experience.

For the patient devoid of symptoms, hospitalization and the accompanying testing may be especially difficult, magnifying feelings of disbelief and unreality. A healthy appearance of the patient makes the possibility of cancer particularly difficult for the patient as well as the family to confront.

Communicating the Diagnosis

The telling of the diagnosis of cancer can be a difficult time for the patient as well as the health team [33]. The nurse can provide emotional support for the patient and family as well as the physician when the diagnosis is confirmed. The therapeutic options should be given, and the patient should be included in the treatment alliance. The fear of abandonment many patients may experience may be alleviated by reassurance and by commitment by the health team to the patient even if the treatment goal is palliation rather than cure.

The response of the patient to the notification of disease recurrence or metastases may be similar in kind but more severe in degree than the response to the initial diagnosis [23]. Vacillations in the disease course may wear away at the patient's hopes and, for some, his will to live. The tantalizing hope for cure may become dimmer with each relapse.

During the diagnostic phase, the nurse can act as an advocate for the patient. The nurse can help the patient to formulate and ask questions related to concerns. The nurse can also make the physicians aware of the patient's concerns by direct communication. The ability to listen may be the most important asset the nurse can offer the patient at this time. The nurse can also help the patient sort fantasy from reality in the realm of cancer causation and cancer cure.

Those patients who undergo diagnostic testing procedures but, fortunately, do not have cancer also need assistance. Their experience with the threat of cancer may color their future experience with health care and their adherence to preventive behaviors. Some of these patients may have a greater cancer risk, and may thus face repeated screening and diagnostic testing.

STAGING OF DISEASE

Staging Classification Systems

Diagnostic tests to evaluate the spread of disease are called staging procedures. Tumors, according to their natural history, have relatively predictable patterns of disease progression and metastasis. Classification systems identifying the spread of cancer have some variability [5,12]. An attempt to improve communication about the size and degree of spread of solid tumors in determining appropriate therapy and evaluating tumor response, resulted in the development of the "TNM" system. It is the most widely utilized system to characterize the degree of growth and spread of solid tumors [7]. Basically, it involves evaluation of three distinct parameters:

T̲umor—primary tumor size
N̲ode—regional lymph node involvement
M̲etastasis—distant organ involvement

Each of these areas also is evaluated with numerical subheadings denoting the stage or extent of involvement, zero indicating no involvement. Thus, a tumor with a $T_1 N_0 N_0$ classification would have a small tumor and no evidence of node involvement or distant metastasis. Generally, TNM patterns are grouped into stages reflecting local disease (Stage I), regional disease (Stage II), and metastatic disease (Stage III).

This method of evaluating or staging cancer spread is very useful in determining the need for local or systemic cancer therapy. It also may indicate the disease prognosis.

A variety of techniques may be utilized in order to evaluate cancer spread depending upon tumor type [30]. The physical exam will continue to be important, especially in terms of assessment of lymph node involvement and organ system integrity and function. Less invasive procedures may be scheduled first. Those results may lead to more intrusive tests later. Knowledge of the histologic diagnosis will also dictate the potential for tumor growth and site of distant metastasis. Staging procedures can be scheduled accordingly. Often multiple tests are used to confirm the extent of spread. In some cases, the primary tumor may never be discovered.

Radiologic Staging Procedures

Radiographic examinations are very important in cancer staging [4]. The chest X-ray is the single most important procedure for detecting and following metastatic disease. Other radiographic procedures utilized in staging are summarized in Table 4.6. A positive histologic diagnosis of cancer is essential before radiographic tests can be utilized for staging because the test can only distinguish between normal and abnormal; it cannot diagnose malignancy. False positives and false negatives can be a problem with these procedures because of their varying sensitivity (ability to detect small metastases) as well as varying specificity (capabilities for discrimination of malignant from benign conditions).

Computerized axial tomography of the brain (CAT scan) may be important in diagnosing central nervous system metastases when suspicious symptoms are present. The procedure can be a frightening one unless the patient is adequately prepared. The patient's head is immobilized in the machine while the scanner makes multiple 180° rotations [29].

Clinical Versus Pathologic Stage

Patients may require surgery for adequate assessment of extent of disease [6]. There is a difference between *clinical stage* and *pathologic stage*. The patient's disease may be given a clinical stage designation reflecting clinical signs and symptoms that are detected by staging procedures. True pathologic staging may not be obtainable unless there is surgical investigation of cancer spread. Since not all patients go to surgery for definitive staging procedures, a clinical stage may guide selection of treatment. In evaluating cancer treatment results, patients with clinical staging designations may not accurately represent the true extent of pathology that would be evident in patients with surgical pathologic staging.

TABLE 4.6
Radiologic Cancer Staging Procedures [4]

Type	Clinical Significance
Chest X-ray	Essential for detecting and following metastatic spread to the lungs
Bone X-rays	Detection of boney metastasis in symptomatic and advanced disease
Abdominal X-rays (KUB)	Detection of displaced anatomical landmarks and obstruction secondary to metastatic disease
Barium examination of GI tract	Detection of metastatic spread and direct tumor invasion
Intravenous pyelogram (IVP)	Detection of retroperitoneal metastatic disease
Lymphography	Evaluation of filling defects, deviation and obstruction of retroperitoneal lymph nodes
Bone scans	Detection of bone abnormalities in early stages
Tomography (chest)	Confirmation of questionable chest X-ray lesions
Brain scan	Detection of primary lesions and metastasis
Gallium scan	Total body scintillation test for metastases
Angiography	Ancillary tool to confirm metastases in brain, liver, and kidney
Ultrasound	Adjunct to scans for hepatic, retroperitoneal, abdominal, and pelvic metastasis
Computed tomography (CAT scanning)	Detection of brain or body metastasis by computation of differential radiation (X-ray) absorption by tissue displayed in cross-sectional picture printouts (able to pick up subtle changes not detectable on ordinary X-ray)

Waiting

A patient may know of the diagnosis of his cancer but still have his treatment options and prognosis undefined pending test results. This waiting period can be extremely difficult for the patient who is confronting the diagnosis of cancer but still does not know his chance for cure. Some patients may express the fear that the cancer is growing during that time. The urgency for something to be done and the tumor to be treated will be a dominating influence in the patient's life.

Treatment Evaluation

Studies similar to staging procedures will need to be done to evaluate the existence and extent of disease and to evaluate the response of tumors to the treatment regimen. For patients who experience a remission (disappearance of clinical evidence of disease) or a possible cure of their disease, the same tests may be performed to detect any evidence of recurrence. Thus patients may become very familiar with some of these tests. The anxiety associated with the tests may result from the fear of the results, as well as the actual physical discomfort.

SELECTION OF CANCER TREATMENT

The patient faced with the diagnosis of cancer encounters many confusing and frightening decisions. With often overwhelming feelings of powerlessness and helplessness, the patient may be confronted with a particular cancer treatment as his only hope for survival. In addition to giving permission or "consent" to a treatment that may have significant morbidity and in some cases mortality, the patient may be required to become an active participant in order to maximize the treatment's effectiveness. Comprehension of the rationale for the selection and utilization of cancer treatment may be critical for his well-being.

In order to fully consider a comprehensive approach to patient care during cancer treatment, it is valuable to review the factors that influence the selection of a particular cancer modality over another. The combination and sequencing of multiple modalities of treatment provided for some patients are important for optimal treatment. Two major categories, tumor factors and patient factors, emerge in directing selection of cancer treatment.

Tumor Factors

Though sharing the common definition of cancer, different types of neoplasms may behave very distinctly [6,12,30]. They may differ as to the role of growth and spread of the tumor as well as their potential for and pattern of metastasis. Recognition of this has led to extensive study to elaborate the particular characteristics of individual tumor types. An essential additional component to the recognition of the categorical differences of cancer is the histologic variations within the category. The type of cancer the patient has may have implications for the patient's disease course and prognosis. By understanding the nature of the cancer to be treated, for example, doubling time and propensity for metastasis, the most effective treatment can be selected. These concepts will be discussed further in the following chapters. They are reviewed here to provide a framework for discussing key factors in the selection of treatment.

Additionally, consideration needs to be given to the location of the tumor. The accessibility of the tumor and its relationship to vital organs are critical factors influencing appropriate treatment. The functional and physical impairment resulting from the removal of a significant mass may make surgery an unacceptable option. In some cases, the size of the tumor may be decreased by chemotherapy and/or radiotherapy before surgery.

Some cancers, such as leukemia, are by their nature systemic diseases affecting many parts of the body. Because of this, they require treatment that has a systemic rather than local impact. Other tumors, while single entities, may have a propensity to metastasize or spread throughout the system. Evaluation and scrutiny for evidence of metastasis must be given when cancer lesions are initially detected. Evidence of metastasis will have significant implications for the selection of a treatment geared for systemic versus local control.

Patient Factors

Patients diagnosed with cancer may have other medical problems that are not necessarily related to the malignancy but that may compromise their ability to withstand certain cancer treatment. Vital organ function integrity (for example, renal status and cardiac status) is an important assessment parameter before the institution of any cancer therapy. Elderly patients, pregnant patients, and children may require alterations in a particular cancer treatment program because of physiologic variables [12,21].

Another important factor considered in the selection of treatment is the patient's previous cancer treatment history. Exposure to some types of cancer therapy may alter organ function such that additional cancer treatment must be carefully scrutinized. Some treatment options may be eliminated due to previous toxicity experienced by the patient; efficacy of a particular treatment modality may have been demonstrated to be decreased, in past utilization, requiring different approaches.

Informed Consent

All patients should be informed of the purposes, benefits, and potential consequences of medical therapy and, indeed, nursing action [9, 20]. In cancer treatment, investigational therapy requires a formalized document of patient consent. The informed consent required of many cancer patients undergoing cancer therapy relates the risks and benefits associated with such treatment. Alternative treatments, their advantages and disadvantages, should also be explained [9]. Many patients may feel during this vulnerable time, that they have no choice but to take the gamble for treatment despite the odds against cure. Patient involvement in the decision-making process may decrease resentment when treatment failure occurs. Patients may center or focus on very different items in the "informed" consent ranging from hair loss to loss of life. Sending the informed consent home with the patient has been shown to increase understanding of the potential treatment [18]. For many, clarification of the percentage of patients experiencing the different side effects is helpful in establishing perspective [25]. Many patients, even when faced with grim statistics, may hope that they will be the "lucky" ones. The nurse can support the patient in this selection process. Patient education regarding the nature and frequency of the side effects associated with cancer treatment should focus on the length of time the side effect will be experienced (many of them are disturbing, but transient) as well as the support measures available to help the patient during treatment.

Nursing Role in Selection of Treatment

The nurse's understanding of the rationale and goal of the proposed treatment for the patient is essential. By reinforcing the explanation regarding the treatment, the nurse can assist the patient's comprehension of treatment choices. The patient's cognitive ability and emotional status may influence style of communication [13,33]. The nurse can assess the patient's hopes, fears, and misconceptions in relation to cancer treatment. Information can be individualized to correct misperceptions. The nurse can be an advocate for patient, assuring patient access to correct information [20]. Reassurance of interventions and resources available may allay some of the patient's anxiety regarding side effects of treatment. The nurse can provide emotional support despite the acceptance or refusal of cancer treatment.

Goals of Treatment

The goal of cancer treatment will be a major factor in the selection and administration of any of the modes of therapy [7]. Possible treatment goals would include cure, prolonged survival with cancer control, and relief or palliation of symptoms caused by the malignant process. The patient's knowledge and perception of the goals of treatment are important areas for nursing assessment.

Cure. The concept of cure in cancer treatment is not necessarily a simple one. There may be no clinical evidence of neoplastic disease after a patient has received cancer treatment. Absence of clinical signs of disease may not, however, always be the determining factor in the definition of cure. Cancer cells may continue to be present but be undetectable by current diagnostic assessment procedures. The term for this state, in which the patient has no evidence of cancer but is not necessarily cancer free, is *complete remission*.

The term *5-year disease-free survival* is another frequently used parameter [23]. Since metastasis or recurrence of the primary disease frequently will show up in the first 5 years after diagnosis and treatment, cure in many diseases may be considered probable after that point. The risk of relapse is difficult for many patients and their families to deal with. Patients may feel well but the nagging doubt of whether or not they are cured remains. Cancer treatment for cure may be repeated if there is recurrence of the tumor and still hope for cure.

Adjuvant Therapy. Understanding of the natural course of events after cancer treatment has resulted in refinements of therapy of curative intent. Cancer therapy, specifically chemotherapy and immunotherapy, may be continued after the patient has been treated with "curative" therapy. This "adjuvant" therapy attempts to eliminate possible subclinical disease which may have a possibility of recurrence. This is an area of current research [14].

Toxicity of Treatment

Cancer treatment is unfortunately associated with side effects of varying degrees, some of long-term significance and some which may in themselves be life threatening. The risks of side effects and of potential life-threatening toxicities due to therapy may be more acceptable if there is a strong potential for cure. This may be especially true if the alternative of a lesser treatment may give no hope for cure. Long-term side effects, such as sterility and body changes, may appear insignificant to the patient at the time when his choice is reduced to life-or-death options. The patient's general health status, exposure to previous cancer therapy, and the availability of support services, may be factors that can influence treatment toxicity. The principles in selection of treatment involves an optimal choice of the most effective therapy with the least toxicity. Rehabilitative efforts may be directed at the consequences of curative cancer therapy.

─── OVERVIEW OF CURRENT CANCER TREATMENT ───

After a definitive diagnostic and staging work-up, cancer treatment can begin. The goal of the treatment will be considered in terms of its potential effectiveness as well as the potential side effects for the patient. Cancer therapy can be classified into local and systemic modalities. These treatments will be explored at greater depth in future chapters.

Surgery

Cancer surgery is intended primarily for localized cure of primary tumor or solitary metastasis. While it can provide short-term relief of symptoms, generally extensive surgery is only done with curative intent. The side effects of surgical treatment may range from minimal scarring to significant body alteration in appearance and function. The risk of surgery also may pose a threat to life. While some patients may be frightened and distressed by the prospect of surgery and the impact of the losses it incurs on their life, others will have a great hope and sense of relief when the surgeon is able to "get it all." Due to the nature of some cancers, the patient will not know until after the surgery whether or not the procedure has a possibility of cure. In some cases, even the diagnosis may not be determined until after the procedure.

Radiation Therapy

Generally radiation therapy, like cancer surgery, is for local treatment. It can be utilized with curative intent but is more frequently used for palliative therapy. Its major advantage over surgery is that it can encompass a large area of cancer treatment without the drastic side effects that would result if surgery was attempted. Radiation therapy can also be utilized when surgical treatment is not possible due to the anatomical location of the tumor and when the patient refuses or is unable to undergo a surgical procedure.

Radiation therapy is not, however, without side effects. Acute side effects during the treatment phase are generally specific to the site irradiated and are self-limiting. Unfortunately, some side effects may emerge months to years later, affecting the quality of life, and, in some cases, leading to lethal complications. An important consideration for the patient may be the length of time involved in radiation therapy, which may last weeks.

Chemotherapy

Chemotherapy is utilized to treat systemic spread of malignant cells. It may be used with curative intent in some malignancies (for instance, lymphoma), but generally it is used for long- or short-term palliation. Side effects occur during treatment and may include some potentially life-threatening toxicities. The quality of the patient's life may also be affected by the results of chemotherapy, for example, sterility in some cases. For the patient, chemotherapy may represent the last hope for containment after surgical and/or radiation therapy failures. Other patients with systemic disease may confront chemotherapy as their first experience with cancer treatment.

Immunotherapy

Immunotherapy attempts to take advantage of the protective ability of the immune system to resist and destroy malignant cells. Cancer patients often have compromised immune systems. Immunotherapy utilizes experimental techniques in an attempt to stimulate, augment, or replace the patient's own immune capabilities. Side effects of the specific treatment efforts, as well as the danger of tumor enhancement through manipulation of the immune system, must be evaluated. Immunotherapy may be most effective in small tumor masses, decreased by previous treatment.

Multimodality Cancer Therapy

Treatment of cancer today may involve a variety of therapeutic options combined or sequenced in different ways. Thus, the treatment of some tumors may be most effective with a combination of modalities such as surgery, radiotherapy, chemotherapy, and immunotherapy. The different modalities may be given in a particular sequence—for example, surgery first, chemotherapy second. They may also be given concurrently. The variations in sequence and combination may be the focus of clinical research trials. Dose alteration in chemotherapy and radiation therapy may occur when a combined approach is utilized to offset cumulative toxicity.

When To Stop Treatment

The point may come in cancer treatment when the goal of cure or even palliation is not appropriate. Active therapy may be decreasing the quality of the patient's life while not offering him substantial gains. The point at which to stop cancer treatment varies from individual to individual, with concerns for the patient's struggle for survival, as well as his desire for peace. The nurse is often in a situation where the assessment of the patient's hopes and desires may be possible. At times the family's wishes may not be congruent with the patient's. An understanding of the patient's desires as well as the family's will help the health team involved in cancer treatment. Misinformation or lack of understanding regarding the side effects as well as other treatment options may be factors influencing the patient's and family's perspectives.

The patient may rely on the nurse's perspective and counsel in treatment decisions [20]. The careful initial assessments and care plans can elucidate the patient's cancer experience, concerns, fears, and importantly, strengths. Consideration of the patient's previous experiences with illness and hospitalizations may be an important dimension in understanding his wishes in treatment cessation or, in some cases, prolongation.

All of the treatment methods discussed may be utilized in relief of symptoms. A change in goal of the therapy may be a difficult one for the patient to comprehend. Honest and continued communication by all members of the health team is critical in this situation where fear of abandonment may excede fear of death. The support-ive caring activities of the nurse in controlling physical pain and emotional discomfort may be the central therapeutic domain in this final stage. The nurse can provide consultation in decision making by the patient and family regarding the setting for terminal care—whether it will take place in a hospice, for example, or at home or in a convalescent facility.

Experimental Cancer Treatment

Many patients with cancer today may be treated at some point in their disease course with experimental therapy. Both patients and those caring for them in major research centers may encounter this situation more frequently.

The essence of experimental cancer therapy is the testing of new treatment options. The comparison of the standard approach with a new but promising treatment will hopefully offer the patient im-proved results [23]. As with any other therapy, the patient must give consent to participate.

The testing of a new treatment when the existing one is effective is an often considered ethical question. Without effective research one cannot determine which treatment is really the best for a given situation. The advancement of cancer treatment relies heavily on further cancer research.

In the selection of cancer treatment, the option of experimental treatment might be pursued by a method of randomization with two patient groups compared for response to standardized and experi-mental therapy. The analysis of the groups for compatability as to key variables will be critical for the interpretation of the results. In order to obtain even further objectivity research studies may be carried out in a double blind fashion. That is, investigators and clinicians involved will not know which therapy is delivered until the results are analyzed.

Nursing staff response to experimental therapy can have a signifi-cant impact on the therapeutic milieu. Lack of information about the research, inadequate data, and misinformation about the ef-ficacy of the treatment program can create anxiety and hostility toward the program. While these feelings may be based on clinical experiences, generally they are very limited and lead to faulty generalizations of the treatment plan.

The question of whether to take a possibly higher risk in decreas-ing the quality of life for a possibly prolonged existence is a personal and individual question. While some patients may be eager to grasp at any hope for survival, others may not wish to pursue unchartered therapy.

Nonapproved Medical Treatment

Untested and nonapproved methods of cancer treatment are considered by some patients and their families [34]. These options may appear more acceptable than the proposed treatment option for a variety of reasons. The fear of debilitating side effects and toxicities of standard therapy may be based on gross misunderstandings. The appeal of many of the nonapproved treatments is that they seem to be devoid of any harmful side effects. Unfortunately, this is often not the case. A grim prognosis without any known effective medical treatment can also make the patient very vulnerable to the nonapproved or quack treatment.

Patients frequently may ask for information, advice, and support for nonapproved treatment. Education of the patient regarding what cancer is and the purpose and goal of treatment may be a critical nursing intervention [12]. However, education alone may not be adequate. The quality of communication between the patient and the health team, the inclusion of the patient in treatment decisions, and continued symptomatic relief and emotional support for the patient may be as important factors.

An evaluation of the nonproven cancer treatment by the health team should include its side effects and potential toxicities for the patient. The financial cost and travel time involved in obtaining the treatment may pose significant hardships for both the patient and his family. In some instances, nonapproved therapeutic techniques for cancer treatment, such as health food diets, may be used in combination with traditional therapy. In the event the patient does opt for nonapproved treatment, the nurse can still provide support to the patient without supporting his decision. This may facilitate later return for conventional therapy if the patient has this need and desire.

REFERENCES

[1] AMERICAN CANCER SOCIETY. Press release, Friday, March 21, 1980.

[2] ANTONOVSKY, A., and HARTMAN, H. Delay in the Detection of Cancer: A Review of the Literature. In *Cancer: Pathophysiology, Etiology, and Management,* ed. L. Kruse, J. Reese, and L. Hart, pp. 104–122. St. Louis: C.V. Mosby, 1979.

[3] BAHNSON, C. Psychologic and Emotional Issues in Cancer: The Psychotherapeutic Care of the Cancer Patient. *Seminars in Oncology*, 2:293–309, 1975.

[4] BASSIT, L., and STECKEL, R. Imaging Techniques in the Detection of Metastatic Disease. *Seminars in Oncology*, 4:39–52, 1977.

[5] COMMITTEE ON PROFESSIONAL EDUCATION OF UICC, INTERNATIONAL UNION AGAINST CANCER. *Clinical Oncology*. New York: Springer-Verlag, 1973.

[6] del REGATO, J., and SPJUT, H. Pathology of Cancer. In *Ackerman and del Regato's Cancer Diagnosis, Treatment, and Prognosis*, ed. J. del Regato and H. Spjut, 5th ed., pp. 31–62. St. Louis: C.V. Mosby, 1977.

[7] FRAUMENI, J. *Persons at High Risk of Cancer*. New York: Academic Press, 1975.

[8] GARFINKEL, L., POINDEXTER, C., and SILVERBERG, E. Cancer in Black Americans. *Ca: A Cancer Journal for Clinicians*, 30:39–44, 1980.

[9] GARGARO, W. Informed Consent, Part I. *Cancer Nursing*, 1:81–82; Part II, 1:167–168; Part III, 1:249–250, 1978.

[10] HALL, T. The Paraneoplastic Syndromes. In *Clinical Oncology for Medical Students and Physicians*, 4th ed., ed. P. Rubin and R. Bakemeir, pp. 119–128. Rochester: American Cancer Society, 1974.

[11] HARTMAN, J. Breast Exams: What You Should Know. U.S. Department of Health, Education and Welfare, Pub. No. (NIH) 80-2000, 1980.

[12] HASKELL, C. *Cancer Treatment*. Philadelphia: Saunders, 1980.

[13] HOLLAND, J. Psychological Aspects of Oncology. *Medical Clinics of North America*, 61:737–748, 1977.

[14] JONES, S., and SALMON, S. *Adjuvant Therapy of Cancer II*. New York: Grune & Stratton, 1979.

[15] LYNCH, H.; LYNCH, P.; ALBANO, W.; EDNEY, J.; ORGAN, C.; and LYNCH, J. Hereditary Cancer: Ascertainment and Management. *Ca: A Cancer Journal for Clinicians*, 29:216–232, 1979.

[16] MERRILL, J., and DEWYS, W. The Paraneoplastic Syndromes. In *Clinical Oncology for Medical Students and Physicians*, 5th ed., ed. P. Rubin and R. Bakemeier, pp. 56–62. Rochester: American Cancer Society, 1978.

[17] MILLER, A. Risk Benefit in Mass Screening Programs for Breast Cancer. *Seminars in Oncology*, 5:351–359, 1978.

[18] MORROW, G.; GOOTNICK, J.; and SCHMALE, A. A Simple Technique for Increasing Cancer Patients' Knowledge of Informed Consent to Treatment. *Cancer*, 42:793–799, 1978.

[19] MOSES, M. Cancer and the Work Place. *American Journal of Nursing*, 79:1985–1988, 1979.

[20] ONCOLOGY NURSING SOCIETY AND AMERICAN NURSES' ASSOCIATION DIVISION ON MEDICAL-SURGICAL NURSING PRACTICE. *Outcome Standards for Cancer Nursing Practice*, Kansas City, Mo.: American Nurses' Association, 1979.

[21] PETERSON, B., and KENNEDY, B. Aging and Cancer Management, Part I: Clinical Observations. *Ca: A Cancer Journal for Clinicians,* 29:322–332, 1979.

[22] ROVINSKI, C. Nurses and Cancer's Seven Warning Signals. *Cancer Nursing,* 3:53–55, 1980.

[23] RUBIN, P. Statement of the Clinical Oncologic Problem. In *Clinical Oncology for Medical Students and Physicians,* 5th ed., ed. P. Rubin and R. Bakemeier, pp. 1–10. Rochester: American Cancer Society, 1978.

[24] SARNA, G. Screening for Lung, Breast, and Colorectal Cancers. In *Practical Oncology,* ed. G. Sarna. Boston: Houghton Mifflin, 1980.

[25] SCHMALE, A. Psychological Reactions to Recurrences, Metastasis or Disseminated Cancer. *International Journal of Radiation Oncology,* 1:515–520, 1976.

[26] SCHOTTENFELD, D., and HAAS, J. Carcinogens in the Workplace. *Ca: A Cancer Journal for Clinicians,* CA 29:144–168, 1979.

[27] SCHOTTENFELD, D. Cancer Detection Programs. In *Persons at High Risk of Cancer,* ed. J. Fraumeni, pp. 399–413. New York: Academic Press, 1975.

[28] SILVERBERG, C. Cancer Statistics, 1980. *Cancer,* 30:23–38, 1980.

[29] STONE, B. Computerized Transaxial Brain Scan. *American Journal of Nursing,* 77:1601–1604.

[30] TERRY, R. The Pathology of Cancer. In *Clinical Oncology for Medical Students and Physicians,* 4th ed., ed. P. Rubin and R. Bakemeier, pp. 26–47. Rochester: American Cancer Society, 1974.

[31] WHITE, L.; CORNELIUS, J.; JUDKINS, A.; and PATTERSON, J. Screening of Cancer by Nurses. *Cancer Nursing,* 1:15–20, 1978.

[32] WHITE, L.; PATTERSON, J.; CORNELIUS, J.; and JUDKINS, A. *Cancer Screening and Detection Manual for Nurses.* New York: McGraw-Hill, 1979.

[33] VETTESE, J. The Problems of the Patient Confronting the Diagnosis of Cancer. In *Cancer: The Behavioral Dimensions,* ed. J. Cullen, pp. 275–282. New York: Raven Press, 1976.

[34] *Unproven Methods of Cancer Management—1976.* American Cancer Society, 1975.

chapter
five

LINDA PATTI SARNA, R.N., M.N.
Assistant Clinical Professor
Teaching in Graduate Nursing
Oncology Program
School of Nursing, UCLA

Concepts in the nursing management of patients receiving cancer chemotherapy and immunotherapy

---

INTRODUCTION

The nursing care of patients receiving chemotherapy or immuno-therapy for treatment of cancer requires understanding of the need for and rationale of medical intervention. A perceptive and sophis-ticated knowledge of the problems implicit to a patient's accepting and tolerating this form of therapy is critical for the nurse. Addi-tionally, the nurse must have the ability to assist patients in adapting to adjustments in life-style that may be necessary in the midst and the aftermath of cancer chemotherapy or immunotherapy. Sys-tematic observation and sensitive appraisal of the patient can provide the necessary data base from which to diagnose nursing problems and to make plans for effective interventions. This assessment, how-ever, cannot be adequate unless the nurse caring for the patient has a thorough knowledge of the scientific principles that underly the rationale, function, and purpose of the treatment mode as well as knowledge of the potential impact of such therapy on the patient's quality of life.

PRINCIPLES OF CANCER CHEMOTHERAPY

Cell Kinetics

The utilization of particular drugs for the destruction of cancer involves many considerations. Since the neoplastic process is manifest at the cellular level, attempts to destroy malignancies may relate to assessment of the cancer cell itself. There are certain distinctive differences and similarities between cancer cells and normal cells which are relevant to the use of chemotherapeutic agents [5,16]. Drugs used in chemotherapy generally have the potential for interfering with cellular function and replication, thus causing cell death. While these drugs do not discriminate between normal cells and cancer cells, certain characteristics may make cancer cells more vulnerable to effective antineoplastic agents. Maximum therapeutic response with minimal toxicity to the patient is a major factor in the evaluation of the therapeutic potential and the usefulness of any drug utilized in chemotherapy [16]. Drug efficacy varies according to tumor type and from tumor to tumor within a given type.

Cell Cycle. Normal cells and cancer cells both replicate in a similar pattern. This pattern is termed the *cell cycle* [16]. It basically consists of four distinct divisions or phases: mitosis (M phase), postmitotic gap (G_1), DNA synthesis (S phase), premitotic gap(G_2). In mitosis, the cell is physically dividing, reproducing two daughter cells. During this phase a number of discrete activities take place to facilitate separation of the replicated chromosomes and the emergence of two new cells. G_1 is the time following cell division where RNA and protein synthesis occur to ready the cell for DNA synthesis. The end of G_1 is defined by the beginning of the S phase in which DNA is synthesized and the chromosomal content is doubled. The G_2 phase is a premitotic phase; here preparation for cell division occurs, including RNA and protein synthesis and the preparation of a mitotic spindle. An understanding of the characteristics of the cell cycle is important in appreciating the theoretical role of kinetics in the administration of cancer chemotherapy[5,16]. (See Fig. 5.1.)

Characteristics of the cell cycle also have implications for growth rate of the tumor and normal tissues. The time interval for the cell cycle to be completed (from mitosis to mitosis) is called the cell cycle time. This time may vary for normal and malignant replicating cell tissues. Normal cell tissues with high growth fractions and short cell cycle times (for example, bone marrow and gastrointestinal mucosa), are particularly vulnerable to antineoplastic drug therapy.

82

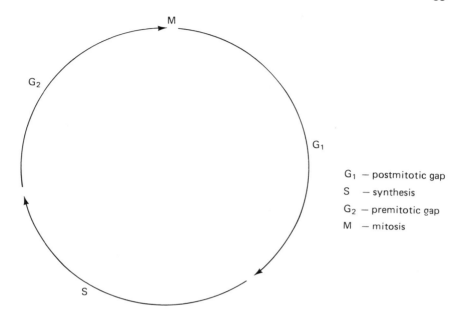

Cell-cycle phase-specific drugs: act only in cycling cells in a
specific cycle phase (e.g., cytosine arabinoside for S phase,
vincristine for M phase)

Cell-cycle phase-nonspecific drugs: act in multiple phases of
the cell cycle and against resting cells (e.g., cyclophosphamide)

FIGURE 5.1 Cell cycle.

Malignancies with high growth fractions and short cell cycle time (for example, leukemia), are most vulnerable to chemotherapy.

Chemotherapy and Tumor Size. Tumor growth represents the net effect of tumor cell production and tumor cell loss. Cell production is a function of what proportion of cells are in active cycle (the growth fraction) and how fast the cycling cells can replicate (cell cycle time). Cell loss is a function of cell death or loss via metastasis. The doubling time is the time it takes for a tumor to double its mass [16].

The Gompertzian growth curve is a mathematical model of a pattern of biological growth that both normal cells and tumor cells follow [16]. It relates tumor size (number of cells) to growth rate. The growth rate is inversely related to the tumor size. When the tumor size is small, rapid growth occurs with a short doubling time (hours, days) related to a high growth fraction, a short cell cycle time and little cell loss. As the mass increases, the growth fraction decreases, and the cell cycle time and cell loss increase. The decreased growth rate is reflected by an increased doubling time (weeks, months, years). Chemotherapy generally works most effectively with rapidly growing, small tumors. Adjuvant therapy is utilized in a curative attempt to eliminate undetectable but present cancer cells while the small tumor mass may maximize their sensitivity to chemotherapy [16,63].

Drug selection, sequencing, and timing are in some instances influenced by the size of tumor and its doubling time. Measures to decrease the tumor bulk may first be implemented before chemotherapy is begun. Radiation therapy and surgery may be utilized, with chemotherapy following, to irradicate remaining tumor cells.

Tumor Cell Kill. The fractional cell-kill hypothesis theorizes that the cancer cell-kill capacity of one time exposure to most chemotherapeutic agents is a variable percent which increases with dose but is less than 100%. An effective drug given to a patient, as a single dose, generally kills from 20% to 99% of cells [16]. This is important in considering chemotherapy protocols requiring long-term administration. Since a single dose of chemotherapy does not have the capacity to kill 100% of the cancer cells, multiple exposures of the cancer cells to the drugs at various time intervals may be necessary to achieve a meaningful therapeutic response. This may be important information to convey in patient teaching to facilitate understanding of prolonged therapy.

Drug Classification and the Cell Cycle. The various chemotherapeutic agents can be categorized as being cell cycle phase specific or cycle phase nonspecific. Agents that are phase specific act on replicating cells during a sensitive phase of the cell cycle. Accordingly, they are selectively more potent if administered when a large number of those cells are passing through that phase [5,16].

An important consideration for phase-specific drugs is that only a certain percentage of cells are cycling at any one time. The S phase of DNA replication is generally the most vulnerable phase of the cell cycle. For certain drugs, this may relate to optimal intervals between doses. Phase-nonspecific chemotherapy drugs destroy the cell by interrupting or destroying cellular functions not limited to a specific phase in the replication cycle. Resting cancer cells (G_0) are cells that are not in active cycle. They may be particularly resistant to irradication by chemotherapy due to their lack of activity and ability to repair cellular damage while resting. The tumor burden may be decreased by surgery, radiation therapy, and chemotherapy. The resting cells can later begin cycling, replacing the killed cells.

Implications for Nursing Care. The cytokinetic characteristics of a tumor and its therapy may have significant implications for nursing care of cancer patients receiving chemotherapy [5,50]. The phenomena produced may relate to the timing, sequencing, and lengths of administration of the various drugs used in treatment. Patient teaching regarding the rationale for administration of drugs in different kinds of ways may be essential in easing patient fears and uncertainties and in improving patient compliance.

Selection of Chemotherapy for Cancer Treatment

Tumor Factors, Patient Factors, Therapeutic Goals. Antineoplastic chemotherapy is generally used as treatment for systemic metastatic malignancies. (See Table 5.1.) Malignancies that have not spread but are not adequately controlled by surgery or radiation therapy may also be treated with chemotherapy [16]. The tumor may be inaccessible for surgical removal due to location and/or size of the mass. Chemotherapy may be utilized alone or in conjunction with radiation therapy to decrease the size of the mass prior to removal by surgery. Chemotherapy may also be used as an adjunct after potentially curative surgery to eliminate likely remaining cancer cells that are too few in number to be clinically apparent. Nursing considerations in planning care for the patient receiving chemotherapy are based on a clear understanding of the goals of the treatment plan (whether cure, palliation, or symptom relief), the toxicity of the treatment as related to the vulnerability of the particular patient (as determined by such factors as age, preexisting diseases, and interaction of chemotherapy side effects with those of the other treatment modalities), and the disease itself. The patient's understanding and interpretation of the purpose of therapy and attitudes toward the potential and expected side effects must be carefully assessed. Previous medical experience with cancer treatment may significantly influence a patient's view of this form of treatment. A nursing assessment prior to chemotherapy, should include an evaluation of the impact of the therapy on the patient's life-style considering the length and time of treatment as well as the potential side effects that might be expected.

Patient factors influencing the use of chemotherapy for cancer treatment include evaluation of baseline physiologic functioning.

TABLE 5.1
Cancer Treatment with Chemotherapy:
Curability and Sensitivity [16]

Potentially Curative (highly responsive)
  Acute lymphoblastic leukemia (childhood)
  Hodgkin's disease
  Gestational choriocarcinoma
  Testicular cancer
  Burkitt's lymphoma
  Wilms's tumor

Long-Term Palliation (moderately responsive)
  Carcinoma of the breast
  Selected lymphomas
  Multiple myleoma
  Ovarian cancer
  Prostate carcinoma
  Chronic leukemia
  Neuroblastoma
  Small-cell carcinoma of the lung
  Osteogenic sarcoma
  Ewing's sarcoma
  Soft-tissue sarcoma

Short-Term Palliation (fairly responsive)
  Lung cancer (non–small cell)
  Head and neck cancer (squamous)
  Colon cancer
  Liver cancer
  Stomach cancer
  Bladder cancer
  Cervical cancer
  Brain tumors
  Gastric carcinoma

Occasional Palliation (poorly responsive)
  Melanoma
  Pancreatic cancer
  Renal cell carcinoma

Note: Results are dependent on individual patient and tumor factors.

Organ integrity of the liver and the kidneys particularly need to be evaluated prior to therapy due to their importance in drug metabolism and excretion. Specific drugs also may have potential toxicity for individual organs, for example, pulmonary toxicity from bleomycin. An evaluation of organ status may alter the treatment plan in terms of drug selection and dosage. Specific methods for clinical evaluation of the potentially vulnerable organs as well as the patient's general physical status need to be implemented. Nursing care adjustments may be dictated by careful and frequent assessment of the patient's clinical status before, during, and after chemotherapy [23,42]. Baseline behavioral and psychological data should also be collected.

Evaluation of Therapeutic Response. As with all cancer treatment, the possible benefit for a patient and the potential toxicities must be carefully evaluated. Evidence of the type and extent of the malignancy must be carefully evaluated prior to treatment (see Chapter 4) and reevaluated during and after chemotherapy to determine therapeutic response [16]. Laboratory tests including complete blood count (CBC), differential and platelet count, bone marrow aspiration and biopsies, lumbar punctures, serum calcium, paraproteins, gonadotropin titer, and presence and degree of clinical symptomatology will be utilized in conjunction with physical findings, X-rays, and scans to determine toxicity and response (tumor size). The nurse should also evaluate the patient's behavioral and psychological response to the stress of chemotherapy in considering the toxicity.

Chemotherapeutic Drugs

Drug Classification. Drugs administered for cancer chemotherapy may be classified in several categories: alkylating agents, antimetabolites, antibiotics, vinca alkaloids, hormones, and miscellaneous drugs. An understanding of the general classification of drugs in terms of mode of action, administration, common side effects, and toxicities will guide specialized nursing care [16,36]. (See Table 5.2.) Individual drugs are highlighted to provide a rationale for nursing assessment and intervention [8,11,21,23,42,58]. Major nursing problems related to side effects of chemotherapy will be discussed in more depth following a discussion of the major drug categories.

Alkylating Agents. Alkylating agents alter the nucleic acids of the DNA molecule, thus interfering with DNA replication. This is

TABLE 5.2
Nursing Care Chemotherapy Guide

Agent	Dose and Administration	Pharmacologic Factors	Significant Side Effects and Toxicity	Nursing Care	Major Uses
		Alkylating Agents			
		(interfere with DNA replication, cell cycle nonspecific)			
Mechlorethamine (Mustargen) (nitrogen mustard) (HN_2)	Intravenous: 0.4 mg/kg once or 0.2 mg/kg for 2 days (dose dependent on patient's bone marrow reserve); 4-week rest period before 2nd dose Vesicant: administer into rapidly running saline I.V. (prepare and use immediately, decomposes quickly); use gloves Intracavitary: 0.2–0.4 mg/kg (change patient's position every 15 min. for 1 hr. after dose for uniform distribution)	Rapid cellular interaction, inactivated in blood within 5 min.	Bone marrow suppression (nadir 7–12 days after 1st dose) Severe nausea, vomiting, diarrhea Alopecia Sterility Birth defects	Avoid extravasation of I.V. Assess signs and symptoms; protect against infection and bleeding Check blood counts Administer antiemetics (sedation if needed) Maintain hydration Adjust diet Assist coping with hair loss Sexual counseling Provide contraceptive information	Hodgkin's disease Lymphomas Malignant effusions

Drug	Dose/Administration	Pharmacokinetics	Side Effects	Nursing Implications	Indications
Melphalan (Alkeran) (L-phenylanaline mustard) (L-PAM)	Oral: 0.25 mg/kg per day for 4 days every 4–6 weeks	Generally slow acting	Bone marrow suppression (nadir may be unpredictable) Immunosuppression Nausea Sterility	Assess signs and symptoms; protect against infection and bleeding Check blood counts Administer antiemetics Sexual counseling	Multiple myeloma Ovarian cancer Breast cancer
Busulfan (Myleran)	Oral: 4–10 mg per day until WBC 15,000 mm^3, then rest, maintenance 2–4 mg per day	Rapid acting Renal excretion	Bone marrow suppression Pulmonary toxicity	Assess signs and symptoms; protect against infection and bleeding Check blood counts (especially platelet count and granulocyte level) Assess signs and symptoms of pulmonary dysfunction	Chronic myelocytic leukemia

TABLE 5.2 (continued)

Agent	Dose and Administration	Pharmacologic Factors	Significant Side Effects and Toxicity	Nursing Care	Major Uses
Chlorambucil (Leukeran)	Oral: 0.1 mg/kg per day in single or divided doses for 3–4 weeks, then maintenance 2–4 mg per day	Slow acting	Minimal, prolonged use: immunosuppression, bone marrow suppression	Assess signs and symptoms; protect against infection and bleeding Check blood counts	Chronic lymphocytic leukemia
Cyclophosphamide (Cytoxan) (Ctx)	Oral: 1–2.5 mg/kg per day in divided doses Intravenous: 20–30 mg/kg IVP into rapidly running I.V.	Must be activated by liver Renal excretion	Bone marrow suppression, immunosuppression Nausea, vomiting Alopecia Hemorrhagic cystitis Sterility Birth defects	Assess signs and symptoms; protect against infection and bleeding Check blood counts Administer antiemetics Assist in coping with hair loss	Multiple myeloma Lymphomas Small-cell lung Breast cancer

Triethylene thiophosphoramide (Thio-Tepa)	Intracavitary: 15–30 mg (depending on effusion size)	Malignant effusions	Bone marrow suppression	Maintain hydration: must have high fluid output (G–U irrigation for patients receiving high dose may be given)
				Watch for signs and symptoms of cystitis
				Sexual counseling
				Provide contraceptive information
				Turn patient every 15 min. for 1 hr. to distribute drug
				Assess signs and symptoms; protect against infection and bleeding
				Check blood counts

91

TABLE 5.2 (continued)

Agent	Dose and Administration	Pharmacologic Factors	Significant Side Effects and Toxicity	Nursing Care	Major Uses
		Nitrosoureas Agents *(alkylating agents, inhibit DNA replication)*			
Carmustine (BCNU)	Intravenous: 200–250 mg/m^2 once every 6–8 weeks (local pain on injection)	Renal, hepatic excretion Crosses blood-brain barrier	Severe nausea, vomiting Bone marrow suppression (nadir 4–6 weeks after dose)	Administer antiemetics Assess signs and symptoms; protect against infection and bleeding Check blood counts (especially platelets and granulocytes)	Brain tumors Gastrointestinal cancer Melanoma
Lomustine (CCNU)	Oral: 100–130 mg/m^2 once every 6–8 weeks	Same as Carmustine	Same as Carmustine	Same as Carmustine	Lymphomas Lung cancer

Vinca Alkaloids
(bind to microtubular proteins necessary for cell division during mitosis, cell cycle phase specific)

Vinblastine (Velban)	Intravenous: 0.1–0.15 mg/kg once weekly Vesicant	Metabolized by liver Slow biliary and renal excretion Crosses blood-brain barrier	Bone marrow suppression (nadir 5–10 weeks after dose) Nausea, vomiting Alopecia Neuropathy (rare)	Avoid I.V. extravasation Assess signs and symptoms; protect against infection and bleeding Check blood counts (especially granulocyte count) Administer anti-emetics Assist in coping with hair loss	Hodgkin's disease Testicular tumors
Vincristine (Oncovin) (VCR)	Intravenous: 1.4 mg/m² (adult dose not to exceed 2 mg) weekly Vesicant	Metabolized by liver Slow biliary and renal excretion	Peripheral neuropathy Autonomic neuropathy: severe constipation, paralytic ileus	Avoid I.V. extravasation Assess signs and symptoms of neurotoxicity: depression of Achilles' tendon reflex (earliest sign), paresthesias in fingers and toes, in-	Acute lymphoblastic leukemia Hodgkin's disease Lymphomas

TABLE 5.2 (continued)

Agent	Dose and Administration	Pharmacologic Factors	Significant Side Effects and Toxicity	Nursing Care	Major Uses
Vincristine (continued)				ability to perform fine motor skills, weakness Assess bowel habits Administer stool softeners, cathartics, and enemas as needed	
Antimetabolites					
(inhibit enzymes of nucleic acid synthesis, generally cell cycle phase specific)					
Cytarbine (Cytosar) (Cytosine arabinoside) (Ara-C)	Intravenous: 100 mg/m² IVP every 12 hours for 5–7 days, or constant infusion over 2–3 days Intrathecal: 4.5–73 mg/m² every 3–7 days Refrigerate unconstituted solution	Rapid acting Minor renal excretion	Bone marrow suppression (nadir 12–14 days after dose) Nausea, vomiting, diarrhea Stomatitis Hepatitis (may occur within 1 week after dose)	Assess signs and symptoms; protect against infection and bleeding Check blood counts Administer antidiarrheal agents, antiemetics	Acute leukemia

| 5-Fluorouracil (Fluorouracil) (5-FU) | Intravenous: 12–15 mg/kg IVP weekly for 4 weeks (halt if toxicity and resume at 5 mg/kg) | Rapid acting Hepatic, renal excretion | Severe bone marrow suppression Severe nausea, vomiting, diarrhea Alopecia (rare) Hyperpigmentation (enhanced photosensitivity) | Assess signs and symptoms; protect against infection and bleeding Check blood counts Administer antiemetics, antidiarrheal agents Maintain hydration Adjust diet Frequent mouth care and assessment Advise patient to avoid sunlight | Breast cancer Gastrointestinal tumors |
| | | | Birth defects | Maintain hydration Adjust diet Frequent mouth care and assessment Assess signs and symptoms of hepatitic dysfunction Provide contraceptive information | |

TABLE 5.2 (continued)

Agent	Dose and Administration	Pharmacologic Factors	Significant Side Effects and Toxicity	Nursing Care	Major Uses
Methotrexate (MTX)	Intravenous: 25–50 mg/m^2 per week; high doses (e.g., over 500 mg/m^2) must be followed by 10–20 mg citrovorum factor I.V. or orally every 6 hr. (dose dependent on renal function and plasma methotrexate level) Oral: 10–30 mg/m^2 twice a week Intrathecal: 6–12 mg/m^2 (dissolved in 10 ml of saline or artificial CSF) twice weekly or monthly for maintenance	Renal excretion Citrovorum factor (Leucovorin) "rescues" cells from cytotoxicity by providing cofactors for DNA synthesis	Bone marrow suppression Stomatitis Severe diarrhea Hepatic toxicity Birth defects Renal toxicity with high doses Neurotoxicity (acute and chronic) with intrathecal administration	Assess signs and symptoms; protect against infection and bleeding Check blood counts Administer antidiarrheal agents Maintain hydration Adjust diet Assess signs and symptoms of hepatic dysfunction Frequent mouth care and assessment Provide contraceptive information For high doses: make sure	Acute leukemia Choriocarcinoma Breast cancer Head and neck cancer Testicular cancer Lung cancer High doses: Osteosarcoma

citrovorum factor ("rescue") has been given

Maintain intravenous hydration (3000 ml/m^2 per day)

Monitor intake and output

Check that drug levels and renal function tests are taken

Keep urine alkaline to augment renal clearance (acetazolamide, sodium bicarbonate)

For intrathecal administration; assess signs and symptoms of neurotoxicity (nausea, vomiting, headache, dementia)

TABLE 5.2 (continued)

Agent	Dose and Administration	Pharmacologic Factors	Significant Side Effects and Toxicity	Nursing Care	Major Uses
6-Mercaptopurine (Purinethol) (6-MP)	Oral: 1.5–2.5 mg/kg daily in divided doses (dose must be reduced 1/4–1/3 when given with Allopurinol)	Metabolized by xanthine oxidase Allopurinol (a xanthine oxidase inhibitor) inhibits drug breakdown Renal excretion	Bone marrow suppression Nausea, vomiting Hepatic dysfunction	Assess signs and symptoms; protect against infection and bleeding Check blood counts Administer antiemetics Adjust diet Assess signs and symptoms of hepatic dysfunction: jaundice	Acute leukemia
6-Thioguanine (Thioguanine) (6-T6)	Oral: 2 mg/kg per day (do not need to alter dose if given with Allopurinol)	Incomplete oral absorption Rapid renal excretion	Bone marrow suppression (may be delayed) Nausea, vomiting Hepatic dysfunction Stomatitis	Assess signs and symptoms; protect against infection and bleeding Check blood counts	Acute leukemia

Drug	Dosage		Side Effects	Nursing Measures	Indications
5-Azacytidine	Intravenous: 150 mg/m² (reconstituted in sterile water and diluted with Ringer's solution) given in continuous 24-hr. infusion for 5 days; solution is unstable (must be reconstituted every 3–4 hr.)	Rapid renal excretion	Severe nausea, vomiting (reduced when given drug as continuous infusion) Diarrhea Bone marrow suppression Hepatic toxicity	Administer antiemetics, antidiarrheal agents Adjust diet Maintain hydration Assess signs and symptoms; protect against infection and bleeding Check blood counts Assess signs and symptoms of hepatic dysfunction Administer antiemetics Adjust diets Assess signs and symptoms of hepatic dysfunction Frequent mouth care and assessment	Acute granulocytic leukemia

TABLE 5.2 (continued)

Agent	Dose and Administration	Pharmacologic Factors	Significant Side Effects and Toxicity	Nursing Care	Major Uses
Hydroxyurea (Hydrea) (OH-urea)	Oral: 20–30 mg/kg per day, or 80 mg/kg every 3 days	Metabolized by liver Renal excretion Inhibits DNA synthesis Cell cycle phase specific	Bone marrow suppression Nausea, vomiting Stomatitis Skin reactions Alopecia	Assess signs and symptoms; protect against infection and bleeding Check blood counts Administer antiemetics Frequent mouth care and assessment Observe skin closely Assist coping with hair loss	Chronic granulocytic leukemia Prostate cancer High leukocyte count in acute leukemia

Antibiotics
(natural products of soil fungi, inhibits DNA, RNA synthesis, generally cell cycle phase nonspecific)

Agent	Dose and Administration	Pharmacologic Factors	Significant Side Effects and Toxicity	Nursing Care	Major Uses
Dactinomycin (Cosmegan) (Actinomycin-D)	Intravenous: 15 mcg/kg for 5 days every 3–4 weeks Vesicant	Prolonged activity Renal, fecal excretion	Bone marrow suppression Nausea, vomiting Diarrhea	Avoid I.V. extravasation Assess signs and symptoms;	Wilms' tumor Rhabdomyosarcomas Choriocar-

Drug	Dosage	Action	Side Effects	Nursing Interventions	Uses
		Increases sensitivity to radiation	Alopecia Stomatitis "Recal phenomenon" Birth defects	protect against infection and bleeding Check blood counts Administer antiemetics, antidiarrheal agents Adjust diet Maintain hydration Assist coping with hair loss Frequent mouth care and assessment Assess skin in previously radiated sites Provide contraceptive information	cinoma Testicular cancer
Doxorubicin (Adriamycin)	Intravenous: 60 mg/m² every 3 weeks; 550 mg/m² total dose limit (450 mg/m² maximum dose limit if risk of cardiac toxicity) Vesicant	Activated by liver Biliary excretion Increases sensitivity to radiation	Severe bone marrow suppression Alopecia Nausea, vomiting Stomatitis Cardiac toxicity Red-colored urine (harmless)	Avoid I.V. extravasation Assess signs and symptoms; protect against infection and bleeding Check blood	Lymphomas Leukemia Sarcomas Breast cancer

TABLE 5.2 (continued)

Agent	Dose and Administration	Pharmacologic Factors	Significant Side Effects and Toxicity	Nursing Care	Major Uses
Doxorubicin (continued)			"Recall phenomenon"	counts Assist coping with hair loss Administer antiemetics Adjust diet Frequent mouth care and assessment Assess signs and symptoms of cardiac toxicity: arrhythmias, dyspnea, edema Inform patient of urine change Assess skin in previously radiated sites	
Daunomycin (Daunorubicin)	Intravenous: 60 mg/m^2 for 1–3 days	Similar to Doxorubicin	Similar to Doxorubicin	Same as Doxorubicin	Acute leukemia

Drug	Dosage	Pharmacology	Side effects/Toxicity	Nursing interventions	Indications
Bleomycin (Blenoxane)	Intravenous: 10–20 units/m² Intramuscular: 10–20 units/m² Subcutaneous: 10–20 units/m² Total dose accumulation over 400 units associated with increased toxicity	Rapid acting Renal excretion	Pulmonary toxicity (pneumonitis, pulmonary fibrosis) Skin reactions (hyperpigmentation, ulceration, erythema) Stomatitis Alopecia Nausea, vomiting Anaphylaxis Fever	Assess signs and symptoms of respiratory distress (especially dyspnea, rales) Assess skin carefully Frequent mouth care and assessment Assist coping with hair loss Administer antiemetics Adjust diet Give test dose (1 mg), and observe for anaphylaxis: fever hypotension, wheezing Take temperature Administer antipyretics	Head and neck cancer Testicular cancer Lymphomas
Mithramycin (Mithracin)	Intravenous: 50 mcg/kg IVP every other day for 3 days each week until toxicity occurs	Little known	Severe bleeding Arterial clotting Hepatic toxicity Renal toxicity	Assess signs and symptoms of bleeding Check platelet	Testicular cancer Hypercalcemia associated

TABLE 5.2 (continued)

Agent	Dose and Administration	Pharmacologic Factors	Significant Side Effects and Toxicity	Nursing Care	Major Uses
Mithramycin (continued)	For treatment of hypercalcemia: 25 mcg/kg IVP daily for 3–4 days, then intermittent weekly doses		Nausea, vomiting Stomatitis Central nervous system reactions (headache, weakness, fatigue) Fever Hypocalcemia	count and coagulation studies Assess signs and symptoms of hepatic, renal dysfunction Administer antiemetics Frequent mouth care and assessment Assess signs and symptoms of central nervous system dysfunction Observe signs and symptoms of hypocalcemia Monitor temperature	with malignancy

| Mitomycin-C (Mutamycin) | Intravenous: 20 mg/m² once or divided doses of 2 mg/m² over 12 days (2-day rest period mid-cycle); repeat every 6–8 weeks as tolerated. Vesicant | Rapid acting. Metabolized by liver. Minor renal excretion | Bone marrow suppression (delayed, serious). Nausea, vomiting. Diarrhea. Stomatitis. Alpecia. Fever | Avoid I.V. extravasation. Assess signs and symptoms; protect against infection and bleeding. Check blood counts (especially WBC and platelet count). Administer antiemetics, antidiarrheal agents. Adjust diet. Frequent mouth care and assessment. Assist coping with hair loss. Monitor fever | Breast cancer. Head and neck cancer. Gastrointestinal tumors |

Hormones
(affect the growth pattern of hormonally responsive tumors)

Estrogen					
Diethylstilbesterol (DES)	Oral: 1 mg per day (prostate); 5 mg 3 times per day (breast)	Slow acting. Metabolized by liver	Nausea, vomiting. Fluid retention. Gynecomastia in males	Administer antiemetics. Adjust diet. Monitor daily weight	Prostate cancer. Breast cancer (postmenopausal)

TABLE 5.2 (continued)

Agent	Dose and Administration	Pharmacologic Factors	Significant Side Effects and Toxicity	Nursing Care	Major Uses
Estrogen (continued)			Uterine bleeding Alterations in libido, impotence Hypercalcemia Hepatic toxicity (high doses)	Intake and output Note edema; observe for uterine bleeding Check radiation to male breast tissue prior to dose Sexual counseling Assess coping with body changes Assist signs and symptoms of hypercalcemia: confusion, polyuria, constipation Assess signs and symptoms of liver dysfunction	

	Dose/Route	Action/Metabolism	Side Effects	Nursing Implications	Indications
Antiestrogen					
Tamoxifen (Nolvadex) (TAM)	Oral: 10 mg twice a day	Slow acting, Competes with estrogen for estrogen receptor	Nausea, vomiting, Uterine bleeding, Hot flashes, Thrombocytopenia (mild), Blurred vision	Administer antiemetics, Assess signs and symptoms of bleeding, Check platelet count, Assess visual changes	Breast cancer
Progestins					
Megestrol acetate (Megace) (MEG)	Oral: 40–320 mg per day (endometrial cancer); 160 mg daily (breast cancer); given in divided doses	Metabolized in liver, Renal excretion	Minimal	Observe for side effects	Endometrial cancer, Breast cancer
Medroxy progesterone acetate (Depoprovera)	Intramuscular	Metabolized in liver, Renal excretion	Fluid retention (minimal)	Daily weights, Note edema	Endometrial cancer, Breast cancer, Renal cell cancer
Androgens					
Testosterone propionate (Neo-Hombreol)	Intramuscular: 50–100 mg 3 days a week	Slow acting, Metabolized by liver, Renal excretion	Fluid retention, Masculinization in women, Altered libido	Dailey weights, Note edema, Sexual counseling, Assist coping with body changes	Breast cancer (post menopausal)

TABLE 5.2 (continued)

Agent	Dose and Administration	Pharmacologic Factors	Significant Side Effects and Toxicity	Nursing Care	Major Uses
Fluoxymesterone (Halotestin)	Oral: 10–40 mg per day in divided doses	Absorbed from gastrointestinal tract	Fluid retention Masculinization in women Hepatic toxicity	Daily weights Note edema Sexual counseling Assist coping with body changes Assess signs and symptoms of hepatic dysfunction	Breast cancer (post menopausal)
		Adrenocorticosteroids			
Prednisone (PRED)	Oral: 15–100 mg on alternate days; take with milk, food, antacid (gradual withdrawal of drug if taken for prolonged period, not necessary for short high-dose courses)	Metabolized by liver Renal excretion	*All Steroids* (prolonged, high doses) Fluid retention, hypertension Hypokalemia Diabetes Immunosuppression Gastrointestinal bleeding Potassium loss	*All Steroids* Daily weights Note edema Monitor blood pressure Assess signs and symptoms: hypokalemia Give potassium replacement (e.g., bananas)	Leukemia Lymphomas multiple myeloma CNS metastases Hypercalcemia

Drug	Dose	Pharmacology	Side Effects	Nursing Considerations	Indications
Dexamethasone (Decadron)	Oral: 0.5–24 mg per day	Slow acting	Mood swing, psychosis; Cushingoid changes; Osteoporosis	Assess signs and symptoms of diabetes: polyuria, polydisia, check urine for sugar/acetone; Assess signs and symptoms; protect against infection; Assist coping with body changes and emotional lability	See Prednisone
Methylprednisone sodium succinate (solu-medrol)	Intravenous: 10–125 mg per day		See Prednisone	See Prednisone	See Prednisone
Podophyllotoxins					
Etoposide (VP-16)	Intravenous: 50–100 mg/m^2 for 5 days every 3 weeks; Oral: 120 mg/m^2 for 5 days every 3 weeks	Renal excretion; Cell cycle specific	Bone marrow suppression; Nausea, vomiting; Diarrhea; Alopecia; Hypotension after rapid I.V. infu-	Assess signs and symptoms; protect against infection and bleeding; Check blood counts	Small-cell lung cancer; Testicular cancer

TABLE 5.2 (continued)

Agent	Dose and Administration	Pharmacologic Factors	Significant Side Effects and Toxicity	Nursing Care	Major Uses
Etoposide (continued)			sion, fever, anaphylactic reactions	Administer antiemetics, antidiarrheal agents Adjust diet Maintain hydration Assist coping with hair loss Monitor temperature Observe for signs and symptoms of anaphylaxis	
(Teneposide, VM-26, similar action used in brain tumors)					

Miscellaneous and Experimental Agents

| L. Asparaginase (L-ASP) (Elspar) | Intravenous: 1,000 IU/kg per day for 10 days; do NOT shake vial—harms enzymes Intramuscular: 6,000 IU/m² 3 times a week for 9 doses | Excreted via reticuloendothelial system Destroys extracellular L-asparagine Cell cycle phase nonspecific | Anaphylaxis Hepatic toxicity Pancreatitis, coagulopathy CNS disturbances: hallucinations, depression | Observe carefully for anaphylaxis (be prepared with emergency supplies) Test dose in patient with prior exposure to drug | Acute lymphoblastic leukemia |

Drug	Dosage	Characteristics	Side Effects/Toxicity	Nursing Implications	Indications
Procarbazine (Matulane) (PROC)	Oral: 100–300 mg daily for 1 week Rest, then 50–100 mg per day when bone marrow recovers	Rapid acting Renal excretion Crosses blood-brain barrier MAO inhibitor Cell cycle phase nonspecific	Bone marrow suppression, immunosuppression Nausea, vomiting Central nervous system toxicity: depression, restlessness, psychosis, somnolence, ataxia, convulsions Birth defects Hemolytic anemia	Assess signs and symptoms of hepatic dysfunction: pancreatitis Check mental status Assess signs and symptoms; protect against bleeding and infection Check blood counts Administer antiemetics Assess mental status for confusion, depression, and drowsiness Inform patient to avoid barbiturates, antihistamines, alcohol, narcotics, sedative antihypotensive agents, sympathomimetic tricycle antidepressant drugs, ripe bananas, and cheese	Lymphomas Hodgkin's disease Lung cancer

TABLE 5.2 (continued)

Agent	Dose and Administration	Pharmacologic Factors	Significant Side Effects and Toxicity	Nursing Care	Major Uses
Procarbazine (continued)				Provide information for contraception	
Dacarbazine (DTIC-Dome)	Intravenous: 150–250 mg/m^2 daily for 5 days; repeat at 3-week intervals Vesicant Cover bottle (solution deteriorates in sunlight)	Activated by liver Cell cycle phase nonspecific	Bone marrow suppression Nausea, vomiting	Assess signs and symptoms; protect against infection and bleeding Check blood counts Administer antiemetics	Malignant melanoma Sarcomas Lymphomas
		Experimental Drugs			
Hexamethylmelamine (HMM)	Oral: 12 mg/kg per day for 21 days, and rest 4 weeks, or 8 mg/kg per day for 90 days Give after meals	Metabolized by liver Renal excretion	Nausea Bone marrow suppression (mild) Neurotoxicity (with prolonged use)	Administer antiemetics Assess signs and symptoms; protect against infection and bleeding	Ovarian cancer Lung cancer Lymphomas

Drug/Dosage	Action	Side Effects	Nursing Considerations	Uses
Cis-d chlorodiammine dichloroplatinum (II) (DDP) (Cisplatin) (Platinol) Intravenous: 20 mg/m² in 2 liters of D$_5$/NS with 37.5 gm of mannitol over 6 hr. for 4–5 days; repeat every 4 weeks for 3–4 times; give Furosemide (Lasix) 40 mg prior to dose	Renal excretion Inhibits DNA synthesis Functions like alkylating agent Cell cycle phase nonspecific	Nausea, vomiting Renal toxicity Hearing loss Anaphylaxis	Check blood counts Assess signs and symptoms of neurologic dysfunction Administer antiemetics Hydrate patient: begin I.V. 12 hr. prior to therapy and continue at 100 ml/hr Assess signs and symptoms of renal dysfunction: monitor intake and output Check for daily serum, creatinine and creatinine clearance tests Assess hearing frequently (audiograph prior to dose) Observe for signs of anaphylaxis	Testicular tumors Ovarian cancer Bladder cancer Head and neck cancer

TABLE 5.2 (continued)

Agent	Dose and Administration	Pharmacologic Factors	Significant Side Effects and Toxicity	Nursing Care	Major Uses
Mitotane (Lysodren) (O,P'-DDD)	Oral: 8–10 gm daily in divided doses	Long-term deposition in fat Renal excretion Interferes with adrenal cortical functioning (avoid use with spironolactone)	Nausea, vomiting Diarrhea Central nervous system effects: depression, lethargy, vertigo Adrenal insufficiency, proteinuria	Administer antiemetics, antidiarrheal agents Adjust diet Assess behavioral, neurological changes Caution patient to avoid tasks requiring mental alertness Stop drug and administer steroids if severe trauma or shock	Inoperable adrenal cortical carcinoma

similar to the effect of ionizing radiation and thus alkylating agents have been called *radiomimetics*. The drugs act by alkylating organic compounds and are generally cell cycle phase nonspecific. These drugs have been utilized for treatment of various types of cancer with varying degrees of success. Particularly important drugs in this group are cyclophosphamide (Cytoxan) and nitrogen mustard. Nitrosoureas also function as alkylating agents. The most common side effects of alkylating agents affecting nursing care are due to the impact of the drugs on the hematopoetic and gastrointestinal systems [16,42,51].

Antimetabolites. Chemotherapy drugs classified as antimetabolites inhibit enzymes involved in nucleic acid synthesis. They act by competing or substituting for other metabolites or binding to them in a way to cause dysfunction. They are generally cell cycle phase specific (except 5-FU). These drugs are also used for a variety of tumors [16]. Patients receiving cytosine arabinoside, 5-fluorouracil, and methotrexate involve close nursing attention [22,23,52].

Antibiotics. Antineoplastic antibiotics are natural products of soil fungi which inhibit DNA and RNA synthesis [16,36]. They are generally cell cycle phase nonspecific. In addition to bone marrow toxicity and gastrointestinal side effects, they have some unusual toxicities requiring skilled nursing assessment and intervention [23,42,52].

Vinca Alkaloids. The plant alkaloids bind to microtubular proteins necessary for cell division during mitosis. They are cell cycle phase specific. Nursing assessment is important in ascertaining the presence of neurotoxicity associated with vincristine [16,42,53].

Hormones. Exogenous hormones may affect the growth pattern of hormonally sensitive tumors [16,36]. Estrogens, antiestrogens, progestational agents and androgens have been utilized for their antineoplastic effect on hormonally responsive tumors. Adrenocorticosteroids can have a cyctotoxic effect which is not well understood. Some of these agents are almost devoid of side effects while others can have a significant impact on the patient's body image and quality of life [62].

Miscellaneous and Experimental Drugs. A variety of chemotherapeutic drugs that are not listed in the previous categories of drug actions are available for investigational purposes. Such drugs may be used in a research setting [16,21,32]. They have varied side effects that may require skilled nursing care. Experimental drugs may be administered according to specific protocols. Patient guidelines specifying who may receive the drug and the factors that will exclude patients will be described in the protocol. Drug administration procedures and important clinical tests to evaluate tumor response and toxicity also will be prescribed. While the patient is on the protocol, the drug therapy will not be altered unless changed in the manner specifically described in the procedure. Patients may come off the protocol if they wish or if there is no adequate tumor response or unacceptable toxicity. Protocols help to establish guidelines for safe and effective therapy.

Clinical Trials. Patients receiving experimental chemotherapy may be participating in clinical trials. Various phases of clinical trials are involved in evaluation of potentially therapeutic drugs. Phase I trials are done to determine the optimal dose and administration schedule of promising antineoplastic drugs and to describe associated side effects and toxicities. Patients in Phase I trials usually have no other effective treatment option. Phase II trials involve the use of the drug in the determined schedule (from Phase I trials) in patients with different types of malignancies to determine effectiveness. Lung, breast, and colon cancer are so-called "signal tumors" used in Phase II studies. Trials also include tumor types that have shown responsiveness in Phase I trials. Patients in Phase II trials have measurable disease and do not have effective standard therapy options. The comparison of experimental therapy with known standard therapy occurs in Phase III clinical trials. Treatment selection between the standard and experimental may be assigned in randomized fashion in order to determine whether or not the investigational therapy is superior to the standard.

Nursing care of patients involved in clinical trials includes careful assessment of signs and symptoms possibly related to the experimental therapy. The nurse may be actively involved in data collection as part of the protocol [31]. Patients may be willing to participate in experimental treatment (Phase I trials) as a last hope for cure or disease regression [57]. Nursing assessment of patients receiving investigational therapy should be attuned to their hopes for the therapy. Informed consent documentation will be required of patients involved in clinical trials. Nurses may be involved in explaining potential side effects of the treatment. The nurse can assure the patient that support and comfort will be given regardless of participation in experimentation. (See section on informed consent in Chapter 4.)

TABLE 5.3
Examples of Impact of Chemotherapy on Granulocytes [16]

Drug	Nadir (days)	Recovery (days)
Mechlorethamine	7–15	21–28
Cyclophosphamide	8–14	18–25
Methotrexate	7–14	14–21

Chemotherapy Schedules

Chemotherapeutic drugs are often given at timed intervals or cycles. The extent of the impact of the antineoplastic drugs on the bone marrow is dose dependent but is generally observed one to two weeks after initial therapy. The nadir (lowest point) of the impact of chemotherapy on the bone marrow components (white cells, red cells, platelets) may be different for the individual marrow elements. The nadir is influenced by the cell cycle and growth fraction of the marrow precursors as well as the availability of components in storage, for example, red cells [25]. Granulocytes, which have a circulating half life of six hours and limited reserve in the bone marrow, often reach their nadir first in response to myelotoxic chemotherapeutic drugs. (See Table 5.3.) Drugs are given for a certain period of time to maximize tumor cell kill and are stopped to minimize toxicity and to allow the patient's hematopoetic and immune systems to recover. Examples of treatment protocol schedules are shown in Table 5.4 [16].

Induction is the term utilized to describe the initial courses of therapy to effect a remission. Once remission is obtained the patient may receive drugs at periodic intervals to maintain the clinically disease-free state. Receiving chemotherapy when the patient is not feeling ill may make compliance difficult. The patient may find it very hard to submit to an uncomfortable treatment when feeling healthy. It interrupts her day and again identifies her as a cancer patient.

Combination Chemotherapy

A combination of antineoplastic drugs may be utilized to optimize tumor destruction while minimizing toxic side effects. Combination chemotherapy has also been found to be substantially superior to single drug cancer therapy for a number of tumors [13]. Drugs with different modes of action and minimal overlapping toxicity are

TABLE 5.4
Selected Chemotherapy Protocols

Uses	Name	Agents	Dose	Administration	Schedule	Cycle
Lung cancer Non–oat-cell carcinoma	CAMP	Cytoxan	300 mg/m^2	I.V.	Days 1, 8	28 days
		Adriamycin	20 mg/m^2	I.V.	Days 1, 8	
		Methotrexate	15 mg/m^2	I.V.	Days 1, 8	
		Procarbazine	100 mg/m^2	Oral	Days 1–10	
Oat-cell carcinoma		*First 6 weeks:*				Alternate cycles every 6 weeks
		Cytoxan	1,000 mg/m^2	I.V.	Every 6 weeks	
		Methotrexate	25 mg/m^2	Oral	Every 2 weeks	
		CCNU	50 mg/m^2	Oral	Every 6 weeks	
		Second 6 weeks:				
		Vincristine	2 mg	I.V.	Every 3 weeks	
		Adriamycin	60 mg/m^2	I.V.	Every 3 weeks	
		Procarbazine	100 mg/m^2	Oral	Days 1–10 every 3 weeks	
Testicular cancer	PVB	Velban	0.15 mg/kg	IVP	Days 1, 2 every 3 weeks, 5 times	
		then	0.30 mg/kg	IVP	Every 4 weeks for 2 years	
		Cis-platinum	20 mg/m^2	I.V. (15-min. infusion)	Days 1–5 every 3 weeks, 5 times	
		Bleomycin	30 units	I.V.	Days 2, 9, 16 of each Cis-platinum course; then every week for 12 weeks	
Lymphomas	BACOP	Cytoxan	650 mg/m^2	I.V.	Days 1, 8	28 days
		Adriamycin	25 mg/m^2	I.V.	Days 1, 8	
		Vincristine	1.4 mg/m^2	I.V.	Days 1, 8	

Disease	Regimen	Drug	Dose	Route	Days	Cycle
		Prednisone	60 mg/m²	Oral	Days 14–28	21 days
		Bleomycin	5 mg/m²	I.V.	Days 14, 21	
	CHOP	Cytoxan	750 mg/m²	I.V.	Day 1	
		Adriamycin	50 mg/m²	I.V.	Day 1	
		Vincristine	1.4 mg/m²	I.V.	Day 1	
		Prednisone	25 mg	Oral	Days 1–5, 4 times per day	
	CVP	Cytoxan	400 mg/m²	Oral	Days 2–6	21 days
		Vincristine	1.4 mg/m²	I.V.	Day 1	
		Prednisone	100 mg/m²	Oral	Days 2–6	
Hodgkin's disease Lymphomas	ABVD	Adriamycin	25 mg/m²	I.V.	Days 1, 15	28 days
		Bleomycin	10 mg/m²	I.V.	Days 1, 15	
		Velban	6 mg/m²	I.V.	Days 1, 15	
		DTIC	150 mg/m²	I.V.	Days 1–5	
	MOPP	Mechlorethamine	6 mg/m²	I.V.	Days 1, 8	
		Vincristine	1.4 mg/m²	I.V.	Days 1, 8	
		Prednisone	40 mg/m²	Oral	Days 1–14	
		Procarbazine	100 mg/m²	Oral	Days 1–14	
Breast cancer	CMF	Cytoxan	100 mg/m²	Oral	Days 1–14	28 days
		Methotrexate	40 mg/m²	I.V.	Days 1–8	
		5-Fluorouracil	650 mg/m²	I.V.	Days 1–8	
	AC	Adriamycin	40 mg/m²	I.V.	Day 1	28 days
		Cytoxan	200 mg/m²	Oral	Days 3–6	
Myeloma	—	Alkeran	0.25 mg/kg		Days 1–4	—
		Prednisone	2 mg/kg		Days 1–4	
Leukemia (AML)	TAD	Cytosine arabinoside (Ara-C)	100 mg/m²	I.V.	Every 12 hours for 7 days	3–4 weeks
		6-Thioguanine	100 mg/m²	Oral	Every 12 hours for 7 days	
		Daunarubycin	60 mg/m²	I.V.	Days 5, 6, 7	

selected to provide a therapeutic synergistic effect. Alterations in sequencing of drug administration and dosage may further minimize side effects. Nursing care of patients undergoing combination chemotherapy will require an understanding of multiple drug side effects.

Multimodality Cancer Therapy

The patient with cancer may require treatment with chemotherapy, radiation therapy, surgery, and immunotherapy at different phases of the illness.These therapies may be done in conjunction or in specific sequences to provide optimal antineoplastic effect and minimize toxicity to the patient. This multimodality approach has definite implications for nursing care. The patient may be exposed to multiple members of the health team. The information provided the patient may differ depending on the source. Coordinated efforts by the health team should minimize confusing or contradictory explanations to the patient. The patient may also be more vulnerable physically and emotionally when experiencing different side effects of the various modalities in a short time interval. Even when therapies are given in sequence the patient may experience unique problems such as the radiation skin reaction "recalled" when certain chemotherapeutic drugs are administered following radiation therapy. (See section on radiation side effects in Chapter 6.) Healing after surgical intervention may require special nursing care if the patient's immune system and bone marrow function have been compromised by chemotherapy. Certain organ functions (for example, cardiac, pulmonary) also may have to be carefully assessed if subject to the side effects of the various modalities. The chapters on surgery and radiation therapy discuss principles of nursing care that must be incorporated when the patient is receiving multimodality cancer therapy.

Adjuvant Chemotherapy

Adjuvant chemotherapy involves the use of antineoplastic agents after the patient has had "curative" cancer therapy (surgery, radiation therapy) [63]. The adjuvant chemotherapy is an attempt to prevent tumor recurrence by eliminating possible micrometastasis. This experimental approach is only used in patients with a significant risk of cancer recurrence. Long-term therapy is usually acceptable only if the side effects experienced by the patients are minimal or well controlled. Examples of such therapy include CMF (Cytoxan, methotrexate, 5-FU) for premenopausal women with breast cancer and positive lymph nodes, and high-dose methotrexate with citrovorum rescue for osteosarcoma [34,63].

NURSING CARE FOR PATIENTS RECEIVING CHEMOTHERAPY

Nursing Approach to Chemotherapeutic Drugs

In the rapidly growing and changing field of cancer care and treatment, the nurse caring for the patient receiving chemotherapy must be prepared to evaluate the nursing needs of patients receiving unfamiliar or experimental drugs [11,23,42]. The following is a suggested framework for assessing individual drugs in terms of nursing care needs:

1. What is it called (that is, its trade name, generic name, abbreviation, initial used in experimental protocol)?
2. What classification system does its properties best fit (for example, alkylating agent)? What is the relation to the cell cycle?
3. How is it metabolized and excreted? How long does this take? What organ functions are critical for proper action and prevention of toxicity?
4. How is it administered and are there any special considerations during administration (as, for example, with vesicants)? How often is it scheduled to be administered?
5. What is the common dosage? Is there alteration of the dose of the drug due to combined chemotherapy or altered physiological variables (such as compromised cardiac status)?
6. What are the common side effects? What is the time frame for occurrence and abatement of these side effects? What variables make the patient more vulnerable to the toxicity? What are the critical signs and symptoms of toxicity? When do they emerge? Can they be prevented?
7. Why is this particular patient receiving this drug (diagnosis, stage of disease)? How does it relate to other drugs or forms of cancer treatment the patient may have or will receive? What is the goal of treatment? How long will the treatment take?
8. How will response to the drug be evaluated (for example, by chest X-ray)? How frequently will it be evaluated?
9. What has the patient been told about the treatment? What does she understand about the goal of treatment and possible side effects?

10. What are the patient's hopes and fears in relation to the treatment?
11. Does the patient know what signs and symptoms are expected side effects and how to manage them?
12. Does the patient know what signs and symptoms signal critical changes and does she know when to notify the physician?
13. Does the drug interact with other agents which may alter its effectiveness or increase toxicity?

Nursing Administration of Chemotherapy Drugs

Regardless of who prepares the drug (pharmacies, nurses, physicians), the nurse administering the drug is responsible for making sure that the exact dose has been calculated. Many doses of chemotherapeutic drugs are determined in relation to body surface area determined from the patient's height and weight [16].

Double checking calculations in dose preparation is a common practice to ensure accuracy. Package inserts for the chemotherapy drugs may be helpful in learning about the drug but sometimes the information may not be relevant to an experimental protocol in which the drug is being used. Rechecking orders with the physician may clarify any alteration or discrepancy.

Chemotherapy drugs may be administered orally, intravenously, intramuscularly, subcutaneously, and intrathecally. Chemotherapy has also been administered in arterial infusions directly to the tumor site. Some agents may be injected directly into pleural or pericardial effusions or ascites.

Nursing Care During Intravenous Therapy. Techniques in intravenous therapy are beyond this chapter; however, certain points are important to keep in mind when administering chemotherapy drugs by the intravenous route [47]. Because of the need for repeated therapeutic administrations of the drugs, careful selection of the vein is very important. Arms can be alternated during treatment; however, chemotherapy should not be administered to extremities with lymphadema, which can hinder absorption of the drug. Some drugs are extremely caustic, causing severe local necrosis if infiltration or leakage of the I.V. occurs during the drug administration (refer to Table 5.2). Careful and close observation of the I.V. site is important, as well as the area proximal to the infusion, since a "blow out" or leakage of the vein may also occur elsewhere. Complaints of burning or pain during the infusion must be carefully considered as an indication of possible infiltration. Some of the vesicants have specific antidotes if infiltrated while others require steroid therapy and prompt application of ice packs to minimize spread of the drug. A slow leakage of fluid may not even be noted during the infusion, but later the patient experiences pain at the infusion site and evidence of extravasation is noted. The patient should be informed of the signs and symptoms of extravasation so that she can quickly inform appropriate health care members if this should occur.

Flushing or irrigating the I.V. between drug administration of combination chemotherapy may be recommended to ensure complete delivery of the drug and to check position of the needle before the next infusion. Some drugs may be administered in large amounts of fluid over time, partly to decrease the pain of infusion.

Patients receiving chemotherapy are often undergoing repetitive bone marrow suppression. Because of this, certain precautions need to be utilized in intravenous drug administration. Sterile technique should be utilized in the injection and careful observation for signs and symptoms of infection in old I.V. sites should be noted. Also, thrombocytopenic patients should have their I.V. site held at the completion of the procedure to ensure that the bleeding stops and that a hematoma does not develop and destroy the possibility for using that vein for future infusions.

When drugs characterized by a threat of anaphylaxis are given, emergency equipment should be available and emergency drugs (Benadryl, adrenalin) close at hand. Test doses may be administered if there is a suspicion of potential allergic response. Patients may be very frightened if aware of this possibility and may need close and supportive observation and care.

Nausea and vomiting may not only be a side effect of the physiologic activity of the drug but may also be a conditioned psychologic response that occurs prior to or during the administration of the drugs [23]. It may even occur when patients see something that reminds them of the drug experience, such as clothing worn to clinic that day. This is an extremely frustrating response for both patient and the nurse. Premedicating the patient with an antiemetic far in advance of the chemotherapy may be helpful. Alteration of food intake prior to the drug administration may also be useful. Systematic relaxation techniques and methods of diversion may also enable the patient to control the nausea. For some severe cases, hypnosis has been utilized to help the patient escape this symptom. Nursing assessment of this problem in the initial stages of treatment and beginning appropriate intervention are very important before a difficult pattern is established.

Alteration of the treatment environment may also be an important nursing intervention. Many patients receive chemotherapy on an outpatient basis. In a clinical setting, chemotherapy may be administered in one large room with little individual patient privacy. These patients may be seated in chairs to receive their drugs. Some patients may respond with less stress and nausea to a more private environment and in a more reclining position. Pictures, mobiles, music, and other stimuli may allow the patient to focus on things other than the injection needle, smell of alcohol, and the emesis basin.

Nursing Care During Intrathecal Administration. Most chemotherapeutic agents will not penetrate the blood-brain barrier. This allows a "sanctuary" or safe place for neoplastic cells to proliferate [16]. In tumors involving the meninges or with a high tendency for such involvement, chemotherapy may be given intrathecally. This may require the use of lumbar puncture which can cause the patient uncomfortable headaches. Frequent access to the central nervous system may be gained by semipermanent placement of an Ommaya Reservoir into the ventricle. The risks of infection and blockage are important nursing considerations [52]. Systemic toxicity may also be seen even though the drugs are administered by the intrathecal route.

Nursing Care During Intraarterial Chemotherapy Infusion. Intraarterial infusion of antineoplastic drugs directly to the tumor requires special nursing care [29]. The patient may receive the drug during a short hospital stay or she may go home with a portable infusion pump for long-term administration. Patients are still vulnerable to the systemic effects of the drug as well as local reactions, particularly if the drug is a vesicant. Surgical placement of the catheter is necessary requiring preoperative education and nursing support. Because the catheter is threaded through an artery, the nurse must closely observe the site for any indication of bleeding or swelling as well as assess the circulation of the distal extremity. Evidence of infection should be frequently assessed. Functioning of the pump apparatus must also be carefully and frequently evaluated for any malfunction that might cause an air embolism. Patient teaching about the equipment and drug side effects will be critically important if the patient is going home with the portable infusion pump.

Nursing Care During Chemotherapy Administration to Effusions. Chemotherapy may also be utilized in recurrent malignant effusions [16,56]. Effusions can severely compromise the patient's ability to carry on her life activities. For pleural effusions the patient may undergo drainage of the fluid and instillation of a drug. The patient will have to assume frequent position changes to provide maximum distribution of the drug. Chest tube drainage will then be required for several days. The patient may still experience systemic side effects of the drug.

Cancer Nursing in the Outpatient Setting

Nursing functions in outpatient settings where chemotherapy and immunotherapy are administered are varied, and often include provision of medical skills (nurse practitioner) and psychosocial support (mental health nurse) [4,14,31,44]. Assessment of the needs of the patient and her family can include a nursing perspective. By assessing the impact of disease and side effects the nurse can elicit the important concerns of the patient. These may be quite different from the medical concerns.

Continuity of care can begin in the outpatient setting with arrangements for home visits and a liaison relationship facilitating entry to the hospital's inpatient setting. Even in private practice, the nurse can facilitate the patient's entry to the hospital by providing a nursing history to accompany the patient upon admission.

——————— SIDE EFFECTS AND TOXICITIES ———————
OF CANCER CHEMOTHERAPY:
IMPLICATIONS FOR NURSING CARE

Bone Marrow Suppression

Cancer patients treated with chemotherapeutic agents frequently have side effects related to the effects of bone marrow suppression. Iatrogenic suppression of the bone marrow may lead to problems of: (1) leukopenia; (2) thrombocytopenia; and (3) anemia. Since chemotherapy generally has an impact on cells in active replication, the high growth fraction of the precursors of platelets and leukocytes make them particularly vulnerable to destruction [16,25]. Thus, by elimination of the precursors, chemotherapy prevents the bone marrow from normal production of elements necessary for hemostastis (platelets) and antimicrobial defenses (white blood cells). Chemotherapy may also affect the precursors of red blood cells. Significant medical management and nursing support are focused on patients treated with chemotherapy who suffer profound bone marrow depression. This toxicity is generally temporary until therapy is halted and the normal bone marrow recovers and resumes production of its essential components. When the hematopoietic system is infiltrated with primary or metastic malignancy, and when combination chemotherapy is used, this resumption is less predictable. Poor marrow reserves due to radiation to the bone marrow can increase myelotoxicity [22].

Assessment of bone marrow function (complete blood count) is essential before beginning chemotherapy and prior to administration of periodic pulses (for example, every 3 weeks) of myelosuppressive drugs. Additional blood counts may be done at the time of an expected nadir or if warranted due to symptoms of bone marrow toxicity such as fever or bleeding. Nurses should be aware of the blood counts since their results may influence nursing actions.

Nursing management of patients experiencing bone marrow suppression is related to the consequences of diminished blood cells. A decrease in functional platelets can cause the patient life-threatening problems due to bleeding. The effects of immunosuppression and granulocytopenia caused by the decrease in leukocytes may have equally disastrous results due to infection. The anemia resulting from marrow suppression may cause constitutional as well as functional problems. Nursing care of such vulnerable patients is focused on the prevention of alleviation of symptoms resulting from the impact of chemotherapy.

Thrombocytopenia. Thrombocytopenia can be a life-threatening side effect of chemotherapy. Decreased production of platelets can result from the marrow suppressive effect of the drugs. Increased destruction of platelets due to a large spleen, infection, disseminated intravascular coagulation, coagulopathy, and other factors also may increase the risk of bleeding [16,25]. Platelets have a particularly rapid cell turnover and life-span (8–9 days) and thus are very vulnerable to chemotherapy. The likelihood of hemorrhage is directly proportionate to the decrease in platelet count.

Nursing assessment of signs and symptoms of bleeding is important in monitoring the patient's clinical status. Normal platelet values are 150,000–300,000/mm^3. Risk of hemorrhage becomes exceedingly dangerous when the platelet count is less than

$20,000/mm^3$. The platelet count, however, is not an absolute indicator of active bleeding. Many variables such as the rate of change in the platelet count or the presence of infection influence the risk of active bleeding [38]. Assessment of clinical symptomatology in conjunction with the platelet count becomes an extremely important indicator for medical management and nursing care.

Nursing care of patients with thrombocytopenia should include careful observation of the patient for signs of bleeding [42]. Evidence of petechiae and ecchymoses should be carefully evaluated. Urine, stool, and emesis should be routinely tested for presence of blood. Active bleeding may be noted in the gums and nasal mucosa (epistaxis). If menstrual suppression has not occurred, prolonged vaginal bleeding may also be noted. Mental status and neurologic integrity should also be carefully evaluated. Central nervous system and gastrointestinal bleeds can be fatal.

Bleeding Precautions. Preventive measures can be taken in the care of the patient with an increased risk of bleeding to minimize the frequency of invasive procedures (such as I.M. injections, and to remove sharp objects in the physical environment. After any procedure that breaks the skin, pressure should be applied for a prolonged period of time until all bleeding stops. If sharp objects cannot be removed, padding may be applied to some of them to protect the patient from accidental injury. Severe injury may result if the patient falls out of bed. Close observation and nursing availability to the patient is particularly important to these patients who often may be in isolation. Aspirin and aspirin-containing drugs should be avoided because that analgesic can impair platelet function as well as irritate the mucosal lining of the gastrointestinal tract [38]. Stool softeners may be given to prevent undue straining and decrease risk of bleeding.

When the patient has a bleeding episode she needs emotional support as well as swift and conscientious interventions. Direct pressure and ice packs may sometimes be applied to the area to decrease the bleeding. Bleeding can be a very frightening symptom for the patient. The physical presence of the nurse can be comforting and reassuring [23].

Platelet Transfusions. Platelet transfusions may be administered to prevent bleeding when the platelet count is less than $10,000/mm^3$ or if the patient is clinically symptomatic [25]. Platelets may also be transfused during episodes of active bleeding. During active bleeding episodes, the patient may require other blood components also. Platelet transfusions are only palliative measures. The risk of bleeding will continue until the bone marrow has recovered.

Cancer patients undergoing chemotherapy may require frequent platelet support. There is an increasing risk of alloimmunization and development of antiplatelet antibodies after multiple transfusions [25,38]. A patient may become refractory to platelet transfusions, making their effectiveness minimal. By limiting the exposure of patients to platelet donors, reactions may be decreased. Family members who are matched for histocompatability locus may become the major donors for the patient. Since platelet freezing is not widely available, donor availability is an important consideration affecting the donor's life-style.

Platelets can be collected separately by centrifugation of whole blood or via pheresis. Platelets can be administered as individual units, as pooled concentrates, or in platelet-rich plasma. Administration of platelets should be done rapidly with a filtered tubing. Nursing measures to facilitate the transfusion flow may be necessary. Patients may be premedicated with Tylenol and Benadryl to prevent or minimize the shaking chills and fever that may accompany a reaction to foreign platelets. Frequent evaluations of the patient's status during the transfusion are essential, with baseline vital signs and subsequent assessments. The patient's own platelets may be collected and frozen in advance in special instances. Platelets, like all blood components, should be irradiated to prevent graft-versus-host disease prior to administration to severely immunosuppressed patients such as bone marrow transplant recipients [12,25,38].

The patient's transfusion history and experiences should be assessed prior to platelet transfusions. The patient's understanding of the purpose and rationale of the transfusion should be assessed as well as the patient's concerns and anxieties related to the platelet administration.

Vulnerability to Infection: Leukopenia. Patients undergoing chemotherapy may also be compromised in their ability to withstand infection [25]. Hematologic malignancy and myelosuppression caused by radiation therapy can compound the impact of chemotherapy. Increased destruction of white blood cells can also occur. White blood cells (specifically granulocytes) play the most important part in cellular defense against infection. The effect of bone marrow suppression by chemotherapy is to drastically reduce and/or temporarily eliminate these infection fighters. White blood cells normally are in the range of 5,000–10,000/mm³. Incidence of infection markedly rises when the granulocyte count is less than 1,000/mm³. This vulnerability particularly affects the patient in every aspect of her interaction with the outside world. Nursing care is important in the prevention, recognition and treatment of infection. The nurse can also help the patient cope with this additional assault.

Immunosuppression. Alteration of the immune system may result from chemotherapy [19]. Malnutrition, advanced age, radiation therapy, surgery, and drugs (for example, corticosteroids) as well as various malignancies (such as Hodgkin's disease or multiple myeloma) may impair cellular and humoral immunity [16,56]. The patient's ability to fight both bacterial and viral infection is further compromised.

Prevention of Infection. Protection of the patient's defense mechanisms is a primary nursing aim. The integrity of the patient's body, particularly skin and mucous membranes, provides a critical barrier to infection. The cancer patient receiving chemotherapy is particularly vulnerable due to easy bruisability and bleeding caused by thrombocytopenia and invasive procedures and treatments (such as the intravenous lines which may be necessary for her care). Meticulous care and observation of any puncture site, wound, indwelling catheter, or intravenous line is a major nursing task. Soaps containing hexachlorophene are effective in reducing staphylococcal infections. Use of iodine containing compounds (povidone-iodine) is necessary for protection from gram-negative organisms and fungi [25]. The prevention of pressure sores and effective pulmonary toilet are especially important in reducing the risk of infection in the bedridden patient [18,19].

Surveillance cultures may be done while the patient is granulocytopenic but before evidence of infection (fever). These cultures may identify the antibiotic sensitivities of the potential pathogens in the normal flora [56]. Cultures are usually taken of stool, urine, sputum, nasopharynx, oropharynx, and skin in a routine schedule (for example, twice a week). Additional cultures are taken of any suspicious site, intravenous lines, or urinary catheters.

In the prevention of transmission of pathogens, thorough handwashing is probably the single most important preventive measure. The patient should not be exposed to staff, visitors, or other patients with chicken pox, herpes zoster, tuberculosis, influenza, pneumocystis, or other contagious diseases [18,25]. If possible,

the reduction of duration of hospital stays may decrease the vulnerable patient's exposure to antibiotic-resistant bacterial infections existing on the hospital wards. While the patient is at home,
she may have to temporarily alter her life-style to reduce exposure
to infection. She may have to avoid crowds and family members
and friends with infections. This may be extremely difficult for
some patients. Adequate nutrition is also important in building
her defenses to infection.

Protective Isolation. Protective isolation may be necessary
for some patients undergoing chemotherapy [18,25]. This may
be isolation in a standard hospital single room with mask and gown
or in a specially designed laminar air flow room. Both environments
are designed to reduce exposure to exogenous pathogens. The
patient may also undergo special procedures, such as pHisoHex
baths, to reduce the bacterial flora on her skin. Endogenous pathogens may be reduced by gut sterilization using various oral antibiotics (such as nystatin, vancomycin, and colistin). Oral and
esophageal candida may be prevented by oral nystatin or clotri-
mazole [56].

The patient's emotional adaptation to the isolation environment
is very important. The sensory deprivation that many patients experience in isolation is well documented [54,30]. The cancer patient
may be particularly vulnerable to perceptual distortions due to side
effects of chemotherapy, the disease process, and relative immobility
influencing perception of meaningful stimuli. She may be able to
participate in the maintenance of the isolation environment. This
may increase her sense of control over an often overwhelming
situation. Some patients get obsessed with sterile technique in their
efforts to prevent invisible germs from harming them. Transfering
out of the protective environment can also cause considerable
anxiety for some patients in their adjustments to human contact.

Signs, Symptoms, and Detection of Infection. Treatment of
infection is critically important in the leukopenic or immunocompromised cancer patient. Locating the source of infection and the
pathogen involved facilitates appropriate and effective treatment.
Common sites of infection include the lungs, urinary tract, skin,
and blood stream (septicemia) [56]. (See Table 5.5.) Careful assessment and evaluation of the patient's symptoms as well as physical
findings are especially important in the presence of fever. Blood
cultures and repeat surveillance cultures are generally done when
fever first presents. These may be negative, but due to factors (such

TABLE 5.5
Common Infections in Granulocytopenic Patients

Pathogens	Treatment
Bacterial	
Gram Positive:	
Staphylococcus	Oxacillin, cephalothin
Gram Negative:	
Pseudomonas aeruginosa	Carbenicillin plus aminoglycosides
Klebsiella penumoniae	(gentamicin, amikacin, or
Escherichia coli	tobramycin)
Fungal	
Candida, Aspergillus	Amphotercin B
Viral	
Herpes zoster	Support measures[a]
Protozoan	
Pneumocystic carinii	Bactrim

[a]No effective treatment.

as ongoing antibiotic treatment) that may obscure the results they are presumed to be infectious in origin [56]. Blood and surveillance cultures may be repeated at intervals to locate the source of infection. When a patient with severe granulocytopenia first presents with fever, broad-spectrum antibiotics are often begun. While there may be other causes for fever (the disease, drug reactions) the risk of infection is too severe to wait for culture verification for patients so compromised in their ability to withstand infections. When the pathogen is identified, drugs can be altered to reflect the sensitivities suggested by the culture. In immunosuppressed patients, evidence of inflammation may be minimal [19]. Nursing observations should be attuned to subtle changes, such as erythema and tenderness, that may indicate an infectious process.

Granulocyte Transfusions. Experimental clinical trials as to the efficacy of white blood cell transfusions are currently underway [25,38]. Granulocytes are collected by various types of cell separators from ABO compatible, HLA matched donors, often family members. The indications for the transfusion are to reduce the risk of infection in the granulocytopenic patient or to assist in the treatment of infection in the compromised patient. The half-life of white blood cells is only about 6 hours so the transfusion must proceed immediately after collection. White blood cells should also be irradiated when administered to an immunocompromised host. The volume of granulocytes may vary from 100 to 300 cc with 10^{11} white blood cells transfused [25,38]. Ideally the patient's white blood cell count would be raised 250-850/mm^3; unfortunately, the response may often be minimal with rapid destruction of the donor white blood cells.

Nursing care of the patient receiving white blood cell transfusions must be carefully attuned to acute observation and management of reactions to the white blood cells. Common side effects include fever and bed shaking chills. Premedication with Benadryl and steroids may alleviate the frightening symptoms. Close observation should also be directed toward potential anaphylactic responses heralded by extreme dyspnea and hypotension. Halting the transfusion and use of epinephrine, antihistamines, and steroids may be utilized in the management of this potentially lethal response. Some patients may also experience pulmonary symptoms of fluid overload or white cell sequestion in the lungs if the transfusion is administered too rapidly [25,38].

Anemia. Anemia may result from the assault of chemotherapy. Decreased production of red blood cells may result from the bone marrow suppression and acute loss may result from bleeding episodes due to thrombocytopenia. The nurse must be aware of the signs and symptoms of anemia (pallor, fatigue, postural hypotension, dyspnea) in altering patient care requirements. Transfusions may be necessary. Acute versus chronic changes in hemaglobin and hematocrit are important indications for transfusion in conjunction with symptomatology [25,38].

Red Blood Cell Transfusions. Whole blood is usually not necessary to treat this form of anemia unless there is an acute blood loss. Packed red blood cells provide the same oxygen-carrying capacity as whole blood but in less volume (without plasma). However, when long-term transfusions are required, the patient may become sensitized to the platelets and granulocytes in packed red cells. This will increase the risk of transfusion reactions and decrease the longevity of the transfusion. Leukocyte poor packed red blood cells (buffy coat poor) are relatively free of white blood cells and platelets. This type of transfusion can provide red blood cell increase with minimal risk of sensitization to the other blood components. This will prevent the febrile reactions associated with previous exposure. It is often the transfusion of choice for cancer patients requiring an increase in red blood cells [38].

Blood Component Therapy for Cancer Patients. Nursing care of the cancer patient receiving a blood transfusion is no different from care of other patients receiving transfusions except for a few important aspects. First, the cancer patient may have a substantially reduced number of adequate veins available for transfusion due to multiple venapunctures and chemotherapy, and those that exist may be less than adequate. Nursing techniques to facilitate the flow may become essential. Frequently, due to a tight schedule of intravenous chemotherapy and antibiotic drugs, red blood cells may have to be delivered in split units or it may be necessary to start another I.V. to accommodate quick administration of the blood product without interrupting other important medications. As has previously been mentioned, irradiation of blood products to destroy potentially replicating stem cells may be necessary in severely immunosuppressed patients. Repeated blood typing and crossmatching are extremely important in these patients who may require multiple transfusions. Additional antigens (HLA, MLC) may be considered in the blood typing for platelet or white blood cell transfusions to ensure the most successful therapeutic result. Lastly the signs and symptoms of hemolytic and nonhemolytic transfusion reactions (fever, chills, nausea, myalgias, hypotension, hematuria, and renal failure) may be clinically present prior to the transfusion due to side effects of chemotherapy and/or the disease process. Expert nursing care is required in observations of subtle symptom changes that may herald a drastic event.

Withholding Chemotherapy. Adjustments in dosage or temporary withholding of the administration of chemotherapy drugs may be necessary when there is evidence of severe bone marrow suppression. This will depend on many variables, for example, the patient's baseline blood counts, chemotherapy protocol, and available blood component support [16,42]. Generally, guidelines for these changes would be a white blood cell count less than 4,000/mm^3 and/or platelets less than 100,000/mm^3. The drugs may be withheld for a week or more to allow for bone marrow recovery. Many patients eagerly await the results of the blood counts. This information becomes for some an important source of control or inclusion in the treatment plan. An interruption in schedule may be a major disappointment for the patient who is actively hoping for the success of the treatment. The nurse can help the patient keep perspective during these temporary stops in treatment as well as educate the patient as to what signs and symptoms she should be reporting. Close contact with the patient by telephone may be an important nursing measure [46].

Gastrointestinal Toxicity

Chemotherapy's effect on rapidly replicating cells is seen most dramatically with its effects on the gastrointestinal system. These side effects may also be the most discomforting to the patient. A patient's ability to eat, talk or, indeed, to kiss is severely compromised. These side effects can include mild to severe nausea, vomiting, diarrhea, constipation, esophagitis, and stomatitis [27,49]. The patient receiving chemotherapy may have had only minor, manageable symptoms prior to the drug administration. These disrupting side effects will often confirm the devastating diagnosis and will account for the perception that chemotherapy drugs are poisonous. While discomforting to the patient, the impact of the chemotherapy on the gastrointestinal tract is generally short term and controllable. It is an expected side effect with many drugs and unless severely compromising the patient's physical status, not a reason for discontinuing successful drug therapy. The patient's ability to cope and endure these side effects may be very dependent on early nursing measures to assess and plan interventions.

Individual Variation. Prior to chemotherapy, the patient's understanding and feelings about the drug therapy need to be carefully evaluated. Not all chemotherapy drugs cause severe nausea and vomiting. The presence and severity of these symptoms can have tremendous individual variability. Patient education regarding drug therapy should stress this fact. The patient's previous experience with nausea, vomiting, and diarrhea should all be evaluated, particularly in relationship to her feelings about these symptoms and use of successful interventions [21]. The patient may also know what techniques or medications have not been helpful. At the same time the patient is informed of the possibility of a distressful symptom, she should know what measures she can take to achieve comfort. Parameters for informing the health team should be given. Family members also should be included in any information sessions if possible.

Anorexia. Cachexia and malnutrition may result from the nausea, vomiting, diarrhea, and stomatitis caused by chemotherapy. The presence of malignancy may have an effect on the patient causing unexplained weight loss. Compounded with the presence of chemotherapy, the wasting may be accelerated by decreased appetite, poor absorption, and the pain and discomfort associated with eating [49]. Depression may also contribute to a loss of appetite. Malnutrition can be a major concern increasing general morbidity [22].

Nutrition. Attempts can be made to encourage the patient to maintain good nutritional status. Selection of the patient's favorite foods prepared and presented in an appetizing way is important. Sometimes, however, the patient may complain of change in taste sensations or exhibit such painful stomatitis that even her old favorites become unpalatable [3,10,29]. Nutritional supplements are available that can be taken in small amounts between meals. If the patient is at home, her eating at the table with other family members can be helpful. In the hospital setting, home-cooked meals can often be negotiated. Nursing assessment should be done of the patient's dietary habits, preferences, and cultural influences early in the treatment program. Some patients attach significance to the healing properties of certain foods and food supplements [21]. These should be evaluated for potential interaction with the drug program and allowed if possible.

The patient's nutritional status may be difficult to evaluate precisely. The patient's weight is an important measure, though fluid retention may mask a loss in weight. Laboratory testing can evaluate electrolyte balance.

Nausea and Vomiting. Nausea and vomiting can occur with many of the chemotherapy drugs but have wide personal variation [27]. For many patients, medication prior to chemotherapy with an antiemetic or sedative is the most critical intervention. Diversion and relaxation techniques may be utilized prior, during and after chemotherapy to stem the feelings of nausea [20]. Dietary manipulation may also be useful for the patient. Some patients prefer light meals prior to or after chemotherapy, snacking until nausea subsides. Patients should be encouraged to maintain a good fluid intake following chemotherapy. Severe nausea and vomiting can plague some patients. Hypnosis may be considered for this problem. Manipulation of the environment may also be useful in decreasing stressful stimuli as has been discussed previously. Tetrahydrylcannabinal (the active ingredient in marijuana) is currently being evaluated for its potential as an antiemetic [1].

Stomatitis. Stomatitis, oral ulcerations, cheilosis, glossitis, and pharyngitis may occur as early side effects to the impact of chemotherapy [3,10]. The severity of the side effect may be dose related and may be a factor limiting the amount of drug administered. Stomatitis can severely decrease a patient's oral intake and cause dehydration while further compromising her nutritional status.

For the patient, oropharyngeal pain is a primary consideration. Topical anesthetics may be utilized prior to meals to facilitate eating. Sometimes these alter the taste sensations and do not offer adequate relief. Analgesics also may be offered, with care given that the patient does not become somnolent or confused, further interfering with her ability to eat. Bland foods of moderate temperature and soft consistency may be offered in small portions to facilitate food intake.

Mouth care, especially in the form of gentle but thorough irrigations, may help to prevent infection. These irrigations can also provide comfort to the patient. Mouth care prior to meals may also increase the patient's ability to eat. Special care should be taken after meal times to decrease the risk of opportunistic infections [3].

The patient with stomatitis is not only affected at meal times, the discomfort may also limit her ability to communicate. In severe cases of stomatitis, alternate forms of communication (for example, writing) may be necessary. Anticipating the patient's needs, and minimizing the demands for her verbal response may be important nursing measures.

Diarrhea. The patient's bowel habits may be severely altered due to chemotherapy [49]. Diarrhea is commonly seen due to the mucosal toxicity of various chemotherapy drugs. In the most severe cases, the patient may have ulceration, bleeding, and perforation. Dehydration and electrolyte imbalances may also result from unabated diarrhea. Needless to say, this symptom can significantly alter the patient's daily pattern of activities. Comprehensive supportive care is essential for these patients.

Antidiarrheal medications may be carefully utilized when diarrhea is caused by chemotherapy. Dietary manipulation of low-roughage, bland meals in small, frequent feedings may also be attempted. For some patients, however, bowel rest must be obtained by placing the patient on a liquid diet or on total intravenous replacement. Mucosal irritation resulting from frequent diarrhea should be carefully assessed and treated early with meticulous perianal care (for example, sitz baths) due to the severe risk of compromising infection [23].

Constipation. Constipation may occur as a side effect with the vinca alkaloids [16]. At its most severe, this symptom may result in paralytic ileus. Narcotic analgesics can further complicate the problem of constipation. Prophylactic use of high-fiber foods, laxatives, and stool softeners may prevent such complications [39].

Renal Toxicity

Metabolism and excretion of certain chemotherapeutic drugs is dependent on the functioning and integrity of various organs. The kidneys are extremely important in the role of excretion of both chemotherapeutic drugs and cellular breakdown products resulting from the destruction of cancer cells [16]. The patient's hydration status is an important clinical concern. The nurse should carefully monitor the patient's intake and output when renal toxicity is a risk [42]. The patient's baseline renal function must be evaluated to determine if her system can handle a particular drug, at a certain dosage. With renal insufficiency, adjustments or alterations in drug dose may have to be made [22]. The patient may require hydration intravenously prior to the administration of chemotherapy to ensure an adequate urine output. The use of allopurinol (started in advance) generally will prevent the complication of hyperuricemia.

Hepatic Toxicity

Liver function tests (such as serum glutamic-oxaloacetic transaminase, serum alkaline phosphatase, and serum bilirubin) are often part of pre-chemotherapy treatment evaluation as well as utilized in follow-up care. The liver is involved in the biotransformation or metabolism of many drugs. Malfunction can cause a build up of drug in the system and increase the risks of toxicity [16]. Hepatitis also can occur after successful chemotherapy treatment of cancer. This complication, while not directly influencing the disease prognosis, can significantly affect the speed of the patient's recovery and ability to resume normal life activities. The nurse should carefully observe indications of hepatotoxicity: jaundice, right upper quadrant pain, bleeding.

Neurotoxicity

Neurotoxicity can be a serious sequala of the chemotherapy drugs classified as vinca alkaloids. This disturbing side effect (involving muscle weakness, parasthesia, and loss of tendon reflexes) usually disappears after the completion of therapy [16]. In some cases, permanent damage may result requiring rehabilitation (braces, walker, cane). At the earliest sign of peripheral neuropathy, therapy may be discontinued. Steroids will also cause muscle wasting and atrophy which can contribute to the impact of cancer on the patient's vulnerable body image [20].

Cardiotoxicity

Cardiotoxicity due to chemotherapy can be lethal. Careful monitoring of the patient's vital signs and frequent assessment of signs and symptoms of fluid retention or other cardiopulmonary manifestations may be necessary with certain drugs (Adriamycin, Daunorubicin) [16,22].

Pulmonary Toxicity

Pulmonary effects may be seen in patients receiving chemotherapy. Risk of pulmonary fibrosis, permanently compromising respiratory function, is a rare but potentially fatal side effect of drugs such as bleomycin [16,22].

Dermatologic Reactions

Some chemotherapeutic agents can cause skin reactions [37]. Sensitivity type reactions can occur with the uncomfortable symptoms of erythema, urticaria and pruritis. Hyperpigmentation of the skin and nail beds can also be unusual side effects. Additional symptoms include skin dryness and photosensitivity. These symptoms can be very confusing to the patient. While not lethal, these toxicities need careful nursing assessment and intervention to assist the patient in coping with these body changes.

Disruptions in Sexuality

Cancer patients receiving chemotherapy may have significant alterations in their sexual functioning and ability to express affection. Chemotherapy may directly affect fertility on a short- or long-term basis [17]. When there is a risk of sterility, men can store sperm in a sperm bank prior to initiation of therapy for later artificial insemination. Women may have their menses suppressed by the drugs or may require artificial suppression to avoid the increased risk of prolonged menstrual bleeding due to bone marrow suppression and to avoid the risk of pregnancy. Short-term impotence may also be a side effect for men receiving certain types of chemotherapy. In addition to impotence and sterility, patients may experience altered libido while on drug therapy [16]. While some patients may conceive and deliver normal babies while on chemotherapy, there is a risk of severe birth defects associated with the use of certain drugs during the first trimester [16].

Expression of affection may be hampered by precautions (such as protective isolation) that are taken to prevent infection in the immunosuppressed patient [30]. The existence of infection and of thrombocytopenia may preclude certain types of sexual activities [21]. Even kissing may become impossible with the stomatitis resulting from chemotherapy. Gastrointestinal irritation and general malaise and fatigue, as well as existing pain, may all add to the difficulties for the patient in expressing and sometimes receiving affection.

Alopecia

The patient's feelings of attractiveness and sexual desirability may be severely compromised by the side effects of chemotherapy in addition to the psychological impact of being a cancer patient. Hair loss may result from chemotherapeutic drugs such as Adriamycin and Cytoxan. (See Table 5.2.) This occurs around two weeks after the beginning of treatment. The alopecia is experienced differently by individual patients. The pattern of hair loss is often gradual over several days, and hair may litter the patient's bed and room. Some patients with very long hair may prefer to have their hair cut short to decrease the debris and anxiety related to watching their hair slowly fall out. While some patients may lose all their hair, others may lose patches or bands of hair. Hair loss may also occur in other parts of the body, involving pubic hair or eyebrows, for example.

A nursing assessment of a patient at risk for hair loss due to chemotherapy should include some plan for intervention acceptable to the patient if hair loss should occur. Some patients would like wigs prepared in advance of the hair loss. Wigs can be uncomfortable due to scalp irritation and some patients may prefer scarves or hats. Some men may prefer remaining bald until the hair returns.

When the hair does return 2–3 months after treatment, it may be of a different color, texture, and consistency from the hair prior to treatment. This can be very disconcerting for patients even if they have been warned in advance.

Other important variables to assess in relation to the patient's hair loss are the understanding and support of significant others and peers in relation to this change in the patient's appearance [35]. While a wig may improve the patient's outward appearance, it will not resolve the anguish some patients experience in grieving the loss of a treasured object. The patient can adapt to this loss with minimal disruption [61]. Appearance may be shifted in importance due to perspective of living with cancer.

Decreasing the hair loss caused by chemotherapy has been a subject of controversy. Scalp tourniquets, scalp freezing, and other maneuvers have been attempted to decrease the impact of the drug on the hair follicles [16,40]. Currently, opinions are mixed as to the feasibility, efficacy, and advisability of protecting the hair but possibly interfering with the treatment goals. When the option is available for these techniques to decrease alopecia, the patient should be included in the decision making. Hopefully in the future there will be a clear answer to this problem.

Secondary Neoplasms

Secondary neoplasms may be a complication of cancer chemotherapy [9,11]. Chemotherapy drugs may be directly carcinogenic or enhance the development of neoplasms due to suppression of the immune system. Prolonged survival may also result in the development of a secondary cancer due to a primary defect allowing oncogenesis [15,59]. In patients who have received chemotherapy and who are able to achieve a long-term disease-free survival, careful follow-up care for the emergence of another cancer is important.

The role of maintenance and adjuvant chemotherapy are being carefully scrutinized in light of the apparent risk.

Pain Relief

Patients receiving chemotherapy may be plagued by pain caused by the effects of primary or metastatic disease. The character of cancer pain depends on the anatomical location of the tumor, particularly involvement of the bones, viscera, and nerves [2]. The cancer treatment itself can also cause pain. Chemotherapy is associated with the pain of stomatitis, pain resulting from infection, as well as the pain caused by organ disruptions as with hepatitis or myocarditis [26].

Individual pain perception and behavioral response have been well documented [33,40]. Attempts at pain relief must be based on consideration of the variables of physiologic pain conduction as well as variables influencing perception of the pain event. Nursing assessment of pain behavior must be sensitive to individual variation influenced by factors such as, age, culture, sex, and the impact of the pain on the patient's daily life. The hope for relief of pain may be a factor influencing patient acceptance of chemotherapy when "cure" is not the goal of treatment.

Chemotherapy may be utilized for systemic pain relief due to its ability to reduce tumor size. Reduction in tumor size may also decrease or eliminate pain caused by nerve involvement. Treatment of the painful consequences of chemotherapy (for example, giving antibiotics for infection), may reverse the triggering pathophysiological event [2].

Drug therapy can alter the perception of pain. The first preference for analgesia is oral nonnarcotic medication. Oral analgesia is prefered for physical, psychological, and social reasons. Both aspirin (not acceptable for thrombocytopenic patients) and acetominophen have been shown to be effective in pain relief [16,39]. If relief is not obtained from nonnarcotics, oral narcotics are then preferred. Methadone can be very effective for severe pain without inducing significant sedation. The use of pain elixirs such as Schlessinger's solution and the Brompton cocktail (morphine sulfate, codeine, ethyl alcohol, flavored syrup, and water) have recently been shown to have no advantage over oral morphine [39]. Phenothiazines (such as Compazine or Phenergan) are used as adjuncts to control the nausea sometimes produced with narcotics and enhance the decrease in pain perception.

There are three important considerations for drug therapy in severe chronic cancer pain. Recurring cancer pain should be treated with a schedule for continual drug therapy independent of whether the patient is experiencing pain at each administration. PRN schedules have been shown to be less effective [39]. The anxiety caused by anticipating the next pain experience may increase the need for pain medication. The nurse can be involved in individual dose titration of the drug until relief is reached. The nurse can also evaluate the types of pain the patient experienced in the past and assess the types of measures that were effective in alleviating the pain [41]. For the patient receiving chemotherapy, the nurse might evaluate potential pain-producing side effects in order to prepare the patient emotionally while reassuring her of the availability of relief measures. The patient's metabolic ability to handle the drug may be compromised by organ damage due to disease or cancer therapy (for example, liver damage due to methotrexate) [16].

Constipation, a frequent side effect of narcotics, can be exacerbated by the patient's decreased activity level (fatigue due to disease or chemotherapy), disrupted nutritional and fluid intake (nausea and vomiting from chemotherapy), and altered bowel motility (as with vincristine therapy, for example), potential consequences of some chemotherapeutic agents. The nurse's involvement in preventive teaching and frequent assessment of bowel function will be extremely important [21]. A diet of high fiber, adequate hydration, and cathartic stimulation in conjunction with stool softeners can prevent much of this side effect.

Many nondrug interventions are also available. Probably the most important is caring, sympathetic involvement with the patient. The nurse can evaluate the patient's "pain story" for additional stressors that might increase pain perception [39,41]. Assessment of the patient's ability to cope with diagnosis of cancer may uncover reasons that might influence the meaning and significance of the pain. Many sources are available detailing nursing interventions for acute and chronic pain relief [33,41].

Addiction should not be a concern for severe chronic cancer pain [39]. Quality of life is the central issue in providing a pain-free existence.

BONE MARROW TRANSPLANTATION

Bone marrow transplantation is an option currently being evaluated for cancer patients requiring intensive therapy in order to attempt cure. The patient's bone marrow is obliterated with vigorous chemotherapy and total body radiation. (See section on total body radiation in Chapter 6.) This is an attempt to eradicate tumor cells prior to the transplant [12].

Transplantation of bone marrow from a carefully matched donor to a patient with diseased or deficient bone marrow, (as in acute leukemia or aplastic anemia for example), can restore bone marrow function. Recipients and related donors (usually siblings) are matched using tests (such as HLA locus testing and mixed leukocyte culture) to minimize the possibility of rejection of the transplant. Immunosuppressive agents are also given following transplant to reduce the risk of rejection.

The bone marrow is obtained from the donor through bone marrow aspirates while the donor is under general anesthesia. Approximately 700 ml of filtered bone marrow is then infused into the patient. Until the bone marrow engrafts, the patient is extremely vulnerable to infection, bleeding, and the side effects of the vigorous pretransplant chemotherapy and total body radiation. In addition to failure of engraftment due to rejection, the patient may also be subject to graft-versus-host disease (GVHD). In this situation, the immunocompetent lymphocytes of the graft recognize the patient as "foreign." This reaction is manifest by mild to severe skin reactions, severe diarrhea, and liver damage. This syndrome can be fatal for the patient. Prolonged immunosuppression even after engraftment of the bone marrow can make the patient vulnerable to infections, particularly viral infections such as cytomegalic virus [12].

This can be an emotionally stressful and life-threatening procedure for the patient. The family, particularly the donor member, needs nursing comfort and support [9]. Bone marrow transplantation can also be the patient's only hope for cure. Expert nursing care is essential to prevent or minimize potential side effects and to provide adequate emotional support [12]. Nursing care involvement is also vital in the rehabilitation of the patient in the aftermath of successful transplantation. Hyperalimentation may be necessary to offset posttransplant malnutrition.

PRINCIPLES OF IMMUNOTHERAPY

The relationship of the immune system to malignancy, and the basic principles and assumptions of immunotherapy, have been explored in previous chapters. Nursing care aspects of immunotherapy will be addressed in this section.

Basically, immunotherapy is administered to stimulate the immune system in general and/or direct the immune response toward a specific tumor. Immunotherapy is more efficient against a small tumor cell burden than a large one. Clinical trials are underway to investigate the efficacy and the place of immunotherapy in cancer treatment [28,48].

Current agents include active, specific agents such as modified tumor cells (vaccines) and active, nonspecific immunostimulators such as BCG, *C. parvum,* and Levamisole. (See Table 5.6.) Thymosin fractions also are being investigated as immunorestorers [43]. Interferons, agents currently receiving much attention, may act on tumors directly or by enhancing lymphocyte and macrophage cytoxicity [7]. Antisera are being utilized in the passive transfer of immunity. Various subcellular and cellular components are being investigated as adoptive immunotherapeutic agents.

TABLE 5.6
Nursing Care—Immunotherapy

Agents	Mode of Action	Common Mode of Administration	Side Effects	Special Nursing Considerations
Active	Host plays active role in the capacity of the immune response			
Specific	Manipulation of immune system toward specific tumor			
Tumor cells (modified)	Tumor specific	Subcutaneous (irradiated prior to administration to stop growth)	Localized erythematous reaction; systemic flu-like syndrome, fever, chills	Assess site for inflammation Keep site clean and dry Administer antipyretics Encourage rest
Nonspecific	General stimulation of immune system			
BCG (Bacillus Calmette Guerin)	Attenuated live bovine tubercule bacillus	Scarification, tine technique on axilla, groin, tumor site; *intradermal; intrapleural* (given over weeks to years)	Local erythematous reactions, fatigue, malaise, fever, chills, hepatic dysfunction, danger of disseminated BCG infection	Keep area dry 24 hours Rotate sites Assess site for erythema, induration, macopapular rash, lymphadenopathy (may have to alter dose if severe local reaction) Avoid clothing constriction, chafing on site Prevent dry skin with oil, lotion

Agent	Action	Route	Side Effects	Nursing Interventions
MER (methanol extracted residue of BCG)		Subcutaneous	Skin reactions, ulcers, fever	Decrease pruritis with calamine, talc Premedicate with benadryl if sensitivity Administer antipyretics Encourage rest Assess signs and symptoms of hepatic dysfunction
C. parvum (Corynebacterium parvum)	Formalin fixed gram + rads; activates macrophages; lung cancer	Intravenous intra-lesional, or intra-dermal (test dose may be given)	Flulike syndrome, chills, fever, hypotension, headache, nausea and vomiting, local inflammation	Halt administration if severe hypotension Administer antipyretics Medicate for nausea and vomiting Assess site for inflammation
Levamisole	Antihelmenthic; increases cell activity	Oral (bitter taste, take with meals)	Nausea and vomiting, headache, pancytopenia	Medicate for nausea and vomiting Administer antipyretics Provide pain relief Assess signs and symptoms of infection, bleeding, anemia Check blood counts

TABLE 5.6 (continued)

Agents	Mode of Action	Common Mode of Administration	Side Effects	Special Nursing Considerations
Passive	Transfer of antibodies does not directly involve host response			
Antisera	Antitumor antibodies	Intravenous	Possible immune reactions	Observe for signs and symptoms of serum sickness (arthritis, renal dysfunction, fever)
Adoptive	Immunocompetent cells adopted by patient as part of immune defense mechanism	Intravenous, subcutaneous		

Subcellular components			
Transfer factor	White cell extract (nonimmunogenic)		
Immune RNA	Lymphoid extract (nonimmunogenic)		
Cellular components			
Leukocytes, lymphocytes	Sensitized in vivo or in vitro against specific tumors; immune or nonimmune	Risk of graft-versus-host disease (skin rash, hepatitis, diarrhea)	If patient has graft-versus-host disease: Provide meticulous skin care and frequent turning to avoid pressure points; Medicate for pain and itching; Assess signs and symptoms of hepatic dysfunction: jaundice, right upper quadrant pain, bleeding; Administer antidiarrhea agents; Manipulate diet

Nursing Care

Nursing care to minimize the side effects of immunotherapy is crucial in facilitating acceptance of treatment [6,45]. Active, passive, and adoptive immunotherapeutic agents are examined in relation to nursing care needs in Table 5.4. General guidelines for nursing care of patients receiving adoptive immunotherapy are noted also. Use of immunotherapy is being investigated in a variety of tumors with various modes of administration. Patients often can be premedicated if they have uncomfortable systemic reactions. Measures can be taken to reduce significant local reactions. Care should be taken when administering live bacteria, such as BCG or *C. parvum,* to prevent contamination and infection in susceptible body sites.

The nurse can assist the patient in making adjustments in her daily life when interruptions are caused by the treatment schedule and side effects. The nurse's careful assessment of the patient's response should include changes or disruption of quality of life as well as clinical response and side effects of immunotherapy. While degree of severity of individual physical side effects will vary, so will individual perception of the severity of the problem. Evaluation of the patient's own methods for problem solving and coping with various problems should be frequently assessed. The nurse's clinical perspective of common behavioral responses and solutions to the anticipated side effects can be an effective intervention for patients anxious about the treatment.

The patient should be aware of potential side effects and know how to manage them. Indications for seeking medical attention should be clarified in advance [14]. By anticipating common fears and anxieties, the nurse can be available to support the patient while maintaining the patient's involvement and participation in her own care.

Body Image Disturbances

The patient's feelings about herself and her appearance can be severely threatened during and in the aftermath of immunotherapy administered by scarification or the tine technique [14]. The numerous scars are permanent reminders of the diagnosis of cancer. The patient may be able to minimize the obvious appearance of the scars by assisting in the selection of less visible administration sites and wearing more occlusive clothing. For some patients though, the knowledge of their personal disfigurement, no matter how well concealed from the public, is a heavy burden. Sexual intimacy and the frequency of other occasions requiring body exposure, such as swimming, may be altered severely by the impact of immunotherapy on the patient's body image. Evaluating the patient's view of her appearance prior to her treatment may be important to consider. It must be stressed that a *patient's* view of the body alteration may be significantly different from the view of her appearance held by those around her [35]. For this reason, sex, age, and attractiveness should not be considered as the sole critical variables in evaluating the potential risk to the patient's body image. The patient's hope for immunotherapy as an effective treatment maneuver should be weighed against the potential impact of the clinical and psychological side effects.

Adjuvant Therapy

The purpose of adjuvant immunotherapy is to activate the immune system to destroy clinically undetectable cancer cells after the patient has received supposedly curative treatment [63]. Compliance with uncomfortable treatments that interrupt a patient's daily life may be difficult without the presence of overt signs of cancer. Because immunotherapy is still investigational, participation in a treatment with only a promise but no assurance of benefit may not be acceptable to some patients. Currently, adjuvant immunotherapy is being attempted in patients with Stage I lung cancer with intrapleural BCG and with melanoma patients with BCG as well as other investigations [63].

QUALITY OF LIFE

Patients undergoing chemotherapy or immunotherapy may experience many changes in their lives. The diagnosis of cancer alone has brought new fears and anxieties, often causing disruptions in daily life activities and relationships with others. While chemotherapy and immunotherapy may bring life-threatening side effects they also offer a promise and hope for the future. For many patients there is seemingly no alternative in their fight against cancer. Their ability to cope with the experience of cancer treatment is dependent upon many factors. Individualized, supportive nursing care is essential in protecting patients against stressors in the environment and facilitating the patient's own emotional and physical defense mechanisms.

Fatigue and Malaise

Many patients experience varying degrees of fatigue and malaise while on chemotherapy and immunotherapy, which interfere in their interest and willingness to participate in life activities. Priorities need to be established in determining how the patient's energy will be expended [21]. Eliminating or alternating some activities may help the patient in coping with a decreased energy reserve. The assistance of family and friends may be important in accomplishing tasks from housework to grocery shopping. This side effect can also alter the patient's perception of body image and quality of life.

Patient Education

Many patients receiving cancer drug therapy are in the outpatient setting. They do not have the opportunity for around-the-clock nursing surveillance and attention. The home setting can provide familiarity, stability, and nurturance. It can also be a very lonely and frightening place to be when the patient is experiencing untoward side effects of chemotherapy and immunotherapy. Patient and family education is essential in providing the necessary information, explaining and predicting the symptoms, as well as directing care activities. Educational programs in the hospital setting as well as informational booklets have been developed to provide the patient with the necessary knowledge to cope with the impact of chemotherapy [24,55,60].

REFERENCES

[1] ANDRYSIAK, T.; CARROLL, R.M.; and UNGERLEIDER, J.T. Marijuana for the Oncology Patient. *American Journal of Nursing,* 79:1396–1398, 1979.

[2] BATZDORF, U. Pain Syndromes in Malignant Disease. In *Cancer Treatment,* ed. C. Haskell, pp. 1009-1021. Philadelphia: Saunders, 1980.

[3] BECK, S. Impact of a Systematic Oral Care Protocol on Stomatitis after Chemotherapy. *Cancer Nursing,* 2:185–199, 1979.

[4] BELIS, L.; WEISS, R.; and THUSH, D. The Oncology Clinic: A Primary Care Facility. *Cancer Nursing,* 3:47–52, 1980.

[5] BINGHAM, C.A. The Cell Cycle and Cancer Chemotherapy. *American Journal of Nursing,* 78:1201–1205, 1978.

[6] BOCHOW, A. Cancer Immunotherapy: What Promise Does It Hold? *Nursing 76,* 6(10): 50–56, 1976.

[7] BORDEN, E.C. Interferons: Rationale for Clinical Trials in Neoplastic Disease. *Annals of Internal Medicine*, 91:472–479, 1979.

[8] BOUCHARD, R., and OWENS, N. Nursing Care of the Patient Receiving Chemotherapy. In *Nursing Care of the Cancer Patients*, ed. R. Bouchard and N. Owens, pp. 74–85. St. Louis: C.V. Mosby, 1976.

[9] BROWN, H., and M.J. KELLEY. Stages of Bone Marrow Transplantation: A Psychiatric Perspective. *Psychosomatic Medicine*, 38, (6):439–446, 1976.

[10] BRUYA, M., and MADEIRA, N. Stomatitis after Chemotherapy. *American Journal of Nursing*, 75:1349–1352, 1975.

[11] BURNS, N. Cancer Chemotherapy: A Systematic Approach. *Nursing 78*, 8:57–63, 1978.

[12] CAHAN, M., and LYDDANE, N. Bone Marrow Transplantation at UCLA. *Cancer Nursing*, 1:47–51, 1978.

[13] CAPIZZI, R. Combination Chemotherapy—Theory and Practice. *Seminars in Oncology*, 4:227–253, 1977.

[14] CARROLL, R.M. BCG Immunotherapy by the Tine Technique: The Nurse's Role. *Cancer Nursing*, 1:241–246, 1978.

[15] CHABNER, B. Second Neoplasm: A Complication of Cancer Chemotherapy. *New England Journal of Medicine*, 297:213–214, 1977.

[16] CLINE, M., and HASKELL, C. Cancer Chemotherapy Philadelphia: Saunders, 1980.

[17] D'ANGIO, G.J. Complications of Treatment Encountered in Lymphoma-Leukemia Long-Term Survivors. *Cancer*, 42:1015-1025, 1978.

[18] DILWORTH, J., and MANDELL, G. Infections in Patients with Cancer. *Seminars in Oncology*, 2:349–359, 1975.

[19] DONLEY, D. Nursing the Patient Who is Immunosuppressed. *American Journal of Nursing*, 76:1619–1626, 1976.

[20] DONOVAN, M. Relaxation with Guided Imagery: A Successful Technique. *Cancer Nursing*, 3:27–32, 1980.

[21] DONOVAN, M., and PIERCE, S. *Cancer Care Nursing*. Englewood Cliffs, N.J.: Prentice-Hall, Inc., 1976.

[22] FRIEDMAN, M., and CARTER, S. Serious Toxicities Associated with Chemotherapy. *Seminars in Oncology*, 5:193–202, 1978.

[23] GOLDEN, S. Cancer Chemotherapy and Management of Patient Problems. *Nursing Forum*, 14:279–303, 1975.

[24] GOLDEN, S.; HORWICH, C.; and LOKICH, J. Chemotherapy and You. U.S. Department of Health, Education and Welfare Pub. No. (NIH) 78-1136.

[25] GRAZE, P. Bone Marrow Failure: Management of Anemia, Infections, and Bleeding in the Cancer Patient. In *Cancer Treatment*, ed. C. Haskell, pp. 961–983. Philadelphia: Saunders, 1980.

[26] GUTIERREZ, M., and CROOKE, S. Pediatric Cancer Chemotherapy: An Updated Review I. Cis-Diamminedichloroplatimun II. (cisplatin), VM-26 (teniposide), V-16 (etoposide), MitomycinC. *Cancer Treatment Review*, 6:153–164, 1979.

[27] HARRIS, J. Nausea, Vomiting, and Cancer Treatment. *Ca: A Cancer Journal for Clinicians*, 28:194–201, 1978.

[28] HASKELL, C. Immunologic Aspects of Cancer Chemotherapy. *Annual Review of Pharmacology and Toxicology*, 17:179–195, 1977.

[29] HILKEMEYER, R. Intra-Arterial Cancer Chemotherapy. *Nursing Clinics of North America*, 1:295-307, 1966.

[30] HOLLAND, J.; PLUMB, M.; YATES, J.; HARRIS, S.; TUTTOLOMA-NELO, A.; HOLMES, J.; and HOLLAND, J.F. Psychological Response of Patients with Acute Leukemia to Germ-Free Environments. *Cancer*, 40:871–879, 1977.

[31] HUBBARD, S., and DEVITA, V. Chemotherapy Research Nurse. *American Journal of Nursing*, 76:560–565, 1976.

[32] ISSELL, B., and CROOKE, S. Etoposide (VP-16-213), *Cancer Treatment Review*, 6:107–124, 1979.

[33] JACOX, A. *Pain: A Source Book for Nurses and Other Health Professionals.* Boston: Little, Brown, 1977.

[34] JONES, S., and SALMON, S. *Adjuvant Therapy of Cancer II.* New York: Grune & Stratton, 1979.

[35] KLEEMAN, K. Distortions in Body Image in Adulthood. In *Distortions in Body Image in Illness and Disability*, ed. F. Bowen, pp. 73–96. New York: John Wiley, 1977.

[36] KRAKOFF, I. Cancer Chemotherapeutic Agents. *Ca: A Cancer Journal for Clinicians*, 27:130-147, 1977.

[37] LEVINE, M., and GREENWALD, E. Mucocutaneous Side Effects of Cancer Chemotherapy. *Cancer Treatment Review*, 5:67–84, 1978.

[38] LICHTIGER, B. Blood Component Therapy for Cancers. *Ca: A Cancer Journal for Clinicians*, 27:194–200, 1977.

[39] LIPMAN, A. Drug Therapy in Cancer Pain, *Cancer Nursing*, 3:39–46, 1980.

[40] LOVEJOY, N. Preventing Hair Loss during Adriamycin Therapy. *Cancer Nursing* 2:117–121, 1979.

[41] McCAFFERY, M. *Nursing Management of the Patient with Pain.* Philadelphia: Lippincott, 1972.

[42] MARINO, E., and Le BLANC, D. Cancer Chemotherapy. *Nursing 75*, 5:22-33, 1975.

[43] MARSHALL, G.; LOW, T.; THURMAN, G.; HU, S.; ROSSIO, J.; TUVERS, G.; and GOLDSTEIN, A. Overview of Thymosin Activity. *Cancer Treatment Review*, 62:1731–1738, 1978.

[44] MAXWELL, M. Nurse Practioner Chemotherapy Clinic. *Cancer Nursing*, 2:211-218, 1979.

[45] McCALLA, J. Immunotherapy: Concepts and Nursing Implications. In *Cancer: Pathophysiology, Etiology and Management*, ed. L. Kruse, J. Reese, and L. Hart, pp. 239-247. St. Louis: G.V. Mosby, 1979.

[46] MILLER, S. Oncology Nurse and Chemotherapy. *American Journal of Nursing*, 77:989–992, 1977.

[47] MOURAD, L., and DONAHUE, M. P. Guide to the Administration of I.V. Chemotherapeutic Agents. Oregon State University Comprehensive Cancer Center, 1978.

[48] MUGGIA, F. Immunotherapy of Cancer. *Cancer Immunology Immunotherapy*, 3:5–9, 1977.

[49] OHNUMA, T., and HOLLAND, J. Nutritional Consequences of Cancer Chemotherapy and Immunotherapy. *Cancer Research*, 37:2395–2406, 1977.

[50] PILAPIL, F., and STUDVA, K. Cancer Chemotherapy. *Cancer Nursing*, 1:153–164, 1978.

[51] PILAPIL, F., and STUDVA, K. Cancer Chemotherapy: Alkylating Agents. *Cancer Nursing*, 1:260–271, 1978.

[52] PILAPIL, F., and STUDVA, K. Cancer Chemotherapy: Antimetabolites. *Cancer Nursing*, 1:337–346, 1978.

[53] PILAPIL, F., and STUDVA, K. Cancer Chemotherapy: Natural Products. *Cancer Nursing*, 1:409–420, 1978.

[54] ROBERTS, S. Emotional-Touch Deprivation. In *Behavioral Concepts and the Critically Ill Patient*, ed. S. Roberts, pp. 291–309. Englewood Cliffs, N. J.: Prentice-Hall, Inc. 1976.

[55] ROSE, K. A Patient's Guide to Chemotherapy. In: *Current Perspectives in Oncologic Nursing*, ed. C.J. Kellog and B.P. Sullivan pp. 183–190. St. Louis: C.V. Mosby, 1978.

[56] SARNA, G. Oncologic Emergencies and Urgencies: Recognition and Treatment. In *Practical Oncology*, ed. G. Sarna, pp. 53–77. Boston: Houghton Mifflin, 1980.

[57] SARNA, L. An Investigation of the Hopes of Terminally Ill Patients. Master's thesis, University of California, Los Angeles, 1976.

[58] SARNA, L., and FRIEL, M. Nursing Care Guide to Chemotherapy. Unpublished manuscript, 1979.

[59] SCHOENBERG, B. Multiple Primary Neoplasms. In *Persons at High Risk of Cancer*, ed. J. Fraumeni, pp. 103–119. New York: Academic Press, 1975.

[60] Van SCOY-MOSHER, M. Chemotherapy: A Manual for Patients and Their Families. *Cancer Nursing*, 1:234–240, 1978.

[61] WAGNER, L., and GORELY, M. Body Image and Patients Experiencing Alopecia as a Result of Cancer Chemotherapy. *Cancer Nursing*, 2:365–369, 1979.

[62] ZELSKI, L. Cancer Chemotherapy: Steroid Hormones. *Cancer Nursing*, 1:473–482, 1978.

[63] ZIGHELBOIM, J. Adjuvant Chemotherapy and Immunotherapy Following Surgery. In *Practical Oncology*, ed. G. Sarna, pp. 32–41. Boston: Houghton Mifflin, 1980.

chapter six

LINDA PATTI SARNA, R.N., M.N.
Assistant Clinical Professor
Teaching in Graduate Nursing
Oncology Program
School of Nursing, UCLA

Concepts of nursing care for patients receiving radiation therapy

INTRODUCTION

Radiation therapy is the use of ionizing radiations to cause damage and destruction to cancerous growths. Radiation therapy is utilized in the treatment of over 50% of cancer patients. It may be utilized with curative or palliative intent, or to alleviate painful and disruptive manifestations of incurable disease. Radiation therapy may also be used in combination with surgery or chemotherapy to improve patient survival and increase quality of life. Patients confronted with the prospect of radiation treatments are often very vulnerable. The treatment itself, in addition to causing fears and anxieties about physical side effects, may confirm the inescapable diagnosis of cancer. This form of cancer treatment, which cannot be seen or felt, inevitably causes varying degrees of discomfort that are difficult for the patient to comprehend. Sensitive and skilled nursing care of the patient experiencing radiation therapy aimed at prevention of complications, reduction of the severity of the inevitable side effects, and support of the patient's ability to cope with the stresses of illness poses a difficult challenge.

154

This chapter provides a framework for understanding key concepts in radiation therapy as they are related to the nursing care of cancer patients. Parameters are given for assessment of variables that may have physical, emotional, and social consequences as a result of radiation therapy treatment. Nursing problems are identified as they relate to the impact and side effects of the treatment. Interventive actions are also discussed. Since radiation therapy treatment may only be one aspect of the patient's experience with cancer, the reader is referred to chapters on the other treatment modalities and the psychosocial impact of cancer for a more complete perspective.

Knowledge pertaining to the fundamentals of ionizing radiation and the principles of radiation therapy will enable the nurse to provide appropriate and safe care for the patient and protect others involved in care giving. Education for the patient and his family directed at the purpose and use of radiation treatments will help in allaying their anxiety and their fear of this treatment. Dismissing inaccurate information, the nurse can help the patient to gain a perspective and an understanding of his particular treatment course [21]. Fears and fantasies associated with radiation may be openly discussed with the nurse who is accessible and who is able to foster trust and rapport in the intimate nurse-patient relationship. Many patients may be reluctant to risk exposure of their irrational fears to the physician or to discuss these sensitive issues with their family or friends.

FUNDAMENTALS OF RADIATION

Fundamental knowledge about radiation, both naturally occurring and artificially created, and its effects on matter underlie the principles of radiation oncology. Knowledge of variables influencing radiation and its impact on humans is applied in the development of effective cancer treatment programs. Implications for nursing care, from patient teaching to interventions in radiation side effects, are derived from basic information about radiation.

Ionizing radiation can be either electromagnetic (X-rays, gamma rays) or particulate (alpha particles, beta particles, neutrons). It may be generated spontaneously (by radioactive elements) or artifically (for example, by cyclotrons or nuclear reactions).

Unstable Atoms

In a basic model of atomic structure (Fig. 6.1), negatively charged electrons orbit a positively charged nucleus containing protons

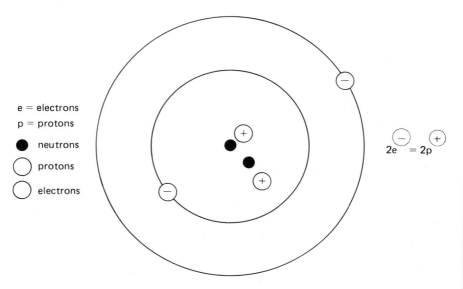

e = electrons
p = protons
● neutrons
○ protons
○ electrons

FIGURE 6.1   Example of a stable atom [16,20].

(positively charged) and neutrons (no electrical charge), maintaining stability when the net positive and negative charges balance [16]. When an atom gains or loses an electron (negative charge), it becomes a chemically unstable *ion*. The unstable atom or molecule (group of atoms sharing electrons) and the resultant charged particle become highly reactive ion pairs capable of further chemical reactions [26]. Radiations capable of producing ions are called ionizing radiations.

Radioactivity

Atomic nuclei with a large number of protons and neutrons are more likely to become unstable or *radioactive*. The generation of particulate energy waves from an atom is called radioactivity. The emission of highly energetic nuclear particles (alpha, beta, gamma rays) is an attempt to gain stability. Elements are fundamental substances (such as carbon or helium) composed of atoms of only one kind which alone or in combination constitute all matter. Elements whose atoms have atomic weights (total number of protons and neutrons) over 209 are naturally radioactive. These elements include but are not limited to uranium, radium, thorium, and actinium. The spontaneous disintegration or expulsion of alpha, beta, or gamma rays from a radioactive nuclide (atomic nucleus) occurs in a particular manner and at a particular rate for each element [16]. The radio-

TABLE 6.1
Half-Lives of Therapeutic
Radionuclides [16, 20]

Radioactive Element	Half-Lives
^{60}Co (Cobalt)	5.3 years
^{137}Cs (Cesium)	30.0 years
^{226}Ra (Radium)[a]	1,602 years
^{32}P (Phosphorus)	14.3 days
^{131}I (Iodine)	8.05 days
^{222}Rn (Radon)[a]	3.8 days

[a] Naturally occurring radioactive nuclides.

activity will decline in intensity over time, from seconds to thousands of years. The *half-life* of a radioactive element is the time required for it to lose 50% of its activity by decay [20]. (See Table 6.1.) Radioactive nuclides can also be artificially induced by bombarding atomic nuclei of various elements with various atomic particles (such as alpha particles).

Ionizing Radiation

Ionizing radiation can cause atomic instability by energizing electrons, enabling them to break their bonds to the atomic nucleus [26]. The collision of ionizing radiation with orbiting electrons, or the nucleus, is random. The considerable distance of electrons from the atomic nucleus is such that there is "empty space" through which the radiations can pass without causing ionization [16]. Atoms are also in constant motion in matter, with speeding orbital electrons making it an unsteady target at best. The radiation may not always result in ionization but may also cause excitation, or the movement of an electron to an orbit further away from the nucleus [26].

Electromagnetic Radiation

High-energy electromagnetic and particulate radiations can cause ionization directly or indirectly by the release of electrons [26]. A spectrum of energy characterized by electrical and magnetic fields is termed *electromagnetic radiation*. This includes radio waves, microwaves, and visible light at the lower end of the spectrum. At the higher-energy levels of the electromagnetic spectrum, X-rays and gamma rays are capable of causing ionization. They can result naturally from radioactive decay or can be made with machines. The impact of this type of radiation on humans, while mediated by effects on atoms or molecules, is subsequently manifest on a cellular level, potentially causing tissue and organ disruption. Such effects on normal tissue imperil life functions and indeed life itself [26]. Effects on malignant tissue can cause regression of growth and tumor necrosis.

Both X-rays and gamma rays are described as photons, discrete bundles (quanta) of energy [16]. Their origins are different. They have no mass or charge. Photon energy is transfered to the absorbing medium when it collides with the orbiting electrons of an atom. Gamma rays are photons emitted from an atomic nucleus, whereas X-rays are photons originating outside the nucleus. They share the same ionizing properties. Photon radiation is used both externally and internally as therapeutic cancer treatment [19,26].

The ionization resulting from photon radiation (X-rays, gamma rays) occurs in various ways (Fig. 6.2). The *photoelectric effect* describes the situation where the photon directly collides with an electron and there is a transfer of energy to the electron, ejecting it from its atomic orbit. This highly charged electron is then capable of provoking further ionization. This occurs most often with lower-energy photons [26].

When the photon gives up only part of its energy to an escaping electron, it is termed *Compton scattering*. As a result of the inter-action, the photon, rather than being absorbed, emerges as a less-energetic photon accompanying the charged electron. They are both capable of further chemical interactions (ionizations). The Compton effect occurs more frequently at medium photon energy levels [26].

High-energy photons are capable of interacting with the atomic nucleus and in doing so their energy is converted to matter. The relationship of mass (m) and energy (E) is characterized in Einstein's famous equation: $E = mc^2$ (c is the velocity of light). Two charged particles (positive and negative electrons) result from the atomic interaction. This *pair production* can only occur at energies higher than 1.02 MeV (million electron volts). It is more likely to occur with larger atoms due to their higher atomic number and subsequently high force-field pull. Electrons from pair production are capable of causing further ionization [16].

Particulate Ionization

Certain atomic particles—alpha particles, beta particles, neutrons, protons, and deuterons—are capable of ionization. They are distinguished from electromagnetic ionizing radiation because they have

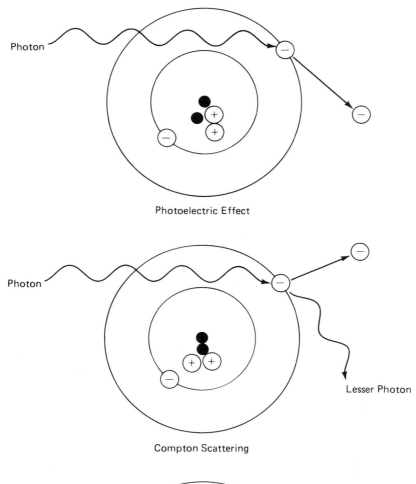

FIGURE 6.2   Ionizing radiation [16].

mass and a capacity for an electrical charge, positive or negative [16,25].

Naturally occurring alpha particles (positively charged nuclei of helium atoms) often result from radioactive decay. They are capable of intense ionization due to their relatively large size and double positive charge and thus quickly lose their energy when absorbed in tissue. Because of this rapid loss of energy they penetrate so poorly that they can be stopped by a sheet of paper [20,26].

Beta particles (negatively or positively charged electrons) are also emitted from an unstable nucleus during radioactive decay [6]. Depending upon its energy, the beta particle is capable of ionization for a considerably longer distance than alpha particles [up to 100 inches in air at 1.7 MeV]. Plastic and aluminum can be used to stop this level of emissions [20].

Other charged particles can be produced in machines. Protons (hydrogen nuclei) and deuterons (heavy hydrogen nuclei) can be produced in cyclotrons and generators [16,26]. Fast neutrons, obtained from cyclotrons and nuclear reactors, rather than directly ionizing, disrupt the atomic nuclei by releasing protons [26]. Negative pi-mesons, produced by high-energy accelerators, are capable of multiple atomic interactions in tissue while penetrating deeply [26]. Nuclei of atoms can also be accelerated and used as ionizing particles [26].

Preferential Bone Absorption

In the photoelectric effect of radiation there is a preferential absorption of photons in material with high atomic numbers (such as bone) when compared to that of lower atomic numbers (such as tissue) [26]. When there is the same exposure of low-energy radiation (150 keV) to the body, bone absorbs significantly more energy than soft tissue. This is the basis of skeletal X-rays. At medium energy levels (200 keV to 10 MeV) the Compton effect occurs, the disparity of absorption of radiation between tissue and bone being much less. At high energy levels (10–50 MeV) bone is twice as receptive as soft tissue to radiation energy. Radiation at this level results in the interaction of photons with atomic nuclei and production of pair products capable of further ionization.

Linear Energy Transfer

Different types of radiation can be compared in terms of their rate of loss of energy along a certain track. This is termed *linear energy transfer* (LET). It is determined by the evaluation of the energy released (usually measured in terms of keV) per micron of absorbing medium (tissue) along the path of a specific ionization and subsequent interactions resulting from radiation [2,26].

The transfer of energy to tissue is affected by mass, velocity, and charge of the ionizing particle or photon. The rate at which energy is lost depends upon the square of the charge of the particle. A more highly charged particle (an alpha particle, for example,) when traveling at the same velocity as lesser-charged particles, will lose energy much more quickly. Highly charged particles are capable of intense ionization due to their strong electrical force field, attracting or repelling electrons from their orbit [26].

The velocity of the radiation is inversely related to the rate of loss of energy. The velocity will determine the amount of time an electrical force field affects the neighboring atoms. Thus, a decrease in velocity will have a higher LET with a higher rate of ionization. The LET will also change as the velocity decreases after collisions causing ionization [20,26].

Radiations capable of high LET include alpha particles, neutrons, and pi-mesons. Particles with higher LET are generally capable of a more profound biologic impact when exposed to tissue because of the dense ionizations as compared with the more sparse ionizations of radiations with lower LET [26]. (See Fig.6.3.) The atoms and molecules in cells generally cannot escape the damage of high LET radiations due to their intense ionization. This is especially important when considering the vulnerability of hypoxic cells to high LET radiations. Lower LET radiations generally require oxygen to produce biologic damage [26]. Higher LET radiations also affect cells regardless of their phase in the cell cycle. These theoretical advantages could be very important in eradication of cancer cells unresponsive to conventional radiation therapy [18,23].

Dimensions of Radiation

Energy in photon radiation (X-rays, gamma rays) is often described in electron volts (eV); 1,000 electron volts (keV); or 1 million electron volts (MeV) [16]. The curie (Ci) describes radioactive disintegrations occurring over time based on the disintegrations of 1 gram of radium (3.7×10^{10} disintegrations/second). It is used to determine the *specific activity* of various radionuclides [20].

Radiation is evaluated in various dimensions. Administering radiation therapy in cancer treatment involves the exposure of a target area (tumor) to a radiation source. The radiation emitted from

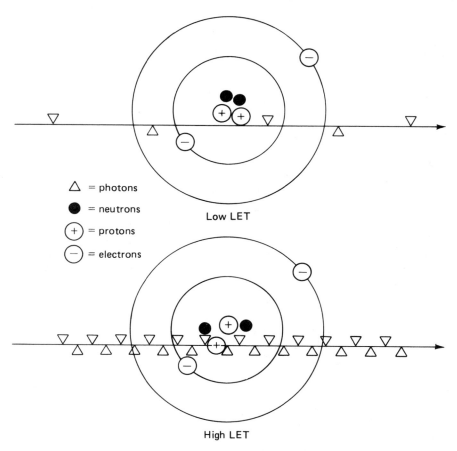

FIGURE 6.3 Ionization in linear energy transfer [26].

a source to the patient is absorbed by the exposed body tissue [12]. The roentgen (R) is the unit of radiation delivered (or exposed) based on the passage of photons in the air [20]. The *rad* is the term utilized to describe the amount of energy absorbed by the tissue irradiated. One rad is equal to 100 ergs of energy (1 erg = 0.625 $\times$ 10^6 MeV) absorbed per gram of tissue. The dose absorbed at various tissue depths depends on the energy level of the administered radiation [25]. The *rem* (*r*oentgen *e*quivalent *m*an) describes the radiation dose required to produce a specific amount of biological damage [36].

At lower energies, the rad and the rem are equivalent. However, not all radiations are identical in their biological effectiveness. *Rel-*

ative biological effectiveness (RBE) is a term utilized to differentiate the biological impact of various types of ionizing radiations. It is derived by comparing the biological damage of a standard radiation (for example ^{60}Co gamma rays) with an unknown radiation. A "quality factor" based on RBE is used as a variable to gain the appropriate rem at higher levels of LET (rad $\times$ quality factor = rem) [36]. The rem level must be determined in order to establish safety levels for radiation protection.

Radiation dose is calculated for each specific site irradiated. The cumulative energy given to all sites is generally less relevant. Various organs and tissues have different sensitivities to ionizing radiation. When considering radiation dose it is important to consider which body area is most affected.

RADIATION CELL DAMAGE

The biological impact of radiation is basically at the cellular level. The damage can range from barely detectable to cell death. The results of the impact can be seen immediately or months, years (carcinogenesis), or even generations later (genetic alteration) [2, 26]. The biological effect of radiation depends on the number and types of cells impaired, not the specific type of radiation used. The degree and permanence of cell loss and the type of function compromised will ultimately determine the extent of biological damage to the body [23,26].

Ionizing radiation can affect the functional and regulatory processes of the cell directly (direct effect), or indirectly (indirect effect). The direct effect is seen when the energy absorbed by the tissues causes atomic or molecular instability (ionization) due to direct collision. The cell also can be affected indirectly as a result of the chemical byproducts resulting from ionization.

Electrons spin in a particular direction around an axis. Electrons rotating in one direction are paired with those rotating in the opposite direction. Ionization can cause an uneven number of electrons. When this happens the disrupted atom or molecule is called a *free radical* [26]. The cell is 70% water. Water molecules are very sensitive to radiation, the resulting ionization creating highly reactive free radicals capable of altering atomic and molecular structure causing cell damage (indirect effect). Oxygen is highly reactive with free radicals due to its own unpaired electrons. Sulfhydryl proteins also found in the cell are capable of reacting with free radicals, preventing reactions with more important molecules [18].

The most critical disruption caused by radiation to the cell is the alteration of the DNA (deoxyribonucleic acid) molecules [2,26]. The DNA molecule is essential for the transfer of genetic material responsible for directing cell function and metabolism. Radiation can cause a strand breakage in the double helix of DNA. Single-strand breakage can be repaired, but double-strand breakage after ionizing radiation is usually fatal to the cell. Radiation can also affect the regulatory processes of the cell, reducing its average or expected life-span. Lethal cell damage may not be seen until the cell attempts to divide (mitosis). Sometimes the injury may not be fatal until the cell has undergone several divisions, death finally coming to the daughter cells [20,26].

Not every cell in an area radiated is lethally damaged or even affected. Nor is every cell or molecule affected by radiation necessary for organ function or survival. Only if cells are lost in large numbers and if they are not replaced quickly is a significant impact seen. The responsiveness of cells to the effects of radiation depends on their vulnerability to damage and their capacity to repair the injuries received [2,23]. The response observed after radiation is influenced by the speed of removal of damaged cells as well as repopulation of cells to fill the loss.

Radiosensitivity

The cells' susceptability to injury from ionizing radiation includes structural or functional deficits and/or death. Radiosensitivity is determined by the amount of energy necessary for producing lethal injuries to the cells radiated and the number of cells lost [26]. (A radiation dose administered over a longer interval of time will generally have less biologic impact than the same dose administered over a shorter period of time.) The resistance of certain cells to the impact of radiation is relative rather than absolute (Table 6.2).

Cells that replicate frequently (that is, cells that have a short cell cycle time), such as mucosal lining, manifest the effects of radiation in a shorter period of time than those with a longer cell cycle time or those at rest, such as muscle. Whether one cell is truly more vulnerable to radiation, or whether the impact is obvious more quickly due to cell loss that occurs during mitosis, is unclear [2].

Oxygenation of the cell enhances the effects of radiation, especially at the lower LET levels [2,26]. The amount of oxygen in the cell is related to the diffusion of oxygen in the tissues. Anatomic and physiologic factors affecting the blood supply can alter oxygenation [2,23]. Hypoxic cells are generally considered more resistant to low-LET radiation.

TABLE 6.2
Radiosensitivity of Normal Tissue [1, 7, 26]

High Sensitivity	Moderate Sensitivity	Low Sensitivity	Radioresistant
Bone marrow	Skin	Heart	Muscle
Lymphatics	Salivary glands	Brain	Mature bone
Gastrointestinal	Kidney	Peripheral nerves	cartilage
epithelium	Liver		Connective tissue
Mucous membrane	Lung		
Gonads	Growing bone		
	cartilage		

While cells can be affected by radiation throughout the cell cycle, they are generally thought to be most vulnerable during the early phases of DNA synthesis and mitosis. A delay in mitosis occurs after radiation to the cell. The amount of delay depends on the radiation dose and the cycle phase during radiation [18,26].

A number of research approaches are being attempted to increase the sensitivity of the cell to radiation [18]. One approach is to increase the number of cells affected by damaging the more radioresistant cells. The use of high-LET particulate radiation which affects normally resistant hypoxic cells is an example. Chemical agents with properties similar to oxygen (for example, metronidazole, Flagyl) are also being examined to increase the vulnerability of hypoxic cells. Hyperthermia and actinomycin-D are being researched because of their apparent abilities to interfere with cell repair following radiation. Increasing the sensitivity of DNA as a radiation target (as with purine starvation) would also increase the impact of radiation. Repeated doses of radiation at intervals (fractionated) are also being examined as an attempt to damage previously resistant cells recruited to replace damaged ones. Synchronization of tumor cells going into mitosis, determining that time, and differentiating it from normal cells could have profound therapeutic implications.

Radiation Recovery

The ability of the cell to recover from the effects of ionizing radiation is very important in determining the ultimate biological impact [18,23]. The cell's capacity for repair of single-strand DNA has been mentioned. The number of lethal double-strand breaks increases with successive exposure to radiation. Fractionated radiation (radiation dose divided over time) generally does not compromise the reproductive capacity of the cell as much as the same dose given at once. A critical factor is the time allowed for recovery between radiations. (See Fig.6.4.) A radiation dose administered over a longer interval of time will generally have less biological impact than the same dose administered over a shorter period of time [23,26].

Cells that were not in active cycle may be recruited after radiation cell loss. This may occur between the intervals of fractionation, redistributing cells throughout the cell cycle. Hypoxic cells, previously resistant to radiation, may be reoxygenated and become viable replacements for the cells lost [26]. Normal cells are generally

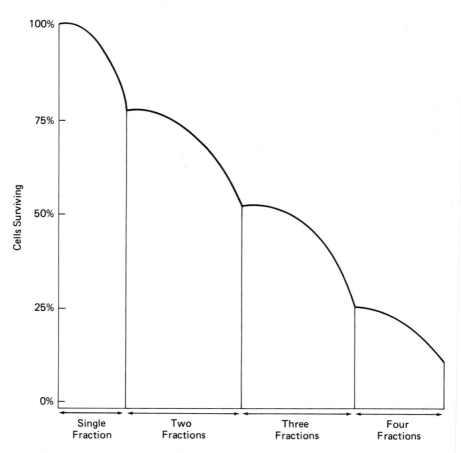

FIGURE 6.4 Example of cell recovery in fractionated radiation [7]. Note that time was not allowed for cell increase from replication.

more efficient than malignant ones in cellular recruitment to offset the depletion caused by radiation [7].

PRINCIPLES OF RADIATION THERAPY

Radiation Therapy in Cancer Treatment

Radiation therapy can be curative for selected cancers today (see Table 6.3). When cure is not possible, it can be utilized to suppress the growth of some tumors. Of vital importance to the patient is the usefulness of radiation therapy in relieving troublesome signs and symptoms caused by the tumor. Radiation therapy is most effective against small, rapidly growing tumors. It is generally not useful for systemic control of metastic cancers.

The goals and objectives of cancer treatment are crucial concerns when considering whether radiation therapy should be utilized. If it is selected, the source (external or internal), and technique (volume irradiated, radiation dose, fractionation) will be selected to best meet the objective, considering tumor factors and other variables influencing the patient. The benefits—the possibilities for cure or control—and the risks—the possibilities of side effects that have associated morbidity and mortality—will have to be carefully evaluated before considering this treatment option.

TABLE 6.3
Malignancies Potentially Curable with Radiation Therapy [1, 7]

Highly Curable	Moderately Curable	Low Rate of Cure
Lymphoma	Head and neck carcinoma	Gastrointestinal
Seminoma of the testes	Bladder cancer	malignancy
Carcinoma of the skin	Prostate adenocarcinoma	Lung cancer
(basal cell epithelium,		Bone sarcomas
squamous cell)		Brain cancer
Vocal cord		Melanoma

Note: Curability rate is related to multiple factors primarily of disease and histologic subtype. It is not directly related to radiosensitivity of the tissue.

Selection of Treatment

Tumor Factors. The success of radiation therapy treatment will depend on multiple factors, an important group being those that characterize the tumor to be irradiated. The histologic type of the cancer is important in predicting the reactive sensitivity of the cancer to ionizing radiation [23]. Generally those cells that are graded as well differentiated are less rapidly responsive to radiation than more anaplastic cell types [26]. Some tumors may have a combination of cell grades making histologic examination less predictive as to the sensitivity to radiation. A tumor with a high growth fraction (cells actively dividing) will have an increased vulnerability to radiation. The most radiosensitive tumors, however, may be the most curative due to other factors (Table 6.3).

The location of the tumor and its degree of extension and/or metastasis is important to determine (through various staging procedures) before therapy is begun. The presence of distant metastasis usually eliminates radiation therapy as a curative treatment option. Rarely, radiation therapy may be utilized as part of a program for cure with few treatable distant metastases [7]. Radiation therapy may be the treatment of choice when the location of a tumor near or on a vital organ (the heart, for instance) makes it surgically unresectable. The radiosensitivity of involved and surrounding tissues and vital structures must also be considered (Table 6.2). The vulnerability of the normal tissue may limit the use of radiation for tumor control due to the risk of unacceptable or intolerable radiation damage [7,26].

Radiation therapy is less successful against bulky neoplasms that have a decreased oxygen supply. The relative resistance of hypoxic cells to radiation and attempts to bypass this therapeutic obstacle was discussed in the section on radiosensitivity. Large tumor masses are also difficult to treat because of the risk of multiple side effects due to radiation encompassing strategic organs and tissues.

Patient Factors. The objective of the therapy will be evaluated in terms of variables influencing the individual treatment considerations for each patient. Since external beam radiation does not require anesthesia, it is less influenced by the patient's physical condition than is surgery [23]. The patient's general constitutional well-being may alter the treatment program. With severely compromised patients, vigorous radiation therapy may be inappropriate if cure or tumor suppression is improbable. The very young and the very old may be more vulnerable to toxic side effects of radiation therapy [23].

The patient's desires and concerns should also be considered. Realistically forewarned of the goals, hopes, and potential side effects of the therapy, the patient can be a participant in the treatment plan. The patient may experience major disruptions in his life due to the frequency (usually 5 days per week), duration (average course 6-8 weeks), and side effects of the treatment. Preexisting physical as well as emotional problems may become even more severe during the treatment time [7,8,24]. Even when curative attempts are successful, the patients treated with radiation therapy may experience irreversible changes affecting their appearance and ability to function normally.

Radiation Therapy and Cancer Surgery

Radiation may be used before or after cancer surgery to optimize efforts for local and regional tumor control [23]. Prior to surgery, radiation can be utilized, especially with rapidly growing tumors, to decrease the size of the tumor. This will, it is hoped, reduce the extent of surgical resection, preventing unnecessary functional and cosmetic damage. Radiation may also decrease the risk of seeding or tumor spread as a result of surgical manipulation [7]. Postoperative radiation therapy can be utilized to control residual but clinically undetectable cancer cells to reduce the risk of recurrence. Unresectable, suspicious lymph nodes may also be irradiated postoperatively.

When radiation therapy precedes surgery there may be a several-week lag period between treatment and surgery to decrease the risk of complications caused by the acute side effects of radiation therapy. This interval varies (usually within 3 months) depending on the type, site, dose, and volume of radiation [7,23]. The extent of proposed surgery is also an important consideration. While this interval will allow for recovery of normal tissue, ideally surgery will take place before tumor regrowth.

A time lapse also occurs with postoperative radiation, allowing for optimal healing of the surgical wound. (The nursing implications of radiation skin reactions and healing will be discussed later in the chapter.)

Radiation Therapy and Cancer Chemotherapy

Radiation therapy can also be utilized in conjunction with systemic cancer chemotherapy. It may have a separate, additive, or interactive effect with the drugs [29]. Increasing the vulnerability of hypoxic cells to radiation and thus improving cancer control has been attempted by the use of drugs such as metronidazole [18,23]. Some agents, such as actinomycin-D, augment the normal tissue response to radiation, enhancing its effects as well as its toxicity [2,23]. Even though a considerable time interval has elapsed, a patient who has received radiation therapy may have an intensified skin reaction if this drug is administered. Adriamycin, as well as actinomycin-D, may provoke a skin or mucosal reaction termed a *recall* phenomenon [13].

Previous radiation to various organ sites will also increase the risk of potential harmful side effects [13]. Examples of this are radiation to the mediastinum potentiating Adriamycin-induced cardiotoxicity and radiation to the chest potentiating bleomycin-induced pulmonary toxicity. In general, previously irradiated bone marrow will increase the risk of myelosuppression due to myelotoxic chemotherapy.

Radiation Therapy and Immunotherapy

Theoretically, stimulation of the immune system may increase the possibility for cancer control by eliminating the clinically undetectable cancer cells present even after curative treatment. Stimulation of the immune system by nonspecific agents such as BCG has been claimed by some to improve the results of radiation therapy in some tumors [12]. Further investigation of the role of adjuvant immunotherapy in radiation treatment is needed [5].

——— TREATMENT WITH RADIATION THERAPY ———

Defining the Treatment Area

Treatment planning involves precise delineation of the target volume (tumor volume to be radiated). This generally includes all contiguous tumor with adequate margins to achieve the desired affect (curative or palliative). Radiation therapy is optimally effective when there is a maximum exposure of tumor and minimum exposure of adjacent and underlying structures to ionizing radiation [19].

Dosimetry. Extensive diagnostic testing and a staging work-up will provide information describing the location and extent of the tumor. Computerized axial tomography (CAT scan) may give more precise information including normal anatomic guidelines as well as tumor location [20]. Different areas in the radiation field will receive different dosages of radiation depending upon the location and density of the anatomical parts. Dosimetry involves the calculation of radiation dose distributions to cancer cells and normal tissue in the radiated field [12]. Since a tumor may extend to different depths, depth-dose curves are calculated to provide guidelines (iso-dose curves) for different penetration levels of radiation. The central axis is the point of maximum absorption. Dosage received by other parts of the tumor irradiated will vary with the various levels of absorption [12]. The patient's normal body contours are evaluated along with the anatomic placement of vital structures and densities of tissues and organs in the treatment field [20]. Calculations of dosimetry can be very complex, in many cases being handled by computer analysis [5].

Skin Markings. After careful calculations of dosimetry have been made, the designated target areas on the patient usually will be outlined with indelible ink which will be removed only after the treatment is ended. Care must be taken by the nursing staff and the patient to preserve the integrity of these markings to assure accuracy of the treatment [20]. Invisible ink and permanent, small tattoo markings have also been used to assure consistent and accurate treatment and to minimize even temporary disfigurement. The invisible ink is still in danger of being washed off by the patient, but the tattoos are permanent marks. Care of radiated skin in treatment area will be discussed in the section involving side effects.

Simulation. In setting up the treatment field, radiographic units called simulators are used to reproduce the exact configuration of the radiation beam and couch angle in therapy [4]. Diagnostic X-rays with radiopaque markers and fluoroscopy will aid in defining the target to be irradiated [20].

Administration of the Radiation Dose

Blocks, Wedges, Filters. Radiation from a source is directed to the target area through a collimator (opening in the therapy machine). In external beam radiation, lead blocks attached to the collimator are placed to block out radiation exposure to normal tissue. Bolus bags (similar in density to tissue) can be placed on the patient in beam pathways to modify penetration of the radiation to certain areas in the treatment field [4,17,20]. Filters can also be placed on the machine to block out lower-energy radiations [17]. Wedge or compensation filters vary the distribution of radiation in the treatment field [17].

Immobilization. Accuracy of the treatment area is critical for optimal and safe treatment. The patient must remain in exactly the same position during each therapy session (usually 1–3 minutes). If patient positioning is a problem, a variety of devices can be utilized to immobilize the particular body part. These restraining devices include plaster casts and molds individually tailored for the patient and treatment needs.

Direction of Radiation Beams. Radiation is delivered in beams with the same characteristics as light (also a form of electromagnetic radiation). Radiation beams may be directed in a number of different intersecting planes and angles to deliver the appropriate dose to the tumor while sparing normal tissue in the pathway [4]. Multiple beam directions may be used in the treatment of any given tumor. The patient may be placed in various positions on the treatment couch angled to maximize appropriate beam direction and absorption. Rotational therapy (encompassing a 360° arc) can provide multiple beam entry points circumscribing the tumor, while sparing normal tissue. The radiation dose is calculated at the point of maximum intensity of absorption of the radiation [9]. Some scattering of radiation known as *backscatter* also occurs after the radiation enters the tissue and must be considered in treatment planning [7,17].

Depth of Penetration. The depth of tissue penetration is directly related to the energy of the radiation. The depth of the tumor will determine the energy of radiation required for optimal treatment and thus, the radiation sources selected [7,20]. Deep-seated tumors are best treated by radiations that can penetrate adequately. Cancers near the surface of the skin will not have the same energy demands. Beams of various energy levels may be utilized in treatment planning. With an increase in penetration, the higher-energy radiations are able to "spare" the skin and subcutaneous tissue in the beam pathway while delivering radiation to deep-seated tumors [23].

Energy Levels and Sources of External Radiation. Orthovoltage is radiation of a relatively low energy level. Thus, its maximum absorption is at the skin or a little below. Because of this, its primary role is in the treatment of some skin cancers [7].

Megavoltage therapy involves higher energy output (over 1 MeV), and thus, deeper tissue penetration. With the greater dose-to-depth ratio, there is significant "skin sparing" or avoidance of normal skin and subcutaneous tissue destruction while the radiation is delivered to the deeper tumor. The capacity for higher output (radiation/minute) makes it possible for larger fields to be treated, with shorter treatment times and less radiation scatter. An additional advantage of this approach is the lack of differential bone absorption allowing a more uniform dose [30]. With the higher energy, more penetrating radiation, there is concern for tissue toxicity on the exit as well as entry side of the beam—for example, in the spinal cord for radiation given anteriorly.

Cobalt therapy (^{60}Co), which produces high-energy gamma rays at the 1.25 MeV level, is an example of frequently used teletherapy (external radiation). Accelerators (VandeGraaff generator, cyclotron, linear accelerator, betatron) produce charged particles that directly or indirectly produce radiation. The multimillion volt betatron and the linear accelerator are utilized to obtain therapy beams with high levels of energy by accelerating electrons to produce high-energy X-rays. In addition to improved skin sparing of superficial tissue, the modern high-energy X-ray machines allow for higher dose rates and shorter treatment times [7]. Accelerators can also provide a more sharply defined radiation beam and thus hit a target (tumor) area more precisely with less lateral scattering of radiation. While cobalt therapy is particularly useful in treatment of head and neck cancer, breast cancer, and cancer metastic to lymph nodes, the betatron may be more effective for tumors requiring deeper treatment such as pelvic irradiation [4].

Machines that emit low-energy electron beams may be superior for some problems to machines that emit photons (X-rays) alone. The low energy level provides a delivery of dose to the skin with minimal radiation to underlying structures, such as the eye or nose [4]. The depth of dose from electrons is again dependent on the energy level. Penetration can be adjusted by varying the energy level of the electron beam. This technique is uniquely useful for large superficial tissues of the scalp and face [4].

High LET Cancer Therapy. Experimental therapy with radiations capable of higher LET is currently underway. These new therapies include neutrons (capable of high LET, but current machines produce poor penetration and wide scattering), negative pimesons (pions with even higher LET but very costly to produce) and various heavy ions [4,20]. The chief potential advantage of radiations of high LET in cancer therapy is their impact on the hypoxic cell, which is relatively resistant to conventional therapy.

Fractionation. Radiation therapy is generally delivered in multiple doses, often daily over a specified period of time [23]. This method of delivering radiation is called fractionation and is usually accomplished in four to eight weeks for curative or suppressive treatment. Rest periods (days without radiation) during therapy vary according to the treatment protocol and objectives and the patient's response to treatment and experience with side effects. The patient will usually not have radiation on the weekend. Treatment with long periods (weeks) of rest is termed *split-course.* Radiation for palliative relief is often accomplished in a period of time shorter than 4-8 weeks. Administration of small doses of radiation over periods of time may, in some cases, increase cancer cell destruction while minimizing the toxic side effects of radiation [2,7,26]. The length of time over which radiation is administered is one of the critical variables affecting radiation recovery. Thus, the intensity of therapy will contribute to the severity of radiation side effects as well as the success of therapy. Protracted administration of radiation will generally decrease the intensity of radiation side effects [7]. Fractionated doses also may be utilized to optimize tumor cell kill by allowing the cells to get into a more sensitive phase of the cell cycle. Radiation doses given over different intervals of time cannot be directly compared biologically [23]. The longer therapy may also prolong the separation of the patient from his family and friends since the therapy can often only be administered in specially equipped hospitals [23].

Individualizing Treatment. The patient's general well-being will influence the application of radiation therapy [9,23]. The morbidity resulting from the cancer as well as previous medical or surgical interventions may influence the vigor of the therapy. Normal tissue limits to radiation may be further compromised by the patient's condition. Tolerance of radiation dose is not absolutely predictable, making sensitive assessment of the patient's reaction to therapy an important guideline to necessary alterations. In conjunction with this, consideration of the goal of treatment is essential. Radiation dosage is tailored as a function of tumor response and patient toxicity.

NURSING CARE DURING
EXTERNAL RADIATION THERAPY

Nursing Assessment

When possible, a thorough nursing assessment prior to the start of radiation therapy treatments should be taken to delineate potential or actual patient problems requiring nursing action [8,20]. Such an assessment can provide information related to the patient's radiation-related fears, anxieties, and educational needs. It also may provide an evaluation of the patient's support systems and coping patterns during stress. A nurse, however, may not be present in the Radiation Therapy Outpatient department. The patient's interactions during therapy may be predominately with technologists as well as the physician. Nursing consultation should be made available by various means to provide input and continuing care.

Tailoring a nursing model for the care of patients undergoing radiation therapy for cancer treatment will involve adaptation of components derived from radiation oncology to guide nursing assessment and intervention. More specifically, the following areas should be included for consideration in assessing the patient's degree of stability or adaptation [8,20,24]:

1. Understanding, fears, and misconceptions about radiation
2. View of radiation therapy as a cancer treatment; sources of information and level of understanding
3. Perception of the intent and goal of the therapy and hope for success
4. Information regarding, and understanding of, potential radiation side effects; concern or anxiety about particular side effects
5. Perception of the impact radiation therapy will have on life activities and social relationships
6. Preexisting physical condition and integrity of area to be irradiated: organ status, function, mobility, cosmetic appearance, presence of pain
7. Importance, significance, and visibility of the site to be irradiated
8. Disease variables: diagnosis, prognosis
9. Treatment variables: past, concurrent, and future radiation therapy, chemotherapy, surgery

Nursing Care During Treatment

Even though radiation may not directly produce discomfort, many patients may be fearful and uncomfortable during treatment. While patients may have received careful explanations of the purpose, rationale, and procedure of radiation therapy, they may need further and repeated explanations during treatment. Fears of the actual radiation may be significant and may vary with the importance and meaning of the site being treated (brain radiation, for example, may be particularly frightening). An opportunity for expression of these fears and anxieties may be especially helpful for the patient. The nurse can acknowledge that these are concerns shared by many patients. Such discussions may also point to areas for nursing intervention in the provision of information, environmental manipulation, symptom relief, and support of the patient's ability to cope with the identified stressors.

The environmental stimuli existing in radiation therapy departments may be particularly unsettling to the already stressed patient [12]. Radiation therapy departments are often in the "bowels" of the hospital due to safety requirements for thick shielding. The patient often experiences awe and fear of the complexities and sheer size of the equipment utilized. The patient may express a concern that such imposing machines will fall on him. The isolation and loneliness of being alone in the treatment room during therapy will be keenly felt by some patients [24]. Communication via intercom can ease the isolation and can provide encouragement and feedback as to the length of treatment time. Visual contact, in some cases by video cameras, is mandatory to provide patient observation, particularly of the very ill and the disoriented and also pediatric patient [19]. The sounds and the noises emitted by the various treatment machines can also be very frightening, especially to the unsuspecting patients. The loud noise of the betatron is frequently sited as a cause for concern by patients under treatment [24].

Many patients receiving radiation therapy may be cachectic or plagued by a general feeling of malaise. For them, lying on a relatively hard table and staying completely still for a period of time is particularly difficult. Premedication with analgesics may make therapy more tolerable. This problem should be frequently assessed so that the patient is aware that comfort measures are available. The same is certainly true for antiemetics. While it may be difficult for the patient to remain still, the prescribed position is vital in obtaining the optimum therapeutic dose and avoiding unnecessary exposure to normal tissue.

Emotional Responses

Patients undergoing radiation therapy also have been noted to have particular emotional reactions in response to their illness and treatment [8,24]. Depression may be manifested by sleep disturbances, decrease in appetite, loss of interest in daily activities, and decreased libido. Patients already coping with the stress of the diagnosis of cancer may be preoccupied with fears of dying and of disability related to the illness and treatment. Anxiety may also be present to various degrees, as patients are fearful of failure of radiation therapy to relieve troublesome symptoms and to cure their disease. Apprehension regarding the side effects of radiation therapy may be increased by misconceptions evolving from alarming information received from family or friends. The effects most feared are radiation "burns," pain, scarring, decrease in libido, and sterility [24]. Many patients also verbalize the fear that radiation treatments may cause additional cancer.

During the radiation treatments, patients may become very irritable and may focus on the technical aspects of the treatment ("Are they doing it right?"). Patients, even if aware of the anticipated radiation side effects, may have difficulty in understanding how a treatment that can make them feel so miserable can have value. Patients may protect the physician (and their good will in hope for cure) by directing their angry feeling to those more available, such as the nurses and radiation technologists. The equipment may also be the focus of scapegoating ("It's not working right") if treatment is unsuccessful. Preexisting psychiatric or emotional problems (alcoholism, marital instability) may increase the intensity of their emotional response to treatment while decreasing their ability to cope [24].

Nursing assessment and intervention in the patient's emotional responses before, during, and after treatment can increase patient compliance with treatment as well as promote maintenance of quality of life. Realistic treatment expectations with specific goals for such treatment course are essential for all patients [21]. Patients who must endure prolonged radiation treatment, such as those with Hodgkin's disease, need particular attention regarding the degree of disruption of their life. Reassurance that the acute side effects will end after the end of treatment will assist the patient in maintaining realistic hopes and perspective.

Radiation Therapy and the Child

For the child, as for the adult, radiation therapy can be particularly frightening [20]. The sights and sounds of the radiation therapy department alone can be terrifying to a young child whose fantasies of monsters and fear of separation may be part of his normal growth and development.

Orientation to the setting for the pediatric patient and his family will be an important part of the introduction to radiation therapy [20]. Depending on the developmental and cognitive level of the child, strategies such as play therapy may be utilized to provide the child with opportunities to cope with the experience.

Nursing assessment of the patient's responses to radiation

therapy will have to include behavioral as well as verbal dimensions. Children suffer from the same side effects of radiation therapy as adults, but may have particular vulnerability in some sites, such as growing bone. They also may exhibit a shorter latent period in certain side effects. Frequent diaper changes (to minimize dermatitis) may be extremely important if the pelvic area is irradiated [20].

In addition to an orientation previsit, other nursing maneuvers may aid in the care of children experiencing radiation therapy. Some children have a favorite toy which can be brought into the treatment room (but not in the field). Consistent caretakers and technicians may also increase the trust and security of the child.

Because radiation therapy requires specific treatment parameters, lying still is crucial for effective treatment. For a child this is no easy request. General anesthesia or milder sedation may be necessary. Immobilization devices also have been developed to allow accurate treatment by securing the immobility of the area to be irradiated [4]. Introduction and use of these devices can also be facilitated by play demonstration, for example, putting the child's teddy bear in the immobilization device. Frequent verbal contact via an intercom system may also be very helpful during treatment. This also needs to be carefully explained so that the "mystery voice" does not increase the child's apprehension. Constant visual surveillance of the child is also important in many situations.

In scheduling radiation treatments, the child's normal day activities and school schedule should be considered to minimize disruption [19]. Peer curiosity regarding the child's treatment and inevitable side effects should be discussed with the parents and teachers. Planning the reentry or continuation of the child in the school setting should include preparation of the fellow students to minimize untoward social consequences.

RADIATION THERAPY SIDE EFFECTS

The effects of radiation therapy on normal tissue exposed during cancer treatment may be seen acutely or after a long period of time [1,3,26]. Side effects may occur days to months or even years after the treatments. The delay will vary with the tissue and organs irradiated and the radiation schedule. The risk of developing complications is an important consideration in the selection and treatment plan of radiation therapy. The goals of the treatment may influence the willingness of the physician and the patient to risk some deleterious side effects. This may be particularly true if the problem can be effectively managed and the likelihood of good therapeutic results with radiation is evident. Alternative treatment options, however, may have to be considered if the therapeutic radiation therapy dose would produce life-threatening side effects for that patient. Consideration of the tolerance dose of normal tissue and the dose necessary for eradication or control of tumor is involved in determining the therapeutic ratio [30]. Lead shielding and various treatment maneuvers can provide optimal tumorcidal dose with maximum protection of normal tissue.

The major variables influencing the nature and severity of the side effects are the following [3,7,26,30]:

1. Volume of normal tissue exposed
2. Radiosensitivity of tissue and organs irradiated
3. Anatomical structures irradiated (organ status)
4. Dose of radiation
5. Time intervals between fractionation (radiation recovery)
6. Speed of delivery of radiation
7. Penetration characteristics (energy level)
8. Patient characteristics (for example, age, health)
9. Previous or concurrent chemotherapy, surgery
10. Individual variability

Acute Side Effects

Acute side effects of radiation therapy are those problems that occur during or shortly after the treatment phase as the result of immediate tissue response to radiation [3]. Acute side effects are primarily related to the rate and fractionation of the dose delivered. Generally, radiation doses are tolerated better when spread over a period of time. In many treatment programs, this is one of the reasons why the patient must return as frequently as daily for small fractionated doses that add up to an optimal therapeutic dose. Discussion of this principle with patients may improve their understanding of the rationale behind their many return visits.

Acute side effects to radiation are often increased in areas of frequent cell turnover. There side effects are related to the failure of proliferation or cell renewal in the areas irradiated [3]. Consequences are acutely seen in the skin, gastrointestinal tract, and the bone marrow. These acute side effects are often anticipated events accompanying the optimum tumorcidal dose of radiation therapy. The symptoms of the side effects are specific to the area irradiated—for example, mucositis in head and neck radiation [12,35]. The presence of side effects per se are not criteria for termination of treatment, but severe patient side effects may warrant daily dose reduction or brief interruption of therapy to allow patient recovery [7,12]. Optimal therapy will provide for maximum tumorcidal dose with minimal side effects. In therapy of curative intent, distressing uncomfortable side effects in the acute period during treatment may be unavoidable if effective therapy is to be given. These side effects, while not necessarily life threatening, may be very difficult for the patient to tolerate.

Nursing management during this acute stage is focused on preventing and minimizing or alleviating the severity of the side effects. An equally important focus is assisting the patient and the family in coping with this stressful time while maintaining hope for the future. The nurse can help the patient cope with these stresses by enabling the patient to keep perspective as to the purpose of the therapy and by giving and reinforcing the information that the side effects do not mean disease progression and that they are generally self-limiting and will subside after the treatment is over.

Careful and frequent assessment during the treatment phase will enable the nurse to monitor the patient when the side effects are beginning. By anticipating the frequent acute reactions of tissue exposed to radiation, the nurse can aid in the prevention of the threatening complications.

Intermediate Side Effects

Intermediate side effects of normal tissue exposed to irradiation may occur weeks to months after the radiation treatments have stopped. This time delay may make it difficult for the patient to relate the symptoms to his past therapy. Symptoms may be confused with worsening of the patient's condition and in fact may be difficult to differentiate from symptoms related to cancer spread or metastasis. Intermediate side effects are generally related to time/dose fractionation and to the total therapeutic dose of radiation received. In tissues that have a slow rate of cell renewal or replication (endothelial tissue, for example), cell death due to radiation injury may not occur until months after the injury (radiation) was delivered [26]. Anticipation and recognition of these side effects, such as radiation pneumonitis, allows for prompt treatment and prevention of serious complications.

Late Effects

Late effects of radiation therapy are related to the total therapeutic dose received by the particular vulnerable or radiosensitive tissue.

They are a limiting factor in effective radiation. Cellular alterations may not be noted until months or years later due to the slow cellular proliferation time. Three debilitating late side effects are: (1) tissue necrosis; (2) fistula development; and (3) dense fibrosis [3]. These complications may be irreversible or become a chronic problem. Their development may have relationship to previous acute or intermediate side effects or radiation [1,3,7]. Carcinogenesis is also a potential effect of radiation not manifested until years after radiation.

NURSING CARE OF RADIATION SIDE EFFECTS

Radiation Syndrome

Patients undergoing radiation therapy may complain of generalized symptoms not related specifically to the site of irradiation. These consist of fatigue, malaise, headache, anorexia, nausea, and vomiting [7]. The symptoms appear to be related to the volume of tissue irradiated and the daily dose delivered. It is theorized that the absorption of breakdown products from rapid tumor cell destruction may be a primary cause [7]. These two variables can be altered to reduce the severity of the symptoms. These symptoms are very important to assess as they may indicate the patient's radiation tolerance level.

Planning rest periods, and providing antiemetics and analgesics, can provide some relief from these symptoms. The distress the particular symptom is causing the patient may not necessarily be due to its physical impact. The increasing dependency on others, which may begin with the onset of therapy, may be particularly difficult for some patients to accept. If prior to treatment the patient experienced minimal distress due to the disease process, the impact of radiation therapy may be the first indication of things to come.

Effects on the Skin

Many patients may begin radiation therapy with the expectation and fear of receiving a radiation "burn" [8,24,20]. The severe skin reactions associated with radiation therapy are rare today [7]. Supervoltage equipment allows for significant "skin sparing" when treatment is given to a deep-seated tumor. Skin in the treatment area is still vulnerable with other types of radiation, but severe damage can be prevented or minimized with newer treatment techniques and nursing care. The quality and method of administration (fractionation) remain the most important variables influencing the severity of the side effect. As previously mentioned, skin effects are often the first reaction seen during radiation therapy due to the skin's rapid rate of cell replication and renewal [3]. Radiation administered to folds of skin, particularly in the groin and axilla, have an increased biological effect. Movement and chafing clothes compound the irritation. The moisture and warmth in the perineal area makes it particularly vulnerable to infections.

Erythema is the first response of skin to radiation. It is not usually seen until the third week of treatment [7]. The initial erythema evolves into a bronzed or tanned appearance of the skin, which may be permanent [20]. The irradiated area may become very dry causing the patient to complain of itching, flaking, and cracking of the skin. This dry desquamation reaction can occur in 2-4 weeks depending on the treatment characteristics (dose/energy level of radiation). It is occasionally followed by a more severe wet desquamation characterized by exudative ulcerations and denudation of the epidermis, similar to a second degree burn. Severe reactions often require halting or reducing the radiation dose temporarily. The skin will eventually heal, but even though it may appear normal, it will have undergone irreversible biological damage [7]. Late effects of radiation can be manifested as fibrotic changes causing obstruction and dysfunction, telangiectasia, and vascular impairment [7].

Care of Radiated Skin. The nurse's initial assessment of the skin in the treatment area is important to provide a baseline for future frequent checks during therapy. Patient involvement in proper skin care will be of critical importance in preventing complications. Various patient education techniques can be utilized to provide information and optimize compliance [21]. The basic fundamentals of skin care involve maintaining skin integrity while preventing irritation due to topical agents, environmental, or mechanical stress [20]. The area should be kept clean and dry without disturbing the treatment markings. Bathing and the use of soap should be approved by the physician. Exposure to sun and infrared lamps should be avoided but the area should be exposed to air when possible. The skin should not be exposed to extremes in temperature, for example, hot water, heating pads, or ice packs. Clothing should be loose and nonconstrictive. Fabric of 100% cotton is usually recommended for clothing in contact with the area [9,20]. Cosmetics, lotions, powders, and other topical agents are avoided unless specifically approved. They may not only cause aggravation of the irritated area, but some may contain metal bases which could augment the absorption of radiation. Shaving should also be avoided. A well-shaven appearance may be an indication of cleanliness for some patients. They may be very disturbed by their seemingly unkept appearance when shaving is not allowed.

If the dry desquamation occurs, cornstarch may decrease the pruritis [20]. The dryness of the skin may be alleviated by the use of white Vaseline or A & D ointment. Meticulous care should be given to prevent skin breakdown and subsequent infections. Signs and symptoms of infection should be carefully assessed. The inflammatory response may be masked by the erythema caused by radiation.

The nurse can support the patient in coping with these expected skin reactions. Symptomatic relief can be provided. Interventions may be dependent on careful and frequent assessment of physical signs and the patient's symptoms. The visibility of irradiated skin as well as its importance to the patient can influence body image. The residual tanning may be a permanent reminder of the cancer experience to the patient and others as well. This may be a small price to pay for effective cancer treatment. But the permanent skin changes may be difficult to integrate into some patients' concepts of a "healthy" appearance.

A moist epidermitis reaction to radiation requires active care. Radiation treatment alterations may also be necessary. Because of the breaks in the skin caused by the blistering, the risk of infection increases. The area needs to be kept clean to promote healing and decrease the risk of infection. Gentle cleansing irrigations and non-constrictive dressings may be necessary. Powder should be avoided in the wet reaction and ointments (including antibiotics and steroids) used only with the approval of the physician. Generally, the wet desquamation subsides within weeks.

The late changes of radiation may involve additional medical intervention as well as rehabilitative efforts to maximize function and preserve appearances. The vasculomusculature may be affected in radiation to such a degree that it is incapable of effective repair. Protracted radiation schedules have reduced this hazard [7]. Fibrosis and atrophy of the skin may gradually appear over the years. The radiated area may be more vulnerable to infection and breakdown after trauma [1].

Recall Phenomenon. Radiation skin reactions can be evoked or "recalled" when certain chemotherapeutic drugs are administered. Adriamycin and actinomycin-D are noted for this [13]. The nurse caring for the patient receiving these chemotherapeutic agents should assess the sites of previous irradiation for the reactivated response. Nursing care of the reaction is the same as for radiation skin responses.

Epilation

Hair loss in the radiated area is usually transitory, but if the dose is large enough it may become permanent [1,7]. It differs from the alopecia associated with chemotherapy in that it occurs only in the treatment field. Hair may fall out or be pulled out painlessly within 2-3 weeks after the start of therapy. Regrowth generally occurs in 2-3 months, but the new hair may be of a different color and texture [20]. The amount of radiation exposure will influence the rate of regrowth. The nurse should discuss the expected hair loss with the patient in advance. By evaluating the patient's needs and concerns, measures can be taken to minimize the change in appearance (for instance, by wearing a wig, or scarf if scalp hair loss). If the scalp is irradiated, irritants such as permanents and hair dyes should be avoided.

Effect on Lymph Nodes

Radiation to the lymph nodes can affect lymph drainage causing fibrosis and constrictive edema [27]. This problem can be compounded when there is surgery to remove lymph nodes in the area. Nursing assessment of the extent of swelling will be important along with measures to optimize drainage. Clothing impeding circulation should be avoided. Support of the affected limb may be necessary. Infection is a significant risk due to the stagnant lymph channel. Any trauma to the extremity should be carefully assessed.

Effects on the Gastrointestinal Tract

Mucositis. Mucosal irritation subsequent to radiation of the digestive tract (including the mouth or esophagus) can cause direct effects such as pain and indirect effects such as nutritional and fluid loss. The signs of mucositis are extremely important to evaluate since they may indicate levels of toxicity approaching radiation tolerance. Initially an inflammatory response is noted in the mucous membranes, then a radioepithelite may develop. This white or yellow glistening membrane covering, not to be confused with *Candida albicans,* should not be removed due to the risk of bleeding [20]. It is self-limited and generally subsides 2-4 weeks after treatment.

Oral mucositis may become extremely uncomfortable for the patient, affecting eating and talking. The patient should avoid all irritants that might aggravate this condition such as alcohol, tobacco, and spicy foods. The patient may be dependent on alcohol and tobacco due to a long-standing habit or may use them as supports to alleviate anxiety and pain. In any case, their absence may require substitutions for support during the stressful treatment time [8]. Dietary manipulation to include nutritious but soft and bland foods can be done in collaboration with the patient. Topical anesthetics prior to meals as well as analgesic relief for pain will hopefully enhance the ability to eat. Alteration of the status of salivary function, especially if the parotids have been radiated, will also affect the patient's ability and desire to eat. Infection can be a significant risk in an area subject to breakdown. Frequent oral hygiene including gentle mouth irrigations can decrease this risk. Dentures may become too painful to wear, further compromising the patient's nutritional status.

Taste Alteration. Alteration of taste occurs after radiation to the head and neck due to damage of the taste buds [11] and alteration of the saliva. Familiar foods may taste unusual due to increased sensation of some dimensions (bitter or acid, for example) and decreased sensation of others. Former favorite foods may become unpalatable. This disquieting symptom may persist until even a year after radiation [11]. Nursing action should include assessment of the symptoms and experimentation to find palatable foods for the patient. The impact of this side effect on the patient's life can be significant.

Dental Care. Radiation to the head and neck area can also affect saliva production. A decrease in saliva occurs, creating a mucus of increased viscosity and acidity [11,34]. Saliva substitutes, hard candies, sherbet, and ginger ale are some of the modalities that may help to counter this dry mouth syndrome [10,34]. Decreased saliva contributes to tooth decay. Frequent mouth care including fluoride application and, if possible, shielding of the teeth during radiation help prevent decay. Assessment of the patient's teeth prior to radiation is essential. Teeth with severe decay may have to be removed prior to treatment [28]. Long-term dental follow-up will be important for these patients.

Late Effects. Late effects of radiation to the head and neck area can result in painful trismus, a dysfunction of the masticating muscles allowing only a small opening of the mouth [11]. The consistent use of appliances created for mouth defects resulting from surgery are necessary to prevent closing and narrowing of the defect. Mouth exercises may also be ordered to maintain optimal function. Fistulas may also develop resulting from ulceration and perforation of the esophagus.

Nausea, Vomiting, and Diarrhea.   Nausea, vomiting, and diarrhea can result from damage to the very radiosensitive mucosal lining of the intestine. This occurs during the first one to three weeks of therapy. It can produce fluid and electrolyte imbalance as well as further compromise the patient's nutritional status. Antiemetics should be provided to decrease the nausea and vomiting. Antispasmodic, anticholinergic, and antidiarrheal medications may be necessary to quiet abdominal cramping and to prevent frequent watery stools. Small, frequent, low-residue feedings also may help. Ultimately, total bowel rest may be ordered until the bowel recovers, with support of the patient with intravenous fluids. The number and character of the stools should be assessed, especially the presence of blood [10].

Fluid and electrolyte balance should be frequently assessed. The patient should be encouraged to drink 2-3 quarts of fluid per day. Caution the patient who is actively vomiting and having diarrhea not to drink just water because of the danger of hyponatremia. Colas, Gatorade, Jello, and apple juice are better choices to correct electrolyte imbalance. The use of steroids as enemas and/or suppositories may relieve the symptoms of proctitis.

Dysphagia. Dysphagia caused by mucositis reaction in the esophagus can be painful enough to severely limit food and fluid intake. It usually begins 2-3 weeks after the start of treatment and subsides several weeks following therapy. Lead shielding of the esophagus can be done if it is in the treatment area but not involved with tumor. The nursing goal during this acute reaction is to alleviate or minimize the pain while providing optimal nutritional and fluid replacement. Analgesics prior to meals and frequent irrigations to decrease secretions may provide comfort. Frequent small feedings of tepid, bland, full liquids may be easier to swallow for some patients. For the patient in the hospital, foods brought from home may be more appetizing. In severe cases, a feeding tube or hyperalimentation may be necessary for support. Difficulty in swallowing may also increase the risk of food aspiration. Availability at meal times of a nurse or family member should be considered with patients having difficulty swallowing [10].

Severe dysphagia can result from the late effects of radiation causing strictures and stenosis. Periodic endoscopic dilatation may be necessary to widen the esophagus to permit swallowing. Surgical intervention may also be attempted. Permanent feeding tubes may be necessary.

Chronic Radiation Enteritis. Chronic radiation enteritis can be a consequence of radiation to the bowel resulting in severe weight loss and megaloblastic anemia. Stricture, ulceration, fistula development, and bowel obstruction are also late effects that can occur with significant radiation damage. Assessment of the nutritional status of the patient as indicated by weight loss and symptoms of avitaminosis will be important in dietary intervention.

Radiation involving the stomach can produce severe loss of appetite and weight [11]. Ulceration can also occur. A bland diet and antacids are preventive interventions.

Nutritional Consequences. Patients beginning radiation therapy may already have a compromised nutritional status. Varied side effects of radiation therapy affecting nutrition have been noted [11]. Anorexia can be a severe problem caused by multiple variables. The physical severity of the symptoms limiting food intake and absorption—nausea, vomiting, diarrhea, stomatitis—must be considered in relation to the patient's own emotional response. The meaning and importance of food with its social and cultural implications should be considered with any attempts at dietary manipulation. Inclusion of the patient and family members in problem solving will be essential. Consultation with a dietician to plan creative and nutritious meals within the limitations resulting from the tissue response to radiation may be helpful. These symptoms, while usually self-limiting, should not be neglected as they can significantly affect the quality of the patient's life. Nutritional build-up prior to radiation may be essential to improve the patient's tolerance to therapy.

Effects on the Respiratory Tract

The most important variable influencing the tolerance of the lung to radiation is the treatment volume and radiation dose [7]. Mild dyspnea and a nonproductive cough are the initial responses to radiation. Radiation pneumonitis can present 2-3 months after therapy. The patient may be asymptomatic with an abnormal chest X-ray. Chronic fibrotic changes can permanently damage the patient's lung capacity [20]. Symptoms of respiratory distress may vary in severity affecting the patient's ability to function and increasing the risk of infection. Administration of the chemotherapy agent bleomycin after irradiation to the lung can increase the risk of pulmonary toxicity [13].

Nursing assessment of symptoms of respiratory dysfunction will be important in individualizing care [10]. The severity of the dysfunction will determine the supportive measures necessary for symptom relief and assistance with daily activities. Steroids may be used to decrease symptoms of pneumonitis while the lung is recovering [3]. Permanent lung damage will require long-term rehabilitative efforts. Infection is a significant risk with a compromised respiratory system. The patient should avoid contact with people with colds. Respiratory distress can cause anxiety in patients, often compounding the symptom. Emotional support along with symptom relief are important nursing interventions. For some patients, their dependency on others due to their physical disability can become an additional source of stress.

Cardiac Side Effects

When the heart is in the treatment field, an acute transient pericarditis can develop [7]. Additionally, pericarditis and myocarditis can present months to years after radiation. Assessment of cardiac symptoms, EKG abnormalities, chest pain, or tachycardia, will be important in evaluating cardiac status. Management of pericarditis involves pain relief and prevention of further problems of cardiac dysfunction, such as constrictive pericarditis or cardiac tamponade. The use of Adriamycin after radiation to the mediastinum can increase the risk of myocardial toxicity.

Bone Marrow Suppression

Depending upon the volume of bone marrow irradiated, radiation can produce mild to severe myelosuppression [1,7,20]. This would result in suppression of the important bone marrow components creating thrombocytopenia (platelet reduction), leukopenia (white blood cell reduction), and anemia (red blood cell reduction). When the precursor stem cells are affected, the suppression could be prolonged or even permanent. The precursors of platelets and white cells are very sensitive to radiation due to short cell-cycle times. Neither platelets nor white blood cells are stored in quantities available for long-term recruitment when the supply is diminished. Red blood cell production is also affected but effects of this are manifest later because of long-term red cell survival. Risk of spontaneous bleeding is significant when platelets drop to less than 20,000/mm^3. Infection almost inevitably occurs when granulocytes are less than 1,000/mm^3. Symptoms of anemia present are variable levels of reduced hemoglobin and hematocrit depending on the acuteness of the change.

Bleeding. Nursing care measures for thrombocytopenic patients involve careful assessment of clinical signs and symptoms in addition to awareness of the platelet count [9,20]. Evidence of bleeding (petechiae, echymosis, nose bleeds, blood in urine or stool), should be frequently evaluated. Nursing measures to reduce the risk of trauma (protection from sharp objects in environment, avoidance of intrusive procedures) should be instituted to prevent hemorrhage. Any breaks in the skin, such as those caused by injections, should be monitored carefully with pressure being applied until bleeding has stopped. Platelet support (see Chapter 5) may be necessary until recovery of the bone marrow.

Infection. Nursing measures to prevent infection involve protection of the patient from exposure to exogenous pathogens [9,20]. Radiotherapy may also be immunosuppressive, further compromising the patient's ability to withstand infection [23]. The patient may be placed in protective isolation, or mask and meticulous hand washing procedures may be instituted to decrease exposure to pathogens. The patient's own hygiene, especially perianal care, should be carefully monitored. Maintenance of the integrity of the patient's skin as the first line of defense is crucial. Routine cultures to screen for infection and attention to signs and symptoms of infection will be important components of care. Antibiotic therapy is used when appropriate. Experimental transfusions of granulocytes are also being utilized to combat infection due to bone marrow suppression. (See section on granulocyte transfusions in Chapter 5 for more details.)

Anemia. Fatigue, dyspnea, orthopnea, and pallor are important clinical signs of anemia. The nurse can provide symptomatic relief by assisting the patient in activities, and allowing for frequent rest periods. Red blood cell transfusions may be indicated along with iron supplements.

Effects on the Urinary Tract

Acute effects of radiation on the mucosal lining of the bladder result in cystitis [7]. Symptoms of frequency, burning, and urgency can be controlled with urinary analgesics and antibiotics if infection is a complication. Hematuria may also occur. The patient should be instructed to drink 2-3 quarts of fluid daily to reduce the risk of infection [20]. Urine cultures should be taken to screen for infection. The urine should be checked for blood. Late effects due to fibrotic and vascular changes can result in contracted bladder necessitating the use of permanent indwelling catheters or cystectomy [7].

Radiation nephritis characterized by proteinuria, hypertension, and anemia can be a side effect presenting three to six months after treatment [1,7]. Chronic nephritis causing azotemia can also evolve [1]. The hypertension can usually be controlled by medications. Surgical removal of the damaged kidney may be necessary. Renal function should be evaluated by the nurse in terms of fluid intake and output, presence of protein in the urine, and blood pressure checks.

Effects on the Central Nervous System

Radiation myelitis can produce a transient syndrome of "electrical parasthesia" affecting upper and lower extremities, particularly with anterior flexion of the hand [7]. This numbness and tingling usually occurs one month to one year after the cessation of therapy and may last for several months, but it is not associated with other neurological findings. The nurse should assess the patient's symptoms and provide reassurance that they are transient and do not indicate irreversible damage.

Occasionally neurological damage leading to progressive weakness and paralysis can occur as a late effect [1,7]. Nursing care should be directed at encouraging the patient to continue long-term medical follow-up.

Radiation to the Eye

Lead shielding may be used to protect the lens during radiation to the head. If the eye is in the treatment field, conjunctivitis can be seen as an acute effect with cataract development and corneal ulceration as late effects [1,7]. Vision should be evaluated at intervals to determine the extent of visual loss resulting from the cataract. Surgical intervention may be necessary [20].

Radiation to the Ear

Otitis media may result from radiation to the ear. Symptoms of tinnitus, earache, and fullness caused by occlusion of the eustachian tube secondary to edema should be evaluated [7].

Radiation to the Liver

Radiation hepatitis is rare but can occur weeks to months after radiation exposure. Abdominal pain, jaundice, hepatomegaly, ascites, and weight gain are symptoms that the nurse should assess.

Effects on Bone and Cartilage

Retardation of epiphysial growth is a late consequence of radiation to children [1,7]. Asymmetrical development and scoliotic deformities may result. The megavoltage therapy has minimal preferential bone absorption and the risk of damage is further decreased with protracted therapy. Frequent long-term assessment of normal growth will be important for children receiving radiation. Rehabilitation, including the use of orthopedic appliances, may be necessary if deformities occur.

Osteoradionecrosis is a late effect rarely seen with current therapy techniques [1,20]. Infection can increase the risk of necrosis. The mandible was particularly vulnerable in the past. Fractures may rarely occur in radiated bones. Assessment of bone pain and function will be important nursing considerations.

Effects on Sexual Function

Sterility. Radiation can have a far-reaching effect on the patient's sexuality. These side effects may be the most threatening to the patient [24]. Gonad function in both the male and female may be affected. The sperm may have a transient decrease in number due to scattered radiation even if not directly in the treatment field. Permanent sterility may also result [1]. Forewarned of the possibility of infertility, the patient may elect to store his sperm if further reproduction is desired [20]. The patient should be informed that destruction of sperm will not affect secondary sex characteristics or sexual drive (due to physical reasons) [1]. Irradiation of the ovaries can cause temporary or permanent cessation of ovulation. Acute manifestation of symptoms of menopause may occur. Oophoropexy, a surgical intervention tucking the ovaries out of the potential treatment field, may preserve fertility. The patient should be reassured that infertility does not affect femininity or sexual drive.

Impotence. Impotence may be a temporary or permanent effect of radiation. This dramatic consequence must be carefully assessed in light of the fact that other variables can cause sexual dysfunction. The loss of the ability to engage in intercourse does not have to prevent the patient from engaging in other satisfying ways of expressing affection. Sexual counseling regarding alternative behaviors should include the patient and his partner for effective problem solving.

Dyspareunia. Irritation of the vaginal mucosa due to pelvic irradiation can cause dryness due to loss of mucous lubrication [33]. Intercourse may be very painful necessitating temporary cessation. Application of a lubricant prior to intercourse may help. Loss of vaginal elasticity and stenosis may be late effects of radiation. Recto-vaginal fistulas may also result from necrosis of damaged tissue [7].

Body Image. The patient's perceptions of attractiveness and desirability will be important for the nurse to assess in determining sexual dysfunction and physical problems. Side effects not directly related to sexual function, such as nausea, pain, diarrhea, and fatigue, may influence the existence and gratification of sexual needs. The patient may experience decrease in libido due to preoccupation with the diagnosis of cancer and fear of death [24]. Supporting the patient's open communication with a partner may be an important nursing intervention in this sensitive area. It may be difficult for the patient to begin the discussion. The nurse should provide an open accepting atmosphere for discussion assuming that the patient may wish to discuss this problem.

Genetic Effects and Fetal Malfunction. Radiation effect on fetal development can be disastrous. The more severe insult is manifested when radiation takes place during the early stages of embryonic development. Spontaneous abortion and fetal malformations may occur due to the effects of radiation [1,7]. Even when the child appears overtly normal, there is a questionable association with later development of cancer, particularly leukemia [26,36]. Genetic mutations in the sperm and the ovum are theoretical possibilities [20]. Genetic counseling regarding the risk of genetic malformations may be necessary to provide information to the patient and provide a forum for the discussion of alternatives to conception. With the possible transient nature of sterility in both the male and female gonads, birth control measures should not be neglected if conception is not desired. Abortion or an undesired pregnancy in addition to the pain of the diagnosis and treatment of cancer may be a tremendous stressor.

Carcinogenesis

All types of ionizing radiation can potentially produce cancer in humans [36]. Clinical experience with people exposed to radiation

TABLE 6.4
Examples of Cancer Associated with Radiation [1, 36]

Type of Cancer	Source(s)
Leukemia[a]	In utero X-ray, Thorotrast, radiation for ankylosing spondylitis, radiation for Hodgkin's disease therapy
Lung[a]	Uranium
Breast[a]	Radiation for benign breast disease and chest fluoroscopy
Thyroid[a]	Childhood radiation for enlarged thymus or acne
Bone	Radium, radiation therapy for retinoblastoma

[a] Associated with atom bomb survivors.

due to the atomic bomb, occupational exposure, diagnostic X-rays and radiation therapy has resulted in evidence of carcinogenesis (see Table 6.4). There is no level of radiation that can be called absolutely harmless [1]. The controversy over levels of background radiation is well documented [36]. In addition to adhering to safety guidelines there should be an attempt to minimize all unnecessary exposure to diagnostic X-rays, carefully evaluating the benefits versus the risk of the exposure. Reduction of a specific dose of radiation required for specific diagnostic X-rays is also being considered [36].

The development of secondary neoplasms in the treatment field has been associated with radiation therapy [20]. While this is rare, the patient should be encouraged to maintain long-term medical follow-up since development may not be noted for years. The patient should be educated regarding suspicious signs and symptoms indicating a possible malignancy. This is a tragic occurrence especially if the patient is presumed cured from the primary neoplasm.

BRACHYTHERAPY

Brachytherapy is the administration of radiation via a radioactive material in close proximity to the patient [7,12]. (See Table 6.5.) This can be accomplished by permanent or temporary implantation of the radioactive sources near or in the tumor. The location and size of the implant must be determined [14]. The radioactive half-life

TABLE 6.5
Examples of Internal Radiation [14, 20]

Source	Type of Radiation	Half-Life	Use in Cancer Treatment
[137] Cesium	Beta, gamma	30.0 years	Gynecological cancers
[226] Radium	Alpha, beta	1,602 years	Head and neck cancer, bladder cancer, gynecological cancer
[32] Phosphorous	Beta	14.3 days[a]	Malignant effusions
[131] Iodine[b]	Gamma	8.05 days[a]	Thyroid
[192] Iridium	Beta, gamma	74.4 days	Head and neck cancer
[222] Radon	Alpha, beta, gamma	3.82 days[a]	Gynecological cancers
[198] Gold	Gamma	2.7 days[a]	Malignant effusions
[125] Iodine	Soft gamma	60.2 days	Head and neck cancer

[a] Permanent implants.
[b] Only used systemically.

of the source is one important consideration in the length of administration of the radiation as well as patient care. High energy level is not a requirement for penetration of the radiation to the tumor due to its close proximity. Intracavity or interstitial radiation is often combined with some form of external beam treatment.

Implantation of needles, seeds, wires, or catheters containing radioactive isotopes may be utilized to obtain optimal, local, therapeutic affect with minimal damage to surrounding tissues and structures. Nursing management of these patients center on comfort and safety measures related to the particular site involved [14,15,20]. Variables of the radioactive substance to evaluate in determining implications for nursing care include: (1) type of radiation—alpha, beta, gamma; (2) energy level or penetration characteristics; and (3) half-life or rate of disintegration [6]. The patient's fears of becoming "radioactive" should be acknowledged with the reassurance that they will be normal once the implant is removed or the substance has decayed.

Intracavitary Implants

Intracavitary implants involve the placement of a radioactive source into a body cavity, for example, the vagina. Applicators are inserted in surgery but the radioactive material is usually not implanted in the patient until after returning to a ward isolation room [14]. This "afterloading" technique reduces unnecessary exposure to the health team. The most frequently used radiation implant is for cervical cancer. Special precautions are taken to prevent it from becoming dislodged [33]. The patient is on strict bedrest during the extent of therapy. The patient is on a regimen (low-residue diet, medications) to prevent bowel movements during the therapy. A Foley catheter may also be inserted. Accurate recording and periodic assessment of the position of the implants is essential. The patient's physical, cognitive, and emotional preparation for this experience can be an important nursing function.

Radioactive substances such as ^{32}P (radioactive phosphorous) are used to treat malignant effusions. Nursing observations should be made for fluid leaks of contaminated material [15].

Interstitial Radiation

Radioactive seeds, such as ^{125}I, and needles, such as, ^{226}Ra, may be implanted directly into the tumor [20]. The nurse should be aware of the exact position and number of such implants. Frequent assessment of their position is essential. Special precautions in patient care and in handling of bed linen and patient supplies are necessary to reduce the risk of displacement and radiation exposure.

Systemic Radiation

Radioactive substances may be administered internally via intravenous or oral routes. Use of ^{131}I (radioactive iodine) is an example of systemic irradiation. In the case of ^{131}I, the patient's bodily fluids—urine, stool, emesis, sweat, and saliva—are considered to be contaminated with radiation. Disposable food tray items are utilized to avoid radioactive spread. The patient also generally avoids taking a bath and employs multiple flushes after using the bathroom to prevent toilet contamination by the principle of dilution. Dilution by washing of the skin is also necessary if there has been contamination of radioactive material. These precautions are generally only necessary for a short time due to the short half-life.

Radiation Safety in Nursing Care

Nursing care management of patients with implants is concerned with optimum comfort of the patient and with maximum safety to the patient, caretakers, and all those in contact with the patient during treatment.

The principles of distance, time, and shielding are the best guides for the safe nursing care of patients with radioactive implants [6,19]. The longer the contact with or the shorter the distance from the radioactive implant, the greater the hazard of radiation exposure for the nurse caring for a patient with an implant. To protect other patients in the hospital setting as well as visitors and health care personnel, precautions should be taken to alert everyone to the fact of danger from radiation exposure. Appropriate use of signs and the use of a designated area or wing of the ward for patients with implants will help to restrict unnecessary exposure.

Generally, patients with implants are located in a single room with the head of the bed against the far wall. The door need not be closed. A wood door would not stop the gamma rays, but the distance from the door to the radiation source is far enough to prevent substantial penetration of radiation. Tape strategically placed on the floor will help to remind visitors and health care personnel to keep a safe distance from the patient. No special procedures are required with bedding or utensils [22].

Since irradiation can harm an unborn fetus, there should be no pregnant visitors or health care personnel attending the patient while the implant is in place. (Diagnostic pelvic irradiation of women of childbearing age is generally recommended only during the 10 days following the menstrual period, prior to ovulation [26].) Visitors under 18 years are also restricted due to the hazards of radiation exposure to growing children. Rotation of nursing personnel caring for patients with implants is also advised to prevent undue exposure.

Time.   Time spent in contact with the patient with a radioactive implant should also be carefully considered. Visits and nursing care are generally restricted to less than 15 minutes per day to ensure safety [19]. The distance from the source will influence the amount of radiation received over any given time [22]. With radioactive substances of short half-life, such as, ^{222}Ra, the amount of time spent with the patient can be increased over time. Radioactive substances with short half-lives such as ^{125}I may be used as permanent implants. An additional notation may be made by the radiation therapist as to the length of time nursing activities can safely be carried out. Quick, organized nursing care can still be effective and comforting. Forewarning the patient of this time necessity may allay some of the feelings of avoidance and rejection that the patient may feel during these short contacts.

Distance.   In nursing care activities, distance from the radioactive source (not merely the patient's body) should be considered.

The intensity of the radiation decreases in proportion to the square of the distance from the radioactive source (Inverse Square Law) [16,33]. Generally, nursing care procedures that require close contact with the implant area should be avoided. Working at the farthest point from the implant should be attempted if possible in most nursing care procedures. Short visits at the doorway can provide reassurance for the patient and an opportunity for nursing assessment.

Shielding. Handling of any radioactive material must be done with forceps. If there is a danger that the implant may become dislodged, there should be an emergency plan with available equipment in which to store the radioactive source. Shielding, in the form of lead aprons, may also provide some safety during patient contact, but it will not shield high-energy radiations (gamma rays) [15]. Contamination of the skin with radioactive material (for instance, with ^{131}I) during patient care, and possible ingestion of the material due to contaminated hands are hazards that may be reduced by wearing gloves during patient contact.

Dislodged Implants. Any dislodged implant should be picked up with special long-handled tongs (never hands) and deposited in a lead-lined container [15,20]. Radioactive seeds can be picked up with a spoon. The type of shielding necessary to protect against radiation is determined by the characteristics and energy level of the radiation. Alpha particles may be stopped by the skin and, thus, when used internally do not create a substantial risk for the caregiver, unless they are ingested, inhaled, or absorbed [20]. Beta particles are generally stopped by tissue. Lucite and aluminum are also used to stop beta particles [20]. Gamma rays can penetrate even when used internally and are still a risk for the caregiver. Gamma rays of higher energy levels ("hard gammas") penetrate further than those of lower energy ("soft gammas") [20]. Lead is used to block gamma rays. The half-value layer (HVL) is the thickness of a material required to reduce radiation penetration by one-half [16]. Penetration characteristics of the radioactive substance are directly related to the energy level.

Detection of Radiation. Radiosensitive film badges that measure radioactivity are required to be worn by health care personnel in contact with patients receiving brachytherapy to measure the amount of radiation exposure [22]. They are best worn at site of maximum exposure, usually the abdomen. Geiger-Muller detectors are used to detect contamination from radiation.

Limits of Radiation Exposure. Safety guidelines designated for individual radiation exposure are limited to less than 500 millirems per year [35]. The maximum permissible dose to minimize potential radiation damage to the individual is five rems for the whole body [35]. Various body sites (the gonads, for example) have individual guidelines for limits of radiation depending upon their sensitivity. Safe limits for environmental radiation exposure for the population are set at 170 millirems per year to reduce the risk of radiation induced genetic damage [35].

PALLIATIVE RADIATION THERAPY

Radiation therapy may be a useful and effective measure in relieving specific distressing symptoms of those cancer patients without hope of curative therapy [28]. It does offer patients hope for quality of survival even though promises cannot be made for quantity. When comfort and support are the major goals of radiation therapy, the method of administration is significantly different than curative treatment.

The objectives of palliative radiation are such that the risk of serious and acute side effects are not tolerated. The risk of long-term side effects is not a major concern. The overall treatment plan will hopefully be as unstressful as possible for the patient. Nursing attention and sensitivity to patient's tolerance and reactions toward the therapy is an important factor in obtaining optimum comfort.

Pain Relief

Relief of pain, depending on the source, may be an important contribution of palliative therapy. Radiation therapy can provide relief of pain due to local causes. The disruptive and degrading nature of malignant pain can plague many cancer patients. Bone metastases are a significant cause of this pain. Local irradiation may provide quick and effective relief in most cases, and also may prevent fracture of the affected area [28]. The effectiveness is primarily related to radiosensitivity of the particular tumor type rather than other factors. Breast cancer, a frequent cause of osseous metastasis, may be sensitive. As the number of lesions increase, systemic chemotherapy treatment may be sought or attempted in combination with localized therapy.

Other causes of malignant pain may also be alleviated with radiation therapy. Reduction of the size of sheer tumor mass may reduce pain associated with bulky disease. Location of tumor (in the pleura, for example) may dictate the nature and severity of the pain.

Nursing assessment, the patient's pain experience, and intervention and evaluation of pain relief measures are central foci in palliative therapy. The patient's perception of pain and interpretation of its meaning will influence symptomatic relief measures [8,32]. The patient's behavioral changes will also be important indications of pain relief. (See the section on pain relief in Chapter 5.)

Obstruction and Effusions

Radiation treatment of splenic infarction, superior vena cava obstruction, spinal cord compression, and malignant effusions may provide the suffering cancer patient dramatic relief. The sudden change, however, may be difficult for both the patient and his family, who may have thought the symptom heralded an immediate end [31]. The hope for cure may be supported by such short treatment successes.

In addition to pain, obstruction of organs (such as the bowel and biliary tree) and of vessels can cause dysfunction and, depending on the nature of the anatomical disruption, death.

Superior Vena Cava Syndrome

Compression of the superior vena cava by tumor is a medical emergency which often responds to radiation therapy [25]. Assessment of symptoms and quick action are critical. The nurse should note the presence of swelling of the face and neck with jugular and thoracic venous distension. The patient may complain of headache, visual disturbances, chest pain, and have loss or alteration of consciousness [31]. The patient's arms may also be distended. Additional treatment with diuretics and steroids is aimed at relieving the symptoms of airway obstruction and increased intracranial pressure [31]. Assessment of respiratory distress, symptomatic relief, and emotional support are important nursing responsibilities. This is a frightening and life-threatening event for the patient.

Spinal Cord Compression

Spinal cord compression resulting from the effects of tumor invasion is manifested by symptoms of motor dysfunction, parathesias, and lower back pain [31]. Symptoms may progress slowly or have a rapid onset. Radiation therapy is used to reverse or prevent progression of symptoms [31]. Steroids are also utilized to decrease edema.

Surgical intervention may be necessary. Radiation therapy can restore some function depending on severity of the compression. Nursing care in addition to supporting the patient during the acute event might also involve rehabilitative efforts. These should be begun, despite the prognosis, to improve the patient's quality of life.

Malignant Effusions

Radiation may be the therapy of choice for malignant effusions. Moderate pericardial effusions of radiosensitive cancers such as lymphoma may be adequately treated by radiation therapy [31]. Nursing assessment of symptoms includes chest pain, dyspnea, cough, fatigue, hoarseness, and dysphagia. Previous irradiation and acute presentation would require other therapeutic alternatives, such as surgery or chemotherapy.

Pleural effusions characterized by pleuritic chest pain, dyspnea, and cough can be treated with the instillation of radioactive isotopes (such as ^{32}P) as a sclerosing agent in the same fashion as some chemotherapeutic agents (nitrogen mustard, for example) [31]. Special precautions will need to be taken with the contaminated pleural drainage.

Hemorrhage

Radiation therapy may be utilized in the suppression of gross hemorrhage [28]. Decreased or complete cessation of the bleeding may occur with radiation to some areas, for example, the bronchus. For many patients and families, profuse bleeding is the most frightening final symptom. It is one for which families may seek help in the form of hospitalization rather than deal with that type of death in the home. Emotional nursing support in conjunction with therapy to stop the hemorrhage can provide significant comfort. Surface lesions that are ulcerated and infected may also be significantly controlled by local radiation.

Quality of Life

The impact of organic disruption due to cancer or complications of treatment on the patient may be influenced by the patient's values and life-style as well as the organs physiologic function. Nursing assessment of the patient's view and feeling toward such disruptions can provide information to help tailor the plan of care.

Tumor masses that disturb mobility, function, and appearance may not necessarily critically affect the quantity of the patient's life-span, though they may seriously affect the patient's ability to carry on and enjoy daily life. Again, assessing the patient for his major life concerns may point to items of a quite different nature from those his medical work-up may reveal.

TOTAL BODY IRRADIATION

Total body irradiation may be utilized in conjunction with chemo-therapeutic agents to obliterate acute leukemia prior to bone marrow transplantation [37]. A dose of radiation, frequently 1,000 rads, is administered to the patient at one time. The patient is then given a transplant of bone marrow in an attempt to prevent otherwise lethal radiation toxicity to the bone marrow. (See section on bone marrow transplantation in Chapter 5.)

The dose is delivered over 2-3 hours, during which time the patient must assume various positions to enable a uniform dosage of radiation to be delivered. The nursing care management of these patients can be divided into three phases: (1) before total body irradiation; (2) during treatment; and (3) after treatment [20].

Prior to total body irradiation, the patient is often debilitated and may be seriously ill from the side effects of vigorous chemo-therapy as well as of disease progression. The hope for cure is a strong motivating factor for those patients opting for bone marrow transplant. They may have experienced numerous treatment failures before this still-experimental therapy is considered. Patients can only tolerate the dose delivered in total body irradiation once. If the transplant should fail it might be attempted again without, however, total body irradiation as part of the preparatory treatment.

Nursing concern in this stage should include attempts to optimize comfort and to minimize fear and apprehension about the treatment. Interventions to reduce pain and discomfort which many patients may be having would involve appropriate premedication and sedation. Assessment of variables, such as positioning, that influence the patient's perception of pain and those, such as diversion, that have been helpful in reducing the perception of pain should be carefully evaluated. This information can be very helpful in planning the patient's care during the total body irradiation [20]. Prior explanation of the procedure, environment, side effects, and feelings the patient may experience with treatment may decrease fears and anxieties related to the treatment. It also may uncover misconceptions and open communication for further discussion of the patient's concerns.

During the actual administration of the total body irradiation, nursing care will be related to the patient's response to the environment and the procedure, and to management of ongoing clinical and symptomatic complaints via such measures as antibiotic administration, pain medication, and measures to alleviate radiation side effects. The isolation during the procedure is very frightening for many patients. Communication with the patient via an intercom may be very comforting. Observation of the patient via a view window or television can be important in assessing the patient's condition as well as reassuring to the patient. Treatment breaks for positioning or symptom relief can also break the monotony of the isolation.

As the dose increases, a prodromal syndrome of nausea, vomiting, and chills and fever may occur. Medication as well as verbal reassurance and support can be very helpful to the patient in providing relief. Acknowledging the expectation of the side effect may also help some patients to keep their feelings in perspective. Diarrhea may also occur during or shortly after irradiation, so preparations should be made to easily accommodate the patient. Again, treatment breaks to assist the patient may be taken. Reverse isolation precautions are generally maintained throughout the supportive care. Usually, they have been initated during the previous chemotherapeutic treatment.

An awareness of the time frame for the resolution of the immediate effects of total body irradiation can be helpful for the nurse caring for the patient. The nausea, vomiting, and chills that occur during or shortly after the irradiation generally subside or resolve in 24 hours. The diarrhea, parotitis, and pancreatitis secondary to radiation generally subside in a few days. The erythema resulting from the inflammatory response of the skin to radiation also will decrease in several days. The mucositis due to the radiation may take weeks to subside, particularly if complicated by infection. Alopecia generally occurs within two weeks and hair regrowth may occur in several months. All of these side effects can certainly be compounded by preexisting or concomitant chemotherapy. The profound vulnerability these patients have to all types of infection due to the bone marrow destruction and immunosuppression has significant implications for nursing care management. Even after successful engraftment of donor bone marrow, susceptibility to infection may exist for a year or more. [20].

The long-term side effects of total body irradiation are hazards accepted in the struggle for cure. As in other forms of radiation treatment, hyperpigmentation of the skin may be permanent. The associated dryness and peeling of the skin and wet desquamation particularly in the skin folds may occur several weeks post treatment and persist for months. Cataracts, sterility, growth retardation, and liver and kidney damage are unfortunate sequalae that may occur months to years after the irradiation.

REFERENCES

[1] ACKERMAN, L., and SPJUT, H. Radiotherapy of Cancer. In *Ackerman and del Regato's Cancer: Diagnosis, Treatment, and Prognosis,* ed. J. del Regato and H. Spjut, 5th ed., pp. 70-98. St. Louis: C.V. Mosby, 1977.

[2] ANDREWS, J. *The Radiobiology of Human Cancer Radiotherapy,* 2nd ed. Baltimore: University Park Press, 1978.

[3] BLOOMER W, and HELLMAN, S. Current Concepts: Normal Tissue Responses to Radiation Therapy. *New England Journal of Medicine,* 293: 80-83, 1975.

[4] BOONE, M.; CONNER, W.; HEUSINKIOELD, R.; and MORGADO, R. New Instrumentation in Radiation Oncology. *Ca: A Cancer Journal for Clinicians* 26:299-309, 1976.

[5] BRADY, L. Radiation Oncology: Present Status and Future Potential. *Ca: A Cancer Journal for Clinicians,* 26:258-259, 1976.

[6] BRAESTRUP, C.B., and VIKTERLOF, K.J. *Manual on Radiation Protection in Hospitals and General Practice: Basic Protection Requirements,* Vol. 1. Geneva: World Health Organization, 1974.

[7] BUSHKE, F., and PARKER, R. *Radiation Therapy in Cancer Management.* New York: Grune & Stratton, 1972.

[8] CREECH, R. The Psychologic Support of the Cancer Patient: A Medical Oncologist's Viewpoint. *Seminars in Oncology,* 2:285-292, 1975.

[9] DIETZ, K. Radiation Therapy: External Radiation. *Cancer Nursing,* 2:129-138, 1979.

[10] DIETZ, K. Radiation Therapy: External Radiation. *Cancer Nursing,* 2:233-244, 1979.

[11] DONALDSON, S. Nutritional Consequences of Radiotherapy. *Cancer Research,* 37:2407-2413, 1977.

[12] FLETCHER, G.; WITHERS, H.; ALMOND, P.; LINDBERG, R.; TAPLEY, N.; HUSSEY, D.; and DELCLOS, L. Modalities of Cancer Treatment: Radiotherapy. In *Cancer Patient Care,* ed. R. Clark and C. Howe, pp. 14-24. Chicago: Year Book Med. Pub., Inc., 1976.

[13] FRIEDMAN, M., and CARTER, S. Serious Toxicities Associated with Chemotherapy. *Seminars in Oncology,* 5:193-202, 1978.

[14] GILLICK, K. Radiation Therapy: Internal Radiation. *Cancer Nursing,* 2:313-325, 1979.

[15] GILLICK, K. Radiation Therapy: Internal Radiation. *Cancer Nursing,* 2:393-402, 1979.

[16] GOODWIN, P.; QUIMBY, E.; and MORGAN, R. *Physical Foundation of Radiology,* 4th ed. New York: Harper & Row, 1970.

[17] HOLLEB, A. A Glossary of Terms Relating to Radiation Therapy. *Ca: A Cancer Journal for Clinicians*, 26:314-320, 1976.

[18] KAPLAN, H. Basic Principles in Radiation Oncology. *Cancer*, 39:689-693, 1977.

[19] KRAMER, S. Definitive Radiation Therapy. *Ca: A Cancer Journal for Clinicians*, 26:269-273, 1976.

[20] LEAHY, D.; ST. GERMAIN, J.; and VARRICHIO, C. *The Nurse and Radiotherapy*. St. Louis: C.V. Mosby, 1979.

[21] MUNTZ, M., and ZUR, B. Patient Education in Chemotherapy and Radiotherapy. In *Current Perspectives in Oncologic Nursing*, ed. C. Kellog and B. Sullivan, pp. 173-182. St. Louis: C.V. Mosby, 1978.

[22] NATIONAL COUNCIL ON RADIATION PROTECTION AND MEASUREMENTS. Protection against Radiation from Brachytherapy Sources. NCRP Report No. 40, March 1972.

[23] PARKER, R. Principles of Radiation Oncology. In *Cancer Treatment*, ed. C. Haskell, pp. 19-27. Philadelphia: Saunders, 1980.

[24] PECK, A., and BOLAND, J. Emotional Reactions to Radiation Treatment. *Cancer*, 40:180-184, 1977.

[25] PEREZ, C.; PRESANT, C.; and VAN AMBURG A., III. Management of Superior Vena Cava Syndrome. *Seminars in Oncology*, 5:123-134, 1978.

[26] PIZZARELLO, D., and WITCOFSKI, R. *Basic Radiation Biology*, 2nd ed. Philadelphia: Lea & Febiger, 1975.

[27] RICHARDS, V. *Cancer, the Wayward Cell*. Los Angeles: University of California Press, 1972.

[28] ROTMAN, M. Supportive and Palliative Radiation Therapy. *Ca: A Cancer Journal for Clinicians*, 26:293-298, 1976.

[29] RUBIN, P., and CARTER, S. Combination Radiation Therapy and Chemotherapy: A Logical Basis for their Clinical Use. *Ca: A Cancer Journal for Clinicians*, 26:274-292, 1976.

[30] RUBIN, P., and POULTER, C. Principles of Radiation Oncology and Cancer Radiotherapy. In *Clinical Oncology for Medical Students and Physicians: A Multidisciplinary Approach*, 5th ed., ed. P. Rubin, pp. 29-41. New York: University of Rochester, American Cancer Society, 1978.

[31] SARNA, G. Oncologic Emergencies and Urgencies: Recognition and Treatment. In *Practical Oncology*, ed. G. Sarna, pp. 53-77. Boston: Houghton Mifflin, 1980.

[32] SCHMALE, A. Psychological Reactions to Recurrences, Metastases, or Disseminated Cancer. *International Journal of Radiation Oncology*, 1:515-520, 1976.

[33] SMITH, D., and CHAMORRO, T. Nursing Care of Patients Undergoing Combination Chemotherapy and Radiotherapy. *Cancer Nursing*, 1:129-134, 1978.

[34] STEIN, J., and MORGAN, J. General Information Concerning Radiation Exposure. *Applied Radiology and Nuclear Medicine*, 4:71-100, 1975.

[35] TROWBRIDGE, J., and CARL, W. Oral Care of the Patient Having Head and Neck Irradiation. *American Journal of Nursing*, 75:2146–2148, 1975.

[36] UPTON, A. Low-Level Radiation. *Ca: A Cancer Journal for Clinicians*, 29:306–315, 1978.

[37] VARRICCHIO, C. Nursing Care During Total Body Irradiation. *American Journal of Nursing*, 77:1314–1317, 1977.

chapter seven

JOSEPHINE A. GATAN SHIPLACOFF,
R.N., M.N.
Clinical Research Nurse Coordinator
Division of Surgical Oncology
Department of Surgery, UCLA

Concepts in surgical oncology

INTRODUCTION

The general principles of surgical nursing care apply to all patients undergoing surgical therapy for cancer. In addition there are certain considerations unique to the cancer patient that require specialized knowledge in surgical oncology. Therefore, in addition to having a solid foundation in basic medical and surgical nursing, the oncology nurse must possess knowledge of both pathophysiologic and psychosocial principles specific to the care of the cancer patient.

Understanding the theoretical concepts supporting a given plan of surgical therapy is essential in anticipating patient needs and planning care. Furthermore, to communicate confidently and interact effectively with the patient, the family, and other members of the multidisciplinary cancer team, the nurse must be able to discuss the planned therapy and its rationale. An appreciation of the rationale behind surgical treatment choices and procedures is essential for the nurse who wishes to succeed in conveying hope to patients and finding satisfaction in her or his own professional practice.

The concepts presented in this chapter are selected to provide the nurse with an understanding of the theory underlying the surgical management of the patient with cancer.

ROLE OF SURGERY IN CANCER TREATMENT

The oldest cure for cancer is surgery. Despite changing concepts regarding the management of cancer, surgical therapy remains the most frequently used and the most successful modality for cancer treatment today. It is widely used not only for primary treatment but also for diagnosis, staging, palliation, and reconstruction. However, it has become clear that surgery alone has not significantly increased cancer cure rates for common neoplasms during the last three to four decades. This realization of the limited effectiveness of surgery has led to a reexamination of the theoretical basis for this treatment mode. Traditionally surgical treatment for cancer was based on the premise that the disease could be cured if every last tumor cell could be removed from the body. The original theory behind this premise was that cancer is a local disease with lawless, autonomous growth that spreads in an orderly and progressive manner from the primary site to adjacent tissues, to regional nodes by lymphatic drainage, and eventually to distant sites through the circulatory system. The type of operation most likely to bring about a cure would be one whereby the entire tumor and regional lymph nodes lying in the path of its lymphatic drainage were widely excised, in continuity or en bloc. Therefore it seemed logical to attempt progressively superradical operations to achieve a wider margin and thereby remove that last cancer cell. This thinking led to the development of surgical procedures such as transectomy or hemicorporectomy in which the body was severed into halves at the level of the umbilicus for neoplasms involving the lower half of the body. While advances in surgical techniques, anesthesia, and the availability of intensive care units and other supportive care have made such radical operations possible, significant increase in cure rates has not been attained from these radical procedures with few exceptions. Sophisticated techniques and supportive care have made cancer surgery widely available. However, it is now recognized that surgery for cancer is effective only in the treatment of localized primary tumor or regional lymphatics. In most neoplasms occult micrometastases already have been established at distant sites when the primary tumor is clinically detectable. At the time of primary tumor treatment the systemic disease has escaped the confines of the operative field. Thus surgical treatment of malignant tumor is considered a limited type of therapy for cancer [2].

Morton [16] recently proposed the concept of surgery as immunotherapy. Enough evidence has accumulated that neoplasms not only can induce specific immunosuppression but also may suppress nonspecifically the host's immune competence. This immunosuppression is directly related to size of the tumor. Removal of the major bulk of tumor decreases the immunosuppression and gives the host's immune defenses the chance to recover and destroy any microscopic foci of disease. It has been established that the host's defenses can destroy from a small number of tumor cells up to 10 million. The role of surgery, then, is to lower tumor burden, thereby decreasing immunosuppression to allow the patient's own immune response to overcome residual disease. Chemotherapy, radiotherapy, and/or immunotherapy may then be utilized as adjuncts to surgery. The greatest chance for success in the management of cancer now appears to be a combination of surgery with other treatment modalities [7].

Surgery for the management of cancer is employed in four major areas: (1) diagnosis and staging; (2) treatment of the primary tumor; (3) treatment of recurrent and metastatic disease; and (4) palliation.

DIAGNOSIS

Before any definitive therapy can be instituted, a histologic diagnosis must be established. To rule out or confirm a diagnosis of malignancy, a biopsy is performed. There are three methods commonly used: (1) incisional; (2) excisional; and (3) needle.

For small discrete masses about 2-3 centimeters in diameter, such as skin lesions, polypoid lesions of the colon, or thyroid and breast nodules, the procedure of choice is excisional biopsy. Complete excision provides the pathologist with the entire tumor from which to make a diagnosis, and minimizes the possibility of tumor seeding. The excisional method may be used subsequent to an incisional biopsy when a definitive diagnosis cannot be made from tissue obtained by subtotal removal of the tumor mass.

When a tumor is so large that total local excision would compromise definitive surgical resection, an incisional biopsy is performed. An incisional biopsy is the removal of only a portion of the tumor mass. This is the procedure usually performed during endoscopic examination of the bronchus, esophagus, rectum, and bladder, when a piece of the tumor visualized is removed for pathologic examination. It is used for deeper subcutaneous or muscular tumor masses when a diagnosis is not established by a needle biopsy. For an incisional biopsy to be useful it should include a sufficient section of tumor and margin of surrounding normal tissue to provide the pathologist with a representative sample of all tissue involved. A frequent objection to this method is the danger of seeding cancer cells into the operative incision and the possibility of the cells spreading to distant sites through exposed lymphatic channels.

The simplest type and easiest method to perform is the needle aspiration biopsy, in which tissue is aspirated by suction from the suspicious nodule or mass. This can be an excellent method of diagnosis in the hands of an expert cytologist. It creates little disturbance to surrounding tissues, causes little tissue reaction, and is inexpensive. However, interpretation of the specimen requires a great deal of experience. The needle may miss the tumor mass and give a false negative result; or the specimen obtained may be too small and not representative of the tumor. Needle biopsy is used mainly to obtain tissue samples from internal organs such as the liver, kidney, and lung. It may be used also for subcutaneous and muscular masses.

In the head and neck area when the primary tumor is not readily apparent, a careful thorough search for the primary site should be made before any lymph node biopsy is done [26]. Cervical node lymphadenopathy is usually due to metastases from laryngeal, oropharyngeal, and nasopharyngeal tumors. Lymph nodes in the lower third of the neck or the supraclavicular area receive metastases from tumor in the thoracic or abdominal cavity. If a positive lymph node has enlarged to 3 centimeters, the tumor usually is confined no longer to the node but has invaded the perinodal tissue [2,16].

The choice of biopsy type and site should take into consideration subsequent methods of treatment. If a needle biopsy is employed, the needle should be positioned in such a way that the entry site is within the area that would be excised during definitive surgery. The incision for an incisional biopsy should be performed within an area encompassed by the planned surgical procedure. Because tumor cells can contaminate biopsy incisions, it is imperative to include the biopsy site within the subsequent operation. In general, the biopsy should not jeopardize the wider en bloc excision required for locally curative resection.

The tissue obtained should be representative of the total lesion. It should include normal tissue at the tumor margin in order that invasiveness can be evaluated.

The tissue sample submitted to the pathologist must meet certain requirements. It must be: (1) large enough to work with—that is, representative of all tissue involved, including normal tissue adjacent to the tumor tissue; (2) carefully handled to prevent crushing, drying out, or tissue distortion; (3) placed in a fixative solution, usually 10 percent formalin unless examined immediately or otherwise specified by the pathologist; and (4) carefully labeled and submitted with the patient's name, age, sex, clinical diagnosis, gross description of the lesion and site from which the specimen was obtained, and a brief clinical history.

Some tissue samples should not be fixed. These include tissue samples to be tested for estrogen receptors and fresh tissue samples for immunological studies and for special histopathological tissue examinations. Other tissue samples that should not be fixed are those used for in vitro studies of descriptive and functional characteristics of tumor cells. Fresh tissue may be placed in saline or simply in a sterile plastic pouch or container and quickly transported to the laboratory. If such dispatch is not possible, and whenever so specified by the laboratory, tissue samples may be quickly frozen in liquid nitrogen and transported (or stored) in the frozen state. When in doubt it is always a wise practice to verify from the processing laboratory or scientist the desired technique of handling a given tissue specimen. Because research techniques are in a constant evolution, laboratory tests and techniques may change more quickly than nursing procedure manuals.

The interpretation of materials submitted for microscopic examination depends on not only the experience of the pathologist and the quality of the material submitted, but also the clinical history and findings on the patient and a review of any previous biopsy material.

Obtaining tissue for diagnosis may require a thoracotomy or laparotomy. When an abdominal syndrome of suspected neoplastic origin cannot be diagnosed by the usual radiologic or endoscopic procedures, a diagnostic exploratory laparotomy may be necessary. Most frequently it is indicated for malignant lymphoma, particularly in the staging of Hodgkin's disease. An accurate description of the degree of intraabdominal involvement determines the choice of therapy.

STAGING

The importance of careful and accurate staging of the extent of a patient's cancer cannot be overestimated. The stage of a disease (a given point in time in the development and progression of a cancer) determines what treatment modalities are considered appropriate. It is also significant as a prognostic indicator.

A system for the classification and staging of cancer has been developed by the American Joint Committee for Cancer Staging and End-Results Reporting [1]. The TNM system is based on the natural history of a life-span of a cancer. These letters designate marker events in the life history of a cancer. T describes the primary tumor growth; N, local spread to regional lymph nodes; M, distant spread or metastasis. In addition, appropriate suffixes or subscripts to these letters are used to indicate increasing tumor size, degrees of spread, or absence of involvement. Other systems, rather than the TNM system, are used for Hodgkin's disease and lymphoma. Different staging terms are employed, depending on the types of information available for evaluating the extent of disease. These include clinical-diagnostic staging, surgical-evaluative staging and postsurgical treatment-pathologic staging.

Staging of cancer may be limited to clinical-diagnostic, which describes the extent of disease that is clinically evident before definitive treatment is carried out. For inaccessible tumors, however, surgical exploration for an open biopsy, if not for complete resection, provides additional information. Surgical exploration alone or with biopsy provides surgical-evaluative staging, which describes the known extent of disease after the exploration. This type of staging helps to determine resectability and to avoid unnecessary surgery. A postsurgical treatment-pathologic staging following resection of the tumor provides the most accurate and complete staging. Careful staging helps identify homogeneous groups and allows comparison of survival statistics and treatment results generated by various institutions. Randomized surgical adjuvant clinical trials require postsurgical pathologic staging since it is only by careful staging that experimental forms of therapy can be evaluated.

TREATMENT OF THE PRIMARY TUMOR

Once the diagnosis of malignant disease is confirmed by diagnostic surgery, a decision must be made about the specific therapy. If the disease is localized without evidence of spread, the goal of treatment is complete eradication of the local tumor. The time interval between primary diagnosis and treatment is a controversial issue. Argument for immediate surgical excision of a primary tumor is based on the premise that the tumor is excised before tumor cells have time to disseminate. But in almost all tumors this time interval is unknown. Some tumors metastasize very early in the preclinical stage, whereas others reach enormous proportions before any metastases become evident.

Since the extent of disease determines subsequent therapy, time should be taken for the patient to undergo the diagnostic work-up necessary to define the stage of disease. An appropriate plan of therapy based on accurate staging can make a difference in ultimate control of the disease. The knowledge gained by waiting for results of a complete staging procedure can rule out inappropriate treatment and therefore be worth the delay. Furthermore the delay between diagnosis and surgery gives the patient and her family some time to prepare for such an anxiety-provoking event.

The primary goal of all cancer surgery is complete removal of the local tumor as well as an adequate surrounding margin of normal tissue. The rationale for adequate tissue margin is based on evidence that surgical excisions with less than a given amount of normal tissue result in a high recurrence rate even though the tumors appear to be grossly excised. The best opportunity for cure is at the time of the first operation [16]. If the tumor is incompletely excised at the initial operative procedure, tissue planes, lymphatics, and blood vessels are violated and tumor cells seed throughout the wound [30]. This could make recurrence difficult to discern from scarring and could rule out or make subsequent surgical procedures much more complicated.

TREATMENT OF METASTATIC DISEASE

Regional Metastasis and Lymphadenopathy

Cancer kills usually because of its ability to metastasize. This propensity for dissemination is particularly vexing from a surgical point of view. Advances in blood replacement, antisepsis, antibiotics, anesthesia, and intensive care have enabled surgeons to extend the anatomic limits of operative procedures and have increased the resectability of primary tumors. However, despite these advances, all too frequently cancer recurs locally, regionally, or systemically. Knowledge of the manner by which different types of cancer spread is important in planning definitive therapy.

Mechanisms by which different types of tumor favor one route of metastasis over another are unknown. Clinically, epithelial cancers such as squamous cell, breast, colon, and skin metastasize primarily by the lymphatic route, while those of mesenchymal tissue origin such as soft-tissue and bone sarcomas tend to enter the blood stream directly.

Cancer cells can gain access readily to lymphatic channels by permeation and reach lymph nodes through the regional lymphatics. Permeation is the growth of a colony of tumor cells along the course of the lymph vessel [16]. Detached cancer cells find their way to lymph nodes, where they lodge. Lymph nodes can act for a time as traps and partial filters for malignant cells, but eventually they become ineffective in doing so [32]. Since many neoplasms have a propensity for spread through the local lymphatics to the regional lymph nodes, surgical procedures have been devised to encompass regional lymph nodes draining the primary tumor area. When a lymph node containing tumor has enlarged to a 3-centimeter size it is assumed to have invaded the surrounding tissue and lymphatic channels [2,16]. It is generally agreed that en bloc regional lymph node dissection should be performed when lymph nodes are clinically involved by metastatic tumor. This dissection consists of removal of the primary tumor and the regional lymph nodes draining the area, in continuity with all tissues between the tumor and regional nodes. Radical resections with en bloc excision of lymphatics have been designed for the neck, axillary, pelvic, and inguinal areas.

The role of regional lymph nodes in metastasis has been a controversial issue. Equally controversial is the concept of elective or prophylactic resection when the regional lymph nodes are not clinically palpable. Those in favor of performing routine dissection of clinically negative regional nodes close to the primary tumor are supported by the finding that on microscopic examination, excised clinically negative nodes reveal evidence of tumor involvement in 20-40% of carcinomas [5,16]. There is a high rate of local recurrence following excision of grossly involved lymph nodes; and some data support a higher five-year survival rate in patients with only microscopic involvement of lymph nodes compared with those in whom lymph node involvement was clinically evident [5].

Elective regional lymphadenectomy is potentially therapeutic [4,5]. It provides valuable staging and prognostic information. But more accurate histologic determination of the stage of disease is necessary to identify those patients at high risk for disease recurrence who may benefit from this procedure.

Concern has been expressed by some surgeons that removal of normal regional lymph nodes may interfere with the patient's immune response to the tumor. This concern originates from experimental results in animals showing that removal of lymph nodes within one to two weeks after tumor transplantation in an extremity hampered the development of tumor immunity [4,16]. Other experiments have shown that if the regional nodes are removed four to six weeks later there is little influence upon host immunity. It has been reported that removal of regional lymph nodes before a methylcholanthrene-induced tumor was clinically evident did not prevent the development of immunologic sensitization at other lymphoreticular sites [22]. These conflicting reports suggest that timing of nodal excision is important.

Most neoplasms in man have been present in the body for some length of time before becoming clinically evident. Patients have had the opportunity to develop an active systemic response to their tumor as evidenced by the presence of killer lymphocytes in the blood and circulating antitumor antibodies. Based on the natural history of tumor growth, tumors may be considered advanced once they are detectable clinically.

If a regional lymphadenectomy is to be performed, appropriate regional nodes must be included. Important considerations specific to two areas should be noted. Some lymph nodes found within the parotid gland drain the forehead, cheek, and scalp area. Therefore removal of potentially involved nodes in the intervening parotid lymphatics requires a superficial parotidectomy [3]. Tumors in the central or inner quadrant of the breast metastasize to the internal mammary group of lymph nodes. Therefore an operation that does not remove these nodes leaves potential malignancy and does not provide accurate staging information essential for appropriate choice of therapy.

Complications of Regional Node Dissection

Complications associated with regional lymph node dissections are a valid concern. These complications are seen more frequently in groin dissection than in axillary or neck dissection [5]. The most common are wound problems, including seromas, hematomas, cellulitis, infection, abscess, and flap necrosis. Sloughing of the skin graft may require secondary skin grafting. Myocardial infarction and pulmonary embolism also have occurred following inguinal node dissection; and phlebitis may occur.

The most common complication of groin dissection, however, is lymphedema, which can be detected by comparing the circumference of the operated leg with the circumference of the opposite leg measured at the ankle, midcalf, or thigh. A difference of less than 1 inch is considered mild lymphedema; greater than 1 inch is significant. The incidence and severity of lymphedema gradually increase over time; one study showed edema increasing despite diuretics and support stockings [21]. As patients live longer there is an increasing incidence of lymphedema. Few patients feel that lymph node dissection seriously alters their life-style, however, and most do make the necessary adaptation to living with some limitation of activity [5].

Distant Metastases

Although the efficacy of surgery is recognized mainly for treatment of localized primary disease, surgical resection has a definite role in treatment of localized recurrent tumor. Surgical resection of a low-grade, slowly growing malignancy may produce a longer period of remission. It is generally thought that once a neoplasm has metastasized it is no longer amenable to surgical treatment, especially when major organs are involved with multiple lesions. However clinical cure occasionally has resulted from the surgical removal of metastatic lesions in the lung [6,15], liver [24], and, rarely, the brain [23,25]. The role of surgery in the management of such metastatic lesions is increasing, largely due to more clearly defined criteria for patient selection and to availability of more effective surgical adjuvant therapy. Patient selection criteria include tumor doubling time, response to prior therapy for the primary tumor or disease-free interval, histologic type of the tumor, surgical accessibility of the lesion, host-tumor factors, and the presence or absence of other metastatic disease. Surgical adjuvant therapies commonly employed are local radiation therapy and systemic chemotherapy and immunotherapy.

Pulmonary Metastases. Surgical resection may be indicated even in the presence of multiple metastases. Results following surgical resection as favorable in patients with multiple pulmonary metastases as in those with solitary lesions have been reported [6,31]. However, indications for resection of pulmonary metastases have been controversial. The concept of tumor doubling time (TDT) has helped establish criteria for selecting patients who might benefit from this procedure. Several studies have demonstrated that measurement of TDT is an accurate and replicable method for quantifying the rate and pattern of tumor growth in individual patients and for predicting response to pulmonary resection for metastatic disease [6,10,15]. Morton et al. [15] demonstrated that patients with a TDT greater than 40 days may have a 63% 5-year survival rate following surgical resection, whereas patients managed by nonoperative treatment usually will not survive more than two years. Conversely, survival in patients with a TDT less than 40 days was shown to be no more than seven months beyond that expected from nonoperative treatment. It is clear that selected patients with lung metastases can benefit from aggressive surgical therapy.

The histologic type of the pulmonary metastasis is another important criterion for resectability [6]. Carcinomas of the breast, colon, and stomach frequently metastasize to the bones or other organs, whereas sarcomas tend to metastasize to the lung before involving other viscera. Patients with pulmonary metastases from osteogenic sarcoma, fibrosarcoma, and other mesenchymal sarcomas are better candidates for resection. Good response to pulmonary resection for metastasis is obtained when there has been good response to prior therapy for the primary tumor. Patients who have the longest disease-free interval respond better to pulmonary resection.

The immune system status of the patient is another consideration for resectability. Patients who are immunocompetent, as shown by a positive response to dinitrochlorobenzene and to one of the recall antigens, respond better than those in whom immune reactivity is depressed.

Unfortunately the results from resection of liver or brain metastases are not as satisfactory as those obtained from resection of pulmonary metastatic lesions.

Brain Metastases. The efficacy of surgical therapy for intracerebral metastasis is not established. Results of surgical removal have been similar to those of radiation therapy. Although there are no reported controlled studies comparing surgery and radiation therapy in the literature, attempts to compare survival in unmatched patients have shown no statistical differences between radiation and surgery]25]. Despite the prospects of an occasional cure, surgery has no reported advantage over radiation therapy in the quality of survival.

However, surgical therapy for intracerebral metastases may be indicated in some instances. The surgical removal of a solitary intracranial metastasis in a patient carefully selected according to the criteria mentioned above can prolong meaningful life. In this case surgical accessibility of the lesion is a deciding factor. Lesions deep in the midportion of the dominant hemisphere are not accessible.

Hepatic Metastases. The only 5-year cures for liver metastases have been attained with surgical resection [24]. Again prognosis is more favorable in patients selected according to the criteria discussed. Carcinoembryonic antigen levels may be helpful in determining earlier surgical intervention.

Gastrointestinal metastatic carcinomas frequently present with multiple foci of disease which preclude surgical resection. Other approaches to the management of hepatic metastases utilizing surgery are hepatic artery ligation and hepatic artery infusion.

The rationale for hepatic artery ligation or dearterialization for the treatment of metastatic liver tumors comes from the observation that tumors of the liver receive their main blood supply from the hepatic artery [24]. Therefore tying the hepatic artery would lead to anoxia and necrosis of the tumor. Normal liver tissue receives blood from the arterial and portal systems and would not be affected. Viable tumor cells often survive this procedure, however. Portal venous ligation to inhibit survival of tumor cells in the margin of hepatic tumors also has been tried on the principle that the core of the tumor is predominantly supplied by arterial blood whereas the periphery of the tumor is supplied by the portal systems [24]. Hepatic dearterialization has not been shown to improve survival significantly [24]. Because some tumor cells remain viable and proliferate, postoperative chemotherapy becomes necessary to help control tumor growth.

Hepatic artery ligation combined with continuous intraarterial infusion of 5-fluorouracil (5-FU) may be more effective than ligation alone, with or without postoperative systemic chemotherapy [24]. Arterial chemoinfusion allows the administration of large doses of the chemotherapeutic agent directly into the tumor, with minimal side effects. Patients with hepatoma have responded well to the continuous intrahepatic artery infusion of 5-FU [24]. This continuous direct delivery appears to increase the drug's effectiveness. Because 5-FU is a phase-specific agent and since the cells of the metastatic tumor are in various stages of cell maturation, only those cells undergoing cell division and DNA synthesis would be susceptible. The continuous presence of 5-FU offers the greatest chance to eventually attack the total cell population as cells take turns passing into their division phase. The high concentration of drug that can be administered also may induce a higher concentration of active metabolites within the target organ.

This approach can be tolerated well by patients. A catheter is placed surgically in the hepatic artery and brought out through a stab wound incision in the left upper quadrant. It is attached to a portable battery-powered compact infusion pump that delivers a steady flow of drug for up to three days without refilling. Patients and their relatives can be taught to refill the pump and cope with minor problems. The pump may be worn in a slinglike holster above the belt or carried in a conveniently placed pocket devised by the patient. Although the catheter can be placed percutaneously via the brachial or femoral route, direct placement into the hepatic artery through laparotomy results in long-term function and less impairment of normal activity. Despite numerous investigations that used hepatic artery ligation combined with infusion and chemotherapy by regional perfusions, these approaches are still experimental, and agreement about their usefulness is not established.

Other Applications of Surgery

Regional Perfusion. Another method of administering increased concentrations of a chemotherapeutic agent involving a surgical procedure is isolated regional perfusion. The artery and veins supplying the region of the body, frequently an extremity, where the tumor is located are cannulated and isolated from the general circulation and connected to a pump oxygenator to provide extracorporeal circulation. Large doses of the chemotherapeutic agent six to ten times that obtainable by systemic administration then can be administered directly into the tumor-bearing area without entering the systemic circulation. The tumor is perfused for a half-hour to an hour with an arterial perfusate of Ringer's lactate, plasma, or whole blood, and heparin containing high drug concentrations normally too toxic if infused systemically. At the end of perfusion, a fluid not containing drug, usually low-molecular-weight dextran, followed by whole blood, is run through the circuit to wash residual drug from the vessels of the limb. Whenever possible perfusion is performed before excisional surgery when the primary tumor is intact, to prevent tumor cell implantation.

Since it has been shown that hyperthermia has a specific tumoricidal effect and that drug activity is greater at higher temperatures, the arterial perfusate may be heated to a maximum of 41°C [12]. The use of hyperthermic perfusion with chemotherapeutic agents has been investigated in the management of satellitosis from malignant melanoma and primary or recurrent sarcomas of the extremities [11, 12]. Adjunctive chemotherapy by hyperthermic perfusion may decrease the necessity of amputation and permit a more conservative surgical resection of primary and recurrent sarcomas. A large fixed tumor normally amenable only to amputation may be reduced to a smaller lesion which then can be locally excised. Cure rates of more than 50% at 5, 10, and 15 years have been reported with the use of this technique in sarcomas of the limbs [12].

Arteriovenous Shunt. Another application of surgical therapy is the creation of an arteriovenous shunt, similar to that used in hemodialysis patients, for long-term chemotherapy [2]. A problem frequently encountered by oncology nurses is the difficulty of finding a suitable vein in a patient whose accessible veins have collapsed after prolonged drug infusion. For some patients with this potential problem who require long-term chemotherapy, creation of an arteriovenous fistula may be indicated.

"Second-Look" Operations. Additional resection may be successful in controlling recurrent soft-tissue sarcomas, colon cancer, and some carcinomas of the skin.

Wangensteen [14] advocated routine second-look operations at designated intervals for patients with gastrointestinal cancers, whether symptomatic or not. Although the purpose for these procedures was to assess the adequacy of the initial surgical operation for the primary tumor, therapeutic results were obtained.

Second-look operations have not gained wide acceptance, however, because of the problem of deciding when the procedure is indicated. Recently serial carcinoembryonic antigen levels have been used to determine reexploration for adenocarcinoma of the colon [14]. Results of this study showed an increase from 27% to 78% in resectable recurrent tumor found at the time of the second-look procedure.

─────────────── **SURGERY FOR PALLIATION** ───────────────

There is a point when surgery fails as the ultimate hope for cure. When cure is no longer possible, surgical procedures may be indicated to relieve the distressing symptoms of cancer, to reduce the severity of the patient's illness, to prolong a useful, comfortable life, or to improve quality of the patient's life. Palliative operations may be performed to relieve pain, control hemorrhage, or remove an obstruction, ulceration, or source of infection. Severe pain may be relieved by permanent nerve blocking, and a cordotomy may be necessary when pain becomes intractable. Depending on the site of the obstruction, a colostomy or gastrojejunostomy may be done. Bleeding such as is seen in tumors of the bladder can be controlled by cystectomy. The removal of an infected, ulcerated breast tumor even in the presence of widespread metastases would contribute definitely to the patient's comfort and might eliminate a source of psychological discomfort.

─────────────── **TECHNICAL CONSIDERATIONS** ───────────────
IN CANCER SURGERY

Although the techniques of cancer surgery are similar to those of general surgery, there are a few techniques and considerations specific to cancer surgery to minimize the "dose" of cancer cells disseminated iatrogenically. These techniques are designed to prevent local recurrence, cancer cell implantation, and vascular dissemination at surgery [8,28,30].

The most important operative technique for cancer is wide excision employing a three-dimensional approach to the tumor. Some neoplasms such as soft-tissue sarcoma and gastric carcinoma may spread widely by infiltration into adjacent tissues. A significant distance may exist between the apparent tumor margin and the microscopic tumor margin [30]. A normal tissue margin wide in length, width, and depth between the line of excision and the tumor mass ensures a complete local excision and prevents violation of the tumor space and its microscopic local extensions. A wide margin therefore acts as a protective barrier against spillage of tumor cells into the open vascular and lymphatic channels. In a wide en bloc excision of tumors previously biopsied, it is especially important to remove prior biopsy incision lines or the needle track from aspiration biopsy.

Incomplete removal or spillage of cancer cells into the operative site may result in local tumor recurrence. Several techniques have been tried to prevent implantation of cancer cells into the operative field. Cytotoxic or cytolytic solutions such as 0.5% formaldehyde, hypotonic saline, sodium hypochloride solution, nitrogen mustard, sterile water, and thiotepa have been used to irrigate the wound following surgery. During the operation the edges of the incisional wound are protected with a plastic drape to prevent cell contamination. When there is a second operative procedure or site involved at the time of tumor excision, all gloves and instruments used for the first procedure are replaced with sterile ones. The operative field is reprepared after a preliminary biopsy before the main operation.

Tumor cells may be transplanted from the primary tumor to a distant site. Instances of tumor transplantation to a distant skin graft site have been reported [16]. Measures to prevent dissemination of tumor cells during operation include: (1) the "no-touch" technique; (2) early ligation of the blood supply; and (3) application of tourniquets to the extremities prior to biopsy.

Although every metastasis grows from a tumor embolus, not every tumor embolus becomes a metastasis. The presence or absence of circulating cancer cells in the blood of cancer patients preoperatively has been demonstrated to have very little effect on prognosis [27,28]. However there is a correlation between prognosis and the presence of circulating tumor cells seen during and after an operation [27].

Manipulation of the tumor mass can release a shower of cells into the lymphatics and blood. Manipulation must be minimized not only during the operative procedure but also in the preparation of the skin prior to actual resection. The size of the incision also can contribute to excess or minimal manipulation. The incision should permit the necessary wide margin without undue handling.

The no-touch technique does not allow the surgeon to see or touch the tumor directly. The surgical excision is performed with a preconceived idea of the margins to obtain adequate normal tissues.

The precise effectiveness of these various techniques is theoretical and controversial. Higher survival rates have been reported, however, in left colon cancer using a combination of wide excision, minimal manipulation, and early ligation of the vascular pedicle [29].

PREOPERATIVE ASSESSMENT OF RESECTABILITY AND RISKS

The preoperative and postoperative care of patients undergoing cancer surgery is basically the same as for all other surgery patients. As with any type of surgery, preoperative assessment includes a complete history and physical examination. The physiological, psychological, and technical parameters influencing the performance and outcome of surgery are evaluated. Some determinants of resectability already have been included in the discussion of metastases. The emphasis here is on general considerations specific to cancer surgery.

The decisions to perform an operation and to what extent are based on several factors related to the tumor, the patient, and the treatment team. These considerations also will determine the goals of treatment.

Tumor Factors

Surgical therapy for cancer cannot be performed rationally without an understanding of the natural history and biologic behavior of the specific tumor. Tumor factors to be considered are the histologic type, stage, size, and anatomical location of the primary tumor. Certain histologic types of tumor are not amenable to surgical resection. For instance, surgeons generally consider undifferentiated small cell carcinoma of the lung as unresectable disease except in very rare situations [19]. This tumor usually is widespread at the time of initial evaluation. However, the availability of multimodal therapy and effective surgical adjuvant therapy may eventually define the role of surgery in the treatment of this disease.

The stage of disease not only has prognostic implications but also determines treatment. Unnecessary surgery can be prevented by knowing the extent of disease spread. In the presence of fixed, large, involved nodes and widespread metastatic disease, surgical therapy alone is not effective. Large tumors tend to have necrotic centers and a poor blood supply. Unlike chemotherapy and radiation therapy, surgical therapy does not require an excellent blood and oxygen supply to maximize its effectiveness. Therefore large localized tumors are best treated with surgical excision.

Anatomical location is another important tumor consideration. Surgery may be inadvisable if major vascularity is suspected in the tumor, as in the brain, or if major blood vessels are involved such as in cancer of the lung involving the aorta. Tumors may be located at a strategic place such as the dominant side of the brain, or may be present at multiple sites in essential organs, for example the liver, so as to render surgery a major threat to function.

Patient and Family Resources

Before any surgical procedure is undertaken, the patient and her family resources are assessed. The patient must be physically able to tolerate an operative procedure. The availability of physical and emotional support from the family constellation needs to be established. The general health of the patient can be assessed from her medical history. Cardiopulmonary problems, recent cerebrovascular accident, or uncontrolled diabetes may preclude surgical intervention due to the associated high postoperative mortality. Age is another important consideration, although in terms of general health and ability to survive an operation physiologic age is much more important than chronologic age. Surgical procedures are better tolerated than radiation or chemotherapy by older patients because the physiologic insult from an operative procedure has a shorter duration.

The meaning of a specific operative procedure to the patient will influence her willingness to undergo the procedure. The different body areas involved carry different qualities of emotion-laden meanings for different patients. The patient's reaction to impending surgery in a given body area will determine her acceptance of the operation and eventual adaptation to her illness.

The patient's nutritional status may adversely affect the outcome of surgery [13]. Nutritional support may be required before and after surgery, especially in debilitated and cachectic patients. Extensive surgical procedures in malnourished patients may be associated with significant complications and death. Enteral or parenteral hyperalimentation is a major advance in providing adequate nutritional support to cachectic patients prior to an operation. The therapeutic value of nutritional support has been established in the long-term management of intestinal fistulas, inflammatory intestinal disease, and following massive resection of the small intestines [9,20]. The use of parenteral hyperalimentation or an elemental diet prior to surgery is primarily intended to prevent wound complications. But whether hyperalimentation, particularly of short-term duration, is truly useful in enhancing wound healing in malnourished subjects is controversial and little information is available. In one experimental animal study, amino acid therapy was associated with a significant improvement in the tensile strength and collagen content of abdominal wounds, but had little effect on the healing of skin wounds or colonic anastomoses [9]. Significant changes in wound healing occurred only in the presence of a severe degree of malnutrition when weight loss was greater than one-third of the normal body weight. Experimental studies have shown that collagen synthesis and wound healing may be delayed in the presence of malnutrition, but the extent to which this occurs in various degrees of malnutrition is not known.

In the past there was some concern that alimentation or a high caloric intake would benefit the tumor more than the host. This fear has not been substantiated by experience. Patients cachectic from carcinoma of the esophagus or those experiencing severe effects following radiation therapy have a lower incidence of complications and death following a surgical operation when supported by enteral or intravenous hyperalimentation [9].

Treatment Team

Once the decision for surgical therapy has been reached on bases of biology and location of the tumor, stage of disease, the patient's age, her general health, and her psychosocial status, the next step in decisionmaking depends on availability of a treatment team to carry out successfully the mandate for operation. Successful management requires surgeons who not only are technically well versed in the complex operative procedures for cancer but also understand tumor biology. Ideally these surgeons should be part of a multidisciplinary team that includes other surgical specialists, medical oncologists, radiotherapists, immunologists, psychologists, oncology nurses, social workers, and others involved in the care of the cancer patient. The outcome of a successful operation should include the eradication of cancer, satisfactory physiologic function, good cosmetic results, and psychologic adjustment to any conditions which may fall short of these ideals.

CONCLUSION

For the first time in several decades there has been a diminution in the death rate for breast cancer patients. Holmes [7] attributes this and other dramatic improvements in nonseminomatous testicular tumors, Wilm's tumor, Hodgkin's disease, lymphomas, osteogenic sarcoma, Ewing's sarcoma and other soft-tissue sarcomas to multi-modality therapy and surgical adjuvant therapy. Surgical oncology plays a central role in cancer management. The acceptance of its limitations has led to recognition that the best chance for cure is through the combined efforts of different disciplines concerned with the problem of cancer and the lives of those afflicted by it.

Total cancer management with curative therapy as the goal is based on a basic knowledge of tumor biology, a clear understanding of the concepts of multimodal therapy and surgical adjuvant therapy, and awareness of rapidly developing concepts in oncology.

REFERENCES

[1] AMERICAN JOINT COMMITTEE FOR CANCER STAGING AND END RESULTS REPORTING. *Manual for Staging of Cancer.* Chicago: American College of Surgeons, 1977.

[2] EILBER, F.R. Principles of Cancer Surgery. In *Cancer Treatment,* ed. C.M. Haskell. Philadelphia: Saunders, 1980.

[3] EILBER, F.R. and STORM, F.K. Surgical Procedures for Diseases of the Neck. In *Head and Neck Surgery and Its Reconstruction,* ed. M.A. Lesavoy. Philadelphia: Saunders, in press.

[4] FORTNER, J.G.; WOODRUFF, J.; SCHOTTENFELD, D.; and McLEAN, B. Biostatistical Basis of Elective Node Dissection for Malignant Melanoma. *Annals of Surgery,* 186:101-103, 1977.

[5] HOLMES, E.C.; MOSELEY, H.S.; MORTON, D.L.; CLARK, W.; ROBINSON, D.; and URIST, M.M. A Rational Approach to the Surgical Management of Melanoma. *Annals of Surgery,* 186:481-490, 1977.

[6] HOLMES, E.C., and MORTON, D.L. Pulmonary Resection for Sarcoma Metastases. *Orthopedic Clinics of North America,* 8:805-810, 1977.

[7] HOLMES, E.C. What's New in Oncology? *Bulletin, American College of Surgeons,* 24-27, 1980.

[8] HOOVER, H.C., Jr., and KETCHAM, A.S. Techniques for Inhibiting Tumor Metastases. *Cancer,* 35:5-14, 1975.

[9] IRVIN, T.T. Effects of Malnutrition and Hyperalimentation on Wound Healing. *Surgery, Gynecology and Obstetrics,* 146:33-37, 1978.

[10] JOSEPH, W.L.; MORTON, D.L.; and ADKINS, P.C. Prognostic Significance of Tumor Doubling Time in Evaluating Operability in Pulmonary Metastatic Disease. *Journal of Cardiovascular Surgery,* 61:23-31, 1971.

[11] KOOPS, H.S.; OLDHOFF, J.; VAN DER PLOEG, E.; VERMEY, A.; EIBERGEN, R.; and BEEKHUIS, H. Some Aspects of the Treatment of

Primary Malignant Melanoma of the Extremities by Isolated Regional Perfusion. *Cancer*, 39:27-33, 1977.

[12] KREMENTZ, E.T.; CARTER, R.D.; SUTHERLAND, C.N.; and HUTTON, I. Chemotherapy of Sarcomas of the Limbs by Regional Perfusion. *Annals of Surgery*, 185:555-564, 1977.

[13] MEGUID, M.M., and MOORE, F.D. Homeostasis and Nutrition in the Surgical Patient: Metabolic and Endocrine Response to Injury. In *Practice of Surgery*. Hagerstown,: Harper & Row, Medical Department, 1978.

[14] MINTON, J.P.; JAMES, K.P.; HURTUBISE, P.E.; RINKER, L.; JOYCE, S.; and MARTIN, E.W., Jr. The Use of Serial Carcinoembryonic Antigen Determinations to Predict Recurrence of Carcinoma of the Colon and the Time for a Second-Look Operation. *Surgery, Gynecology and Obstetrics*, 147:208-210, 1978.

[15] MORTON, D.L.; JOSEPH, W.L.; KETCHAM, A.S.; GEELHOED, G.W.; and ADKINS, P.C. Surgical Resection and Adjunctive Immunotherapy for Selected Patients with Multiple Pulmonary Metastases. *Annals of Surgery*, 178:360-366, 1973.

[16] MORTON, D.L.; SPARKS, F.C.; and HASKELL, C.M. Oncology. In *Principles of Surgery*, ed. S.I. Schwartz, 3rd ed. Philadelphia: Saunders, 1979.

[17] MORTON, D.L. Changing Concepts of Cancer Surgery. *American Journal of Surgery*, 135:367-371, 1978.

[18] McCARTHY, J.G., HAAGENSEN, C.D.; and HERTER, F.P. The Role of Groin Dissection in the Management of Melanoma of the Lower Extremity. *Annals of Surgery*, 179:156-159, 1974.

[19] MOUNTAIN, C.F., McMURTREY, M.J. and FRAZIER, O.H. Current Results of Surgical Treatment for Lung Cancer. *The Cancer Bulletin*, 32:105-108, 1980.

[20] NEALON, T.F.; GROSSI, C.E.; and STERER, M. Use of Elemental Diet to Correct Catabolic States Prior to Surgery. *Annals of Surgery*, 180: 9-13, 1974.

[21] PAPACHRISTOU, D., and FORTNER, J.G. Comparison of Lymphedema Following Incontinuity and Discontinuity Groin Dissection. *Annals of Surgery*, 185:13-16, 1977.

[22] PENDERGRAST, W.J.; SOLOWAY, M.S.; MYERS, G.H.; and FUTRELL, J.W. Regional Lymphadenectomy and Tumor Immunity. *Surgery, Gynecology and Obstetrics*, 142:385, 1976.

[23] POSNER, J.B. Management of Central Nervous System Metastases. *Seminars in Oncology*, 4:81-91, 1977.

[24] RAMMING K.P.; SPARKS, F.C.; EILBER, F.R.; and MORTON, D.L. Management of Hepatic Metastases. *Seminars in Oncology*, 4:71-80, 1977.

[25] RANSOHOFF, J. Surgical Management of Metastatic Tumors. *Seminars in Oncology*, 2:21-27, 1975.

[26] RAZAK, M.S.; SAKO, K.; and MARCHETTA, F.C. Influence of Initial Neck Node Biopsy on the Incidence of Recurrence in the Neck and Survival in Patients Who Subsequently Undergo Curative Resectional Surgery. *Journal of Surgical Oncology*, 9:347–352, 1977.

[27] ROBERTS, S.S.; HENGESH, J.W.; McGRATH, R.G.; VALAITIS, J.; McGREW, E.A.; and COLE, W.H. Prognostic Significance of Cancer Cells in the Circulating Blood. *American Journal of Surgery*, 113:757–762, 1967.

[28] SALISBURY, A.J. The Significance of the Circulating Cancer Cell. *Cancer Treatment Reviews*, 2:55–67, 1975.

[29] STEARNS, M.W., Jr. Surgical Aspects of Colorectal Cancer. *Seminars in Oncology*, 3:399–405, 1976.

[30] SUGARBAKER, E.V., and KETCHAM, A.S. Mechanisms and Prevention of Cancer Dissemination: An Overview. *Seminars in Oncology*, 4:19–32, 1977.

[31] TELANDER, R.L.; PAIROLERO, P.C.; PRITCHARD, D.J.; SIM, F.H.; and GILCHRIST, G.S. Resection of Pulmonary Metastatic Osteogenic Sarcoma in Children. *Surgery*, 84:335–341, 1978.

[32] WEISS, L. A Pathobiologic Overview of Metastasis. *Seminars in Oncology*, 4:5–17, 1977.

chapter eight

MAIRE FRIEL, R.N., M.N.
Assistant Clinical Professor
Teaching in Graduate Nursing
Oncology Program
School of Nursing, UCLA

Concepts related to the nursing care of surgical oncology patients

INTRODUCTION

The comprehensive nursing care of surgical oncology patients is a challenge that requires an integration of theoretical knowledge, sensitivity, and clinical skills. Surgery is exciting because, as a treatment, it can offer the ultimate hope of cure for a variety of cancer patients. The purpose of surgery as a curative treatment is simply to remove every cancer cell. Theoretically, this prevents risk of metastasis. Ideally, this can be achieved most effectively when early diagnosis reveals a very small solid tumor that is surgically accessible. Fears, fantasies, and hopes are intertwined as surgical oncology patients face the reality of cure or palliation and adapt to the changes in their physical appearance, body function, or both. Problems emerge and the nurse is called upon to intervene effectively. What nursing problems face the surgical oncology patient? How does the nurse intervene effectively? Answers to these questions may seem complex and yet are critical in the care of patients today.

This chapter attempts to reduce the complexity of the situation by highlighting concepts related to the nursing care of surgical oncology patients at a variety of time periods. The cancer patient's association with surgery as a treatment modality may include the following time frames: (1) decision-making period (diagnostic work-up and treatment choice); (2) preoperative period; (3) postoperative period; and (4) postdischarge and follow-up. (See Fig. 8.1.) Nursing care will be discussed in each time frame by describing the unique and significant variables confronting the surgical oncology patient, general behavioral responses, general nursing problems, appropriate nursing goals, and selective nursing interventions. Although each time period can be described separately, surgical oncology patients are seen in a variety of settings and must adapt to the changes confronting them at various rates and intensity. Therefore, it is important to keep in mind that these time periods often overlap and are rarely identical for each patient.

Since each patient responds in an individual manner to cancer and surgery as a treatment, the general concepts presented in this chapter can be used only as assessment and interventive guidelines. The surgical nurse faces the charge of tailoring the assessment and interventions to meet each patient's particular needs.

DECISION-MAKING PERIOD

The decision-making period includes both the diagnostic work-up and the treatment choice. When patients enter the work-up period, various diagnostic procedures can be utilized to detect with various degrees of accuracy the presence of cancer, its size, its histological type, and the extent of spread. Therefore, the detection, classification, and staging of primary cancer as well as the monitoring of metastatic disease are components of the diagnostic work-up. These components are essential in deciding whether or not surgery is possible as a treatment choice for patients.

Diagnostic Work-up

During the diagnostic work-up, the first major concern for patients is the possible diagnosis of cancer. The two major questions facing patients at this time are: Do I have cancer? If I do have cancer, can it be removed and can I be cured? These questions and their answers represent a threat of severe loss to patients and trigger a variety of grieving responses. One or more of the following reactions are usually displayed: denial, anxiety, anger, guilt, depression, fear, and dependency.

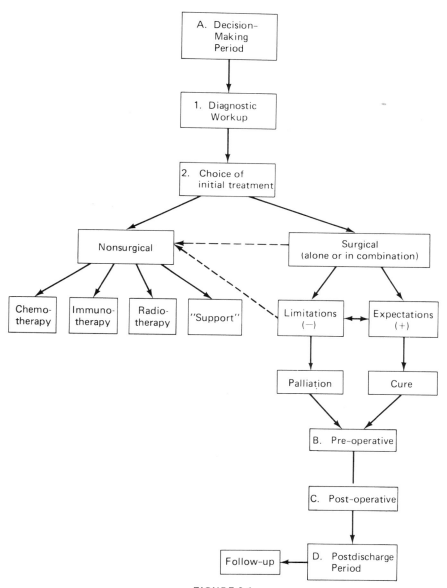

FIGURE 8.1

229

Patients who face the diagnosis of cancer, even with the option of surgical intervention, are apt to present with a variety of physiological, psychological, or social nursing problems. The tumor may be causing physiological problems requiring symptom relief by the nurse. Possible physiological problems include fatigue, pain, change in bowel habits, malnutrition, abnormal changes in mental status and equilibrium, an irritating cough, and decreased use of a limb. A diagnosis of cancer is often considered a direct threat to a patient's self-concept. This threat can be intensified with the additional fear of invasive surgery. Cancer surgery can be quite extensive in order to remove all of the cancer cells locally as well as in sites which are considered high risk for metastasis. Regional lymph nodes are often dissected (see Chapter 7 for more details). The patient's perception of actual threat may be real or be distorted by fear. Grieving is considered a normal behavior prior to an anticipated loss. However, reactions to the potential losses associated with the diagnosis of cancer and surgery can result in disorganized patterns of activity. Strong dependency needs are experienced and, if unmet, will develop into specific nursing problems. During the diagnostic phase, patients must also adapt quickly to a variety of roles including the "cancer patient" role. Patients may anticipate that cancer and its surgical treatment will cause significant losses or changes in family, career, and social roles.

Crisis is commonly assessed as either an actual or potential nursing problem during the diagnostic work-up. The general statement of crisis as an actual nursing problem may be written as follows: situational crisis related to the inability to cope with the diagnosis of cancer and possible surgery resulting in refusal to seek proper surgical or medical treatment. An appropriate nursing goal for this problem is stated in Table 8.1. Nursing interventions based on crisis intervention must be implemented immediately in order to reduce the crisis and increase appropriate coping behavior. The intent of these interventions is not to force patients into accepting treatment but, rather, to allow patients an opportunity to learn about the available medical and surgical options.

Crisis intervention can be utilized effectively to prevent crises from occurring or to resolve a crisis as quickly as possible. Aguilera [1] uses a crisis intervention paradigm that is very practical in clinical situations. Very simply, a person is confronted with a stressful situation (for example, diagnosis of cancer) that disrupts a normal state of equilibrium. The person experiences disequilibrium (for example, severe grieving reaction) and feels the need to restore equilibrium. There are three major factors which influence the person's

TABLE 8.1
General Nursing Problem with a Nursing Goal
during the Diagnostic Work-up Period

Problem

Situational crisis related to the inability to cope with the diagnosis of cancer and possible surgery resulting in refusal to seek proper surgical or medical treatment.

Goal

Patients will demonstrate a decrease in crisis behavior and an increased ability to cope with the diagnosis of cancer as evidenced by seeking proper surgical or medical treatment.

---

ability to regain equilibrium. These factors include: (1) a realistic perception of the event; (2) adequate situational support; and (3) adequate coping mechanisms. If one or more of these factors are missing, disequilibrium continues and crisis ensues. Nursing interventions are aimed at restoring the balancing factors that are absent, strengthening the balancing factors that are weak, and reinforcing the balancing factors that are strong.

In order to implement effective interventions, the nurse needs to assess, plan, and intervene carefully. Simple and direct questions may be asked to *assess* information regarding: (1) the event that is causing the disequilibrium; (2) the patient's perception of the event; (3) the patient's situational supports; (4) the patient's coping mechanisms; and (5) the patient's suicidal and homicidal potential. Next the nurse *plans* and sets goals for intervention based on the analysis of the data obtained in the assessment. In analyzing the plan of action, variables such as the degree of disruption, meaning of the stressful situation, and the patient's strengths are discussed. A tentative explanation as to the cause of the crisis is proposed. After the interventions are carried out, *evaluation* of their effectiveness takes place and any necessary follow-up is provided [1].

How can crisis intervention be used to help patients face the diagnosis of cancer and get them out of crisis as soon as possible? A clinical case study may be useful to answer this question.

Case Study I. This is the first hospitalization for Mr. C., a 38-year-old Jewish male admitted for a diagnostic work-up of a right lung nodule detected 5 days earlier on a routine chest X-ray. Since admission, Mr. C. has undergone several diagnostic tests including chest tomograms, sputum cytologic studies, a bronchoscopy, and biopsy. A very small epidermoid carcinoma of the right lung was found. Additional diagnostic tests to determine metastasis were negative. No chest symptoms are present. Mr. C. has no other medical problems. His physician recommends surgery and is hopeful that a right lobectomy will be a curative treatment. Mr. C. was told a tentative prognosis. A 40–50%, 5-year survival is predicted following surgical resection for early lung lesions detected on chest X-rays without evidence of metastasis. It is hoped that with the use of adjuvant therapy the prognosis will improve. Mr. C. is married and lives with his wife and three children, ranging in age from 5 to 10 years. He is the editor of a successful local community newspaper. His father, who lives out of state, is alive and well. His mother died from metastatic breast cancer two years ago. He has two married brothers who live in the area. They have not been told that Mr. C. is in the hospital because "They will worry too much."

Mr. C. states that he is feeling very depressed and anxious. His symptoms since the X-ray results include insomnia and anorexia, inability to concentrate, and feelings of hopelessness and failure. Mr. C.'s appearance is unkept. His medium-length hair is uncombed. He has not shaved in 4 days. Mr. C. states that he feels really sloppy but he just doesn't have the energy to do anything about it. His hands are shaky and sweaty. He has a dull, depressed facial expression and a rather flat, low tone of voice. His wife works during the day but visits for a short time in the evening. She tries to give Mr. C. support but finds the situation very frustrating and often leaves angry and in tears.

Mr. C. refuses to discuss the possibility of surgery. He is packing his suitcase so that he and his wife can go on a month cruise "to forget it all." He also states, "I'm used to telling others what to do— I'm not about to have someone tell me what to do." He continues, "What's the use of surgery, I'm going to die anyway. I don't have a chance. My mother died of cancer and I will too. What good will I be to my wife or children? The surgery is going to be so painful and I won't be able to breathe very well after the operation. Those breathing machines make so much noise and can explode at any time. I bet if I use one after surgery, my stitches would rupture. No, I don't want to talk to anyone about surgery. I just want to leave."

A *nursing assessment* would reflect a patient who is faced with many diagnostic tests and finally a diagnosis of epidermoid carcinoma of the right lung with a possible 40–50% 5-year survival after surgical resection. Mr. C. experienced a state of disequilibrium (severe anxiety, depression, denial) after the first chest X-ray and it continues without relief. He feels the need to restore some equilibrium but does not have the energy to do so. Mr. C.'s perception of the event is extremely distorted. He appears to believe that any type of cancer, no matter the type, site, or extent of metastasis, means sudden death and even surgery cannot change this. Mr. C. has some situational support from his wife. However, the wife's ability to provide a great amount of support at this time is questionable. Mr. C.'s coping mechanisms do not seem to be working well, probably due to the great fear of cancer. Mr. C.'s suicidal and homicidal potential needs to be assessed.

An *analysis* of the situation determines that there is a great degree of disruption in Mr. C.'s life which is creating a nursing problem. He drifts between acute situational denial, depression, and anxiety. The resulting behavior (refusal to seek proper treatment) is considered maladaptive. For further analysis and planning, the nurse must assess in greater detail several variables which may be contributing to the crisis. The following questions may be asked. What is the meaning of the diagnosis to Mr. C.? Did Mr. C. complete the grieving process after the death of his mother? Are Mr. C.'s culture or value systems contributing to the crisis in any way? What are Mr. C.'s future expectations? (His present expectation is that he will die.) What current or future losses does he perceive and what meaning do these losses have for him? (For example, Mr. C. may feel loss of control, loss of the father and husband role, loss of life.) The goal is set: Mr. C. will demonstrate a decrease in crisis behavior and an increased ability to cope with the diagnosis of cancer as evidenced by: (1) remaining under surgical and medical care; and (2) demonstrating an increased understanding of treatment modalities available to him.

A three-prong *plan* based on crisis intervention was initiated to: (1) educate Mr. C. and his wife regarding his diagnosis, prognosis, and expected outcome of surgical resection; (2) provide support to Mr. C.'s wife so that she can offer more effective support to her husband; and (3) strengthen Mr. C.'s own coping mechanisms. These general interventions will be discussed more comprehensively and in more detail throughout the chapter. In this case, the nurse helped Mr. C. verbalize his fears and sort out what was real and unreal. Mr. C. was then able to learn about his diagnosis, the anticipated result of surgery, and other available treatment modalities. The nurse reinforced Mr. C.'s ability to intellectualize which appeared to be an effective coping mechanism. The nurse also gave Mrs. C. an opportunity to discuss the fears and anxieties she was experiencing because of her husband's illness. The nurse offered Mrs. C. specific suggestions and agreed to meet with her every day. Mrs. C. became more relaxed and was able to spend more time talking with her husband. A decrease in angry outbursts and crying led to a feeling of mutual support.

The nurse *evaluated* the effectiveness of her interventions and observed that Mr. C. was less anxious and depressed (out of crisis) and agreed to remain under his physician's care. Additionally, Mr. C. described a very realistic picture of his disease, found it easier to cope with new stressors, and accepted the support of his wife.

The nurse was very effective in assessing, planning, intervening, and evaluating. At this time she may want to provide follow-up by reinforcing Mr. C.'s more adaptive behavior, especially during times of increased stress.

As seen in the case study, the nurse cannot take away the diagnosis of cancer, nor can the nurse offer surgery as a chance for cure when cancer is metastatic. The nurse can, however, mobilize the balancing factors in the crisis intervention paradigm that are necessary for adaptation to the stress associated with the diagnosis and possible surgical treatment of cancer. Patients who learn how to successfully cope with stress or crisis during the diagnosis period usually demonstrate adaptive behavior more readily during other periods of their treatment course.

Treatment Choice

The second major component of the decision-making period is referred to as the treatment choice. The surgeon may offer patients the hope of cure through surgical treatment, either alone or in combination with other treatment modalities. The factors that the surgeon must consider in making this decision have been discussed in Chapter 7. If the surgeon does propose surgery as a feasible treatment choice, patients move into the second phase of the decision-making period. Now patients evaluate whether or not surgery is the best possible treatment available to meet their individual needs. Patients base this evaluation on the simple concept of benefits versus risks. What are the expected benefits or positive expectations? What are the expected risks or complications? The physician who offers surgery as an option for treatment has already weighed the benefits and risks. The physician's recommendation for surgery is certainly an important influencing factor in the decision made by patients. However, patients should not accept surgery simply because it has been recommended. Patients have a right to be actively involved in the decision-making process. The amount of involvement patients want in the decision-making process varies and is a critical consideration.

The nurse's role complements the physician's role in obtaining an informed consent from patients. The nurse is a key person who can assist patients in making an informed decision regarding a choice of treatment which they feel is in keeping with their individual value system. Oftentimes, patients experience a great amount of ambivalence caused by intense feelings and lack of clear-cut answers. Patients also seem to fear that their families, friends, and even the health team may not support them if there is a difference in opinion about the treatment choice. A general nursing problem that covers this area of concern during treatment choice is identified in Table 8.2. Nursing goals and suggested nursing interventions are also outlined. Further discussion of Interventions 1 through 4 is appropriate.

TABLE 8.2
Nursing Problem during the Treatment Choice Period
with Suggested Nursing Goals and Interventions

Nursing Problem

Acute situational anxiety related to the ambivalence in deciding on the treatment choice which meets individual needs and which will elicit continued support from others.

Nursing Goals

1. Patients will make a rational decision that meets individual needs.
2. Patients will feel support from medical and nursing staff, family, and significant others after the decision regarding surgical treatment is made.
3. Patients will experience a lower level of anxiety.

General Nursing Interventions

1. Explore with patients their expectations related to the benefits and risks of the surgical procedure.
2. Teach the patients about the significant factors necessary to make a rational decision.
3. Reinforce available coping mechanisms so that patients can continue to deal effectively with the inherent emotional reactions and make rational decisions.
4. Support patients and encourage families and significant others to support them after the choice is made.
5. Allow catharsis of feelings associated with the anxiety.

Treatment Choice Period: Nursing Intervention 1. The positive expectations and limitations (benefits and risks) of the proposed surgical treatment must be explored with patients. A nurse cannot effectively do this without a sound understanding of the medical benefits and risks. Patients have a natural tendency to ask general questions about their prognosis. "Is it going to do any good?" It is critical for the nurse to know if the surgery is being done for cure or palliation. Palliation and cure are terms that appear to be very clear, yet in relation to surgical oncology may be confusing and ambiguous to the patient. Cure cannot be guaranteed but certainly can be aimed at. Patients are forced to weigh the past surgical success with their general type and size of tumor against the emotional and physical risks involved. Nurses need to reinforce the positive surgical results and discuss the realistic risks.

Patients also ask questions about their chance for survival. "Can I make it?" The risk of surgery itself is an issue that is carefully considered by the surgeon and yet is often frightening for patients. For example, patients who have had vague symptoms for a long time may be in a debilitated state and feel hesitant to take any more physiological stress.

Concerns about the quality of survival after surgical treatment are both realistic and important. Surgical intervention does offer cancer patients a hope for long-term survival. Some of these surgical procedures, however, cause both immediate and long-term changes that require an alteration in life-style.

The nurse needs to assess how patients perceive the risks involved with surgery and how significant these risks are to them. Problematic areas of change may include: (1) severe physiological alterations which may cause a loss of normal body function (colostomy or ileal conduit, for example); (2) threats to a person's self-concept resulting in fears of mutilation and rejection; (3) an increase in dependent behavior (following an amputation, for example), or a forced increase in independent behavior (such as self-care of a newly acquired colostomy or ileal conduit) that is unacceptable to the patient; (4) loss of roles which are significant to the patient (for example, a boy who gives up his role on the school football team after a disarticulation of a lower extremity).

Patients who take an active part in the decision-making process weigh the benefits and risks differently. Some patients carefully scrutinize the balance between the risks and benefits and are consciously in touch with the possible changes. Other patients gamble the quality of life for the chance of cure. Most patients will probably fall between the two ends of this continuum. There seems to be a fine line between scaring patients about possible changes and giving them information in order to make a conscientious choice. The next intervention discusses the nurse's role in providing pertinent information to the patient.

Treatment Choice Period: Nursing Intervention 2. An individualized teaching plan can be initiated by the nurse to: (1) validate or reinforce what the patient has learned from the physician or other sources regarding the surgical benefits and risks; (2) correct any misunderstanding of information the patient has learned regarding the surgical benefits and risks; and (3) discuss available methods that can help the patient adapt to the changes created by cancer surgery. The last goal of the teaching plan may give patients enough hope to feel that they can adapt to the physiological losses anticipated by the proposed surgery. Frequently, patients know the chance for survival and the likely insult to the body without knowing what is available to counter the insults of surgery. They would be encouraged to know, for example, that breast and limb prosthetics have improved considerably in physical appearance, comfort, and function; that reconstruction surgery for cancer patients is becoming more refined and acceptable; that support groups have rapidly been forming throughout the nation and are available to patients and families who need this type of emotional support; and that more and more health team members are aware of the specific sexual needs of patients following cancer surgery and are qualified and available to do sexual counseling for this patient population.

Treatment Choice Period: Nursing Intervention 3. *Coping* can be defined as individual responses to new situations and challenges that may become potential or actual threats [16]. The nurse assesses what coping mechanisms patients are trying to utilize at this time and evaluates their effectiveness. It is very important that the nurse reinforces the coping mechanisms that are functional. Reinforcement provides feedback and encourages patients to continue coping with the stress felt during the decision making period. Coping mechanisms will be discussed again later in this chapter.

Treatment Choice Period: Nursing Intervention 4. The fourth intervention flows directly from the other three interventions in principle and practice. All patients need emotional support from the health team and significant others after they have made a decision regarding treatment choice. Patients may not always agree with the decision felt to be best by the health team, family, or friends. It is crucial to remember that the health team and significant others need not support the decision but must continue to support and accept the patient. Feelings of abandonment by the health team and family can be quite devastating. Family members may need assistance from the nurse to help them accept and support the patient when the patient's decision is contrary to the family's choice of treatment.

In summary, during the decision-making period, patients are faced with the diagnosis of cancer, the option of surgical treatment, and the decision to accept or reject the proposed surgical treatment. The nurse's role is to mobilize emotional and physical strength so that after a diagnosis of cancer, patients can decide if surgery is the treatment that offers them the highest quality of life.

PREOPERATIVE PERIOD

Patients who accept the option of surgery move at various speeds into the preoperative period. The time spent in the hospital immediately prior to surgical treatment is considered the preoperative period. The time between the decision-making period and the preoperative period varies considerably. Both can occur simultaneously since some patients receive the initial diagnosis of cancer at the time of surgery. Other patients receive an initial diagnosis of cancer prior to the surgical treatment through the use of diagnostic biopsies. Whatever the particular situation, there are similar concerns that confront most cancer patients during the preoperative time.

A major concern for the patient at this time is not knowing the exact extent of invasion. Physical examination, lab tests, radiography tests, and biopsies are certainly valuable in assessing the *possible* extent of local spread and invasion. However, confirmation is often made at the time of surgery. Patients who have negative metastatic diagnostic work-ups may still end up with positive findings during surgery. Preoperatively, therefore, patients not only face the threat of impending surgery, but they also face the uncertainties of the surgical outcome. The extent of spread (local and metastatic) found during the surgery after a thorough examination for tumor invasion and metastasis is a key factor in performing curative, palliative, or simply exploratory surgery.

Emotional responses due to the anticipated surgical losses are very active at this time. Denial may become less effective as the patient physically prepares for the impending surgery in the hospital setting. Fear, anxiety, and depression increase as denial decreases.

Feelings of guilt and anger may also be expressed. Sutherland [24] has studied patients undergoing surgery for cancer. He found that "the initial concern about the nature or seriousness of the illness frequently gives way at the time of hospitalization to anxiety focused on the impending operation" [24]. Patients seem to be concerned with death in surgery, injury from surgery, and the effect of injury on their life-styles. Sutherland also found that "fears of inacceptability and of isolation can be greater sources of depression than fears of recurrence . . ." [24]. He concluded that anxiety appears to be more prevalent with patients who do not have specific and accurate knowledge about the operation [24]. The information presented by Sutherland provides a good basis for selective nursing interventions initiated during the preoperative period. Significant variables that can affect the patient's ability to adapt preoperatively are outlined in Table 8.3. Every preoperative nursing assessment should examine these variables to some degree. Although some of these variables overlap, each variable will be discussed separately.

Available Coping Mechanisms

Assessment of the patient's available coping mechanisms during the preoperative period will be similar to the assessment made during the treatment choice period. The nurse will need to assess the effectiveness of the patient's available coping mechanisms. How did the patient cope with the diagnosis of cancer and the decision to undergo surgical treatment? Were new coping mechanisms initiated at that time; or were past coping mechanisms effective? Are the patient's available coping mechanisms assessible in the hospital preoperatively?

TABLE 8.3
Significant Variables Included in the
Preoperative Nursing Assessment

1. Available coping mechanisms
2. The anticipated purpose of surgery (cure or palliation)
3. The type of proposed surgery (extent of mutilation and anticipated loss of functioning in valued life activities)
4. Expected prognosis
5. Physical well-being (including nutritional status and physical reactions to preoperative chemotherapy and/or radiation therapy)
6. Family support
7. The meaning of the surgery to the patient and family

Are the patient's available coping mechanisms effective against the amount of stress found in the preoperative period?

The Anticipated Purpose of Surgery

As mentioned earlier, cancer surgery can be done with the intent of cure, palliation, or exploration. The nurse must know the anticipated purpose of surgery in order to accurately assess the meaning of surgery for each patient. Both positive and negative behavior may reflect the patient's response to the anticipated surgery and the meaning it takes on. The stakes are high for cancer patients who have a chance at cure. Surgical insult on one's body may be more acceptable when the chance for cure is great. Patients with hope for cure seem to get more in the long run for their surgical incision! On the other hand, cancer patients anticipating palliative surgery may not be thinking about the possible extent of metastasis as much as they are thinking about the relief that surgery may bring. For these patients, palliative surgery is acceptable. A third situation illustrates maladaptive behavior: A male cancer patient in for palliative surgery is extremely depressed. He hides under the sheets and refuses any nursing care. His hope for cure has been shattered by a positive metastatic work-up. Palliative surgery represents a kiss of death to him. The meaning of the proposed surgery is devastating to the patient.

Type of Proposed Surgery

Concerns and fears preoperatively can be associated with the type, site, and extent of mutilation caused by the proposed cancer surgery. Anticipated loss of body function in valued life activities may be very difficult for some patients to cope with. Other fears and concerns, such as fear of pain, inability to manage postoperatively, discontinuance of family support, altered sexuality, and a decreased quality of life, may also be influenced by the type of proposed surgery. Responses by patients to the threat of a particular surgical procedure are greatly influenced by the value they have placed on the effective body part or its function. The greater the value placed on a particular body part, the greater the loss that will probably be experienced when it is altered by surgery. During the preoperative period, patients anticipate this loss and experience anticipatory grieving appropriate to the felt loss. Nursing problems occur when the amount of grieving is not appropriate to the anticipated loss or the patient is unable to cope with the amount of grieving experienced.

Expected Prognosis

In addition to facing the fears of surgery, patients also contend with a statistical prognosis. These patients have already dealt with this variable during the decision-making period. Anxiety may be intensified during the preoperative period since surgical findings may confirm or refute the information used to predict an expected prognosis. Patients may feel caught between optimistic hopes for cure and fear of further metastasis.

Physical Well-Being

Patients enter the preoperative period in a variety of physical conditions. Physical symptoms caused by the malignancy may be present such as bowel obstruction, diarrhea, pain, fatigue, malabsorption, anorexia, weight loss, bleeding, dysphagia, nausea and vomiting, or a decreased function of a body part.

Psychosomatic symptoms related to bereavement following a diagnosis of cancer may occur. Parkes [17] describes such symptoms as "loss of appetite and weight, difficulty in sleeping at night, digestive disturbances, palpitations, headaches, and muscular aches and pains. . . ."

There is still another factor that influences the patient's preoperative physical condition and must be considered. For some disease entities, preoperative chemotherapy or radiation therapy or both are given to reduce the number of cancer cells and consequently decrease tumor bulk in some cases. The side effects caused by such treatment modalities can leave patients with less strength and energy to ward off the other physical and emotional problems confronting them in the preoperative period.

Family Support

During the preoperative period many patients are afraid that needed family support will not be available. Some patients question their ability to be loved by anyone; others fear family rejection. Patients who are accustomed to having family members as support in times of stress will be at lower risk for crisis during the preoperative period if the family members are available and able to be supportive. Patients who do not depend on family members for support will usually need alternative support. The nurse must assess the support available and intervene accordingly.

The Meaning of the Surgery to the Patient and Family

The meaning of the proposed cancer surgery to patients and families will certainly be influenced by all of the six variables discussed above. The nurse continues the assessment by finding out more specifically what the cancer surgery means to patients and their families. Preoperatively, patients probably do not realize the full meaning of cancer surgery, even though they may know the diagnosis, prognosis, and expected surgical procedure. Answers to questions about physical, psychological, and social changes will help patients sort out the meaning of cancer surgery to them. A systematic preoperative nursing assessment based on a model or theoretical framework is useful in providing this information.

Problems and Interventions in Preoperative Period

Problems occur preoperatively when patients are unable to adapt effectively to the changes facing them. Three hypothetical problems and three proposed nursing goals are identified in Table 8.4. Many

TABLE 8.4
Nursing Problems during the Preoperative Period
with Appropriate Nursing Goals

Nursing Problems

1. Acute situational anxiety related to the uncertainties of the impending cancer surgery resulting in an unsatisfactory understanding of the preoperative teaching or treatment plan.
2. Severe loneliness related to the unmet need for family support resulting in feelings of sadness and isolation.
3. Poor nutritional intake related to tumor growth resulting in delay of surgery.

Nursing Goals

1. Patients will decrease their anxiety and increase their coping mechanisms to a level that would enable them to learn the necessary preoperative teaching or treatment plan at a satisfactory level.
2. Patients will experience decreased feelings of loneliness, sadness, and isolation, and increased feelings of support by family members.
3. Patients will increase their nutritional intake to a level that is sufficient for them to undergo surgery.

242

nursing interventions from a variety of disciplines may be utilized to achieve the identified goals. This discussion on nursing interventions during the preoperative period will focus on understanding the problem of anxiety more clearly and serve as a guideline for more specific patient problems.

Nursing interventions may be activated to decrease an *actual* problem of acute anxiety or to prevent a *potential* problem of acute anxiety for patients in the preoperative period. In order to intervene more effectively, an understanding of anxiety is required. Sharon Roberts [20] ties together two ideas about anxiety (Portnoy's and Peplau's) that seem to reflect the type of anxiety often experienced by oncology patients at this time. According to Portnoy [19], anxiety is a natural phenomenon experienced when values essential to one's existence, sense of being, and identity are threatened. Peplau [18] categorizes these threats as: (1) threats to biological integrity; and (2) threats to the self system. As stated earlier, patients, prior to cancer surgery, face threats to their biologic integrity such as loss of normal body function, mutilation, and possible extensive invasion. These biological threats related to cancer surgery often disrupt the patient's self system. Patients may fear that negative changes will damage their body image, self-esteem, personal relations, role function, and amount of desired independence.

No matter how skilled one is, a nurse cannot take away the anxiety from patients who face a potentially significant loss. Anxiety is an appropriate response to this threat. However, the nurse can intervene to help patients keep anxiety at a level which is functional for them. It is functional for patients to understand the essential components of the preoperative teaching and treatment plan. However, as indicated in Table 8.4, high-level anxiety interferes with the ability to learn. The nursing interventions are directed at the problem of coping with the anxiety and the major uncertainties of surgery.

Suggestions for nursing interventions include:

1. Acknowledge to patients the right to have intense feelings at this time.
2. Reassure patients that at times they need to express these feelings (catharsis) and that it is all right to do so.
3. Reassure patients that the nursing staff is sensitive to the general needs of surgical oncology patients and is qualified and available to talk with them about such concerns if and when they would like to discuss them.
4. Begin to establish trust with patients.
5. During the admission assessment, obtain general information

about the meaning of the diagnosis and surgery to the patients. Try to find out what patients know, think they know, and want to know about the diagnosis and the surgical plan. This assessment should be the beginning attempt at identifying the felt threats to biological integrity and the self system.

6. Clear up misconceptions patients have regarding the implications of their diagnosis and proposed treatment regime. Provide information that will give patients hope when appropriate. Although this intervention appears rather simple, it is difficult to achieve without clinical experience and a strong knowledge base in cancer and its treatment.

The next three interventions will be discussed in more detail with general clinical application. Interventions can be applied to other nursing problems.

7. Teach patients pertinent information that may decrease the uncertainties about the diagnosis and treatment in a manner that takes into consideration individual needs. The physician is usually the first person who describes the surgical procedure to patients. The nurse's role is to reinforce what the physician has said about the surgical procedure and to discuss the surgical preparation, immediate postoperative activities, methods to control lost body function after surgery, and goals for rehabilitation. The information must be presented in a manner that elicits realistic hope. Teaching strategies must be tailored to meet patient learning needs and are influenced by several factors as shown in Table 8.5. Suggestions for teaching preoperative cancer patients can be found in Table 8.6.

TABLE 8.5
Factors To Be Considered in the Development
of an Individualized Teaching Plan

1. What the patient knows
2. The patient's intellectual ability
3. What the *patient* feels is important to know
4. What the *nurse* feels is important for the patient to know
5. The patient's coping mechanisms
6. The amount and type of anticipatory grieving the patient is experiencing at the time
7. How the patient is physically feeling at the time

TABLE 8.6
Suggestions for Teaching Patients Prior to Cancer Surgery

1. Establish a rapport with the patient based on trust, honesty, and concern.
2. Assess the patient's learning needs and level of knowledge.
3. Set teaching goals.
4. Create an environment which offers privacy and is free from interruptions by use of learning labs, private guest rooms, offices, pulled curtains, "Do not disturb" signs on the door, and careful timing of visits by team members.
5. Teach in fairly short time periods if attention span is short or if information is emotionally charged and difficult for the patient to comprehend.
6. Use visual aides and provide examples to better explain the information.
7. Attend to emotionally charged issues.
8. Repeat information frequently.
9. Provide frequent positive reinforcement in order to strengthen correct behavior, to give praise, and to provide knowledge of results [4].
10. Evaluate the patient's acquisition of knowledge during the teaching session and after the instruction is completed.

8. Mobilize coping mechanisms, reinforce available coping mechanisms, and try new coping mechanisms that may be more effective for patients in the present situation. It is sometimes necessary for the nurse to point out to patients that they have coping mechanisms. Together, they can identify available coping mechanisms. The nurse can encourage patients to use what has worked for them in the past. The nurse needs to reinforce patients when their coping behavior has been successful. If usual coping mechanisms are ineffective or not feasible in the hospital setting, the nurse must offer alternative methods to patients so they can handle the felt stress. Two examples will illustrate how a nurse can either alter an existing coping mechanism or teach new coping behavior to patients.

Example 1: Ms. A. copes with stress by taking long walks by herself. The nurse obtains patio privileges for Ms. A. The nurse and Ms. A. schedule times when it would be feasible for Ms. A. to be off the floor without interrupting her care. At this time, Ms. A. could walk at least to and around the patio by herself.

Example 2: Mr. B. copes with stress by going to his health spa and relaxing in the sauna. The nurse offers to teach Mr. B. a progressive relaxation exercise that he could do by himself in his room or bath.

9. Identify the members of the patient's support system and encourage them to provide support. The family is frequently the major support system for patients throughout their confrontation with cancer and can be effectively utilized to maintain or restore equilibrium during crises [1]. Barbara Giacquinta [8], however, raises an important point: "But an entire family may be in crisis because one of its members is diagnosed as having cancer." The fears and hopes of surgical treatment add significantly to the stress of the family. Members of the family experience grief themselves, and like the patient, fluctuate between denial, anger, depression, anxiety, guilt, and dependency. If the nurse wants to mobilize family support, the family must avoid going into crisis. What does it mean to the family to have one of its members face surgery for malignancy? An ongoing family assessment can find out the answer to this question. Ideally, a family assessment should be started preoperatively in order to plan for postoperative care and rehabilitation. Information about the family may also be available from nursing assessments made during the decision-making period. Often, the preoperative time is limited and a complete family assessment is impossible. A short family assessment with key questions may be most appropriate for many cases. Since family assessment, mobilization, and support is a continuous process, a preoperative assessment is only one step in the total nursing involvement with the family. Key family assessment questions that may be asked preoperatively are found in Table 8.7. Answers to these questions give the nurse guidelines to work from in order to encourage family support through counseling, reinforcing adaptive or supportive behaviors, problem solving, and teaching.

The nurse's role in family *counseling* varies. Basically, the nurse attempts to establish trust and encourages the family members to express their feelings about the diagnosis and the impending surgery. The nurse: (1) is able to acknowledge understanding and acceptance of the family's feelings; (2) may discuss alternative ways with the family to cope with the stress if present coping mechanisms are not working well; (3) may also need to guide the family members through the process of more effective communication with the patient and the physician. It is extremely important for the nurse to convey a message of concern and support.

The nurse can also positively *reinforce the family* for both

TABLE 8.7
Family Assessment Questions

1. What are the immediate changes confronting the family due to the patient's diagnosis of cancer and impending surgery?
2. How has the family handled stressful situations in the past?
3. What are the individual responses of the family members to the patient's diagnosis of cancer and planned surgical treatment?
4. What is the family's normal interaction pattern? (Focus on the amount of open and honest communication in the family system.)
5. Is the family supportive to the patient at the present time?
6. In what ways would the family members like to be more supportive to the patient?

adaptive or supportive behavior. Reinforcement provides the family with knowledge of results they might not have noticed (for example, a subtle but positive change in the patient's behavior), and also incentive to continue with their support.

Simple problems may become major problems for families during the stressful preoperative period. The nurse is called upon to help prevent or *solve a variety of problems* ranging from recommending local hotels, churches, and restaurants to finding a day-care center for children. Orientation to the hospital facilities and introductions to the health team can prevent unnecessary problems by setting the scene of a caring and competent staff which evokes trust. The family and nurse together can assess how the family's normal coping and supportive behavior can fit into the hospital setting. The nurse can also help prevent communication problems (especially regarding the results of surgery) between family and surgeon by setting up a single communication system for the family while the patient is in surgery. The family should know who they can talk to about the patient's progress during surgery and where they can meet the surgeon for a report immediately following surgery.

When follow-up care involves a family member, it is customary for that family member to get involved in the preoperative *teaching program*. It seems reasonable to expect that good preoperative teaching with the primary family care giver regarding the vague and somewhat complex responsibilities of home care, would increase the patient's sense of support by the family member and may ease to some extent the threat of loss.

In summary, during the preoperative period, oncology patients and their families face the threat of impending surgery and the uncertainties of metastatic spread and the hope for curative surgical treatment. Behavior is affected by significant variables that reflect the overall meaning of the cancer surgery to patients and their families. Nursing interventions are explored with emphasis on reducing anxiety, increasing coping behavior, teaching, and providing support.

POSTOPERATIVE PERIOD

The postoperative period (extending until discharge) brings with it additional problems that require adaptation by patients. During the postoperative period, the nurse cares for patients who have undergone a wide variety of surgical procedures to treat a local, a regional, or in selective cases, a metastatic malignancy. Surgical procedures vary according to the: (1) type, site, and extent of cancer; (2) the capabilities and experience of the surgeon; (3) the health team available to support the surgeon; and (4) the patient's physical and psychological makeup.

Many patients come out of surgery with questions about the malignancy of their tumor, the extent of spread, and the extent of surgery. Did you get it all? did you remove my ___ (breast, bladder, leg, or other organ)? With the use of frozen sections, patients have the opportunity to face the initial surgical results immediately after surgery. Most surgical oncology patients face one of the several surgical findings that are found in Table 8.8. Anxiety sprinkled with denial, hope, and pain pervades this time period in wait for the final pathology report, which is usually available in 3 to 5 days.

TABLE 8.8
Postoperative Surgical Findings

1. A benign tumor
2. An excisible lesion without evidence of metastasis
3. An excisible lesion with questionable metastasis
4. An excisible lesion with lymph node metastasis
5. An unexcisible lesion due to extensive direct invasion
6. An unexcisible lesion due to distant metastasis
7. An excisible metastatic lesion with curative intent
8. An excisible primary or metastatic lesion with palliative intent

Postoperative nursing care is directed toward physiological, psychological, and social adaptation. Patient behavior, nursing problems, goals, and nursing interventions will be integrated into a nursing assessment that covers these three areas of postoperative care.

Physiological adaptation to cancer surgery requires skilled nursing care in order to prevent or minimize postoperative complications. Patients who receive chemotherapy or radiation therapy or both, either preoperatively or postoperatively, may be at higher risk for developing complications such as tissue damage and immunosuppression. Physiological problems are more difficult to detect when a patient's immune system is compromised. Therefore, careful observation for early signs and symptoms of potential problems is an essential nursing task.

Some of the nurse's major postoperative physiological concerns include:

1. Wound assessment
2. Pulmonary assessment
3. Peritoneal assessment
4. Urinary assessment
5. Gastrointestinal assessment
6. Pain assessment
7. Nutritional assessment

A synopsis of these major physiological assessment areas is found in Tables 8.9 through 8.15 [7,10,14,23]. These charts are intended to serve as a guide for implementing quality nursing care following cancer surgery. Information on specific interventions can be found in many nursing texts.

Many factors seem to influence physiologic adaptation following cancer surgery. A nursing assessment should include the following factors:

1. Diagnosis (primary site, cell type, extent of spread)
2. Surgical procedure
3. Other treatment modalities utilized
4. Psychological make-up of patient (including behavior and social changes caused by cancer and surgical treatment)
5. Physiological make-up of patient (for example, nutrition status)

Self-concept is likely to change after experiencing cancer surgery. Self-concept is defined as "The composite of belief and feelings that

TABLE 8.9
Wound Assessment

High Risk Variables	Problems	Signs and Symptoms	General Nursing Interventions
Poor vascularity to surgical incision Bone marrow suppression due to radiation therapy and/or chemotherapy	1. Hematoma	Swelling Pain within first 24 hr. after surgery	Check incisional site for swelling, discoloration Report to physician immediately Apply pressure to surgical site Check patency of drain
Tissue damage and/or poor tissue healing due to chemotherapy, radiation therapy, and/or poor nutritional status	2. Seroma	Swelling Pain	Measure amount of drainage Check for clots and change in color or consistency Check vital signs
Obesity	3. Infection	Usually occur 3–4 days after surgery Increased pulse rate Low grade intermittent fever Edema and redness of wound Undue pain	Check vital signs Check blood count Check wound site Check amount, color, odor, and consistency of drainage Administration of antibiotics Place on wound isolation Check orders for wound care Send specimen for culture and sensitivity

4. Lymphadema secondary to lymph node dissections	Swelling of affected limb	Elevate affected limb No BP or venapuncture on affected arm Encourage progressive exercise of affected limb Check for infection secondary to lymphedema External compression—usually after wound heals and reduction of swelling (e.g., heavy duty, elastic stockings, alternating air compression) Teach importance of good hygiene
5. Dehiscence (disruption of several layers of the wound) Evisceration (escape of viscera from the abdominal or thoracic cavity)	Sudden onset of serosanguineous drainage "Popping sensation"	Check amount and color of drainage Call physician immediately Check vital signs Prepare patient for surgery (after dehiscence or evisceration occurs) After evisceration apply sterile moist towels over extruded intestine or omentum Check use of abdominal binders for prevention in obese patients

TABLE 8.10
Pulmonary Assessment

High Risk Variables	Problems	Signs and Symptoms	General Nursing Interventions
Thoracic and upper abdominal operations Surgical interference with normal respiratory tract History of obstructive pulmonary airway disease Heavy smoking Prolonged immobility, abdominal pain, and abdominal distention Discomfort and fear of chest tubes and other respiratory equipment Bone marrow suppression due to chemotherapy and/or radiation therapy Tissue damage and/or decreased tissue healing due to poor nutrition, radiation therapy, chemotherapy, and/or disease process	1. Atelectasis (collapse of a lung segment or lobe) 2. Aspiration pneumonia	Fever usually within 48 hr. after surgery Tachypnea Moderate tachycardia Fever Dyspnea Tachypnea Tachycardia Hypotension Frothy and blood tinged sputum Decreased lung sounds	Check splitting, rales, and breath sounds Encourage coughing and deep breathing Change positions, mobilization Perform nasotracheal suctioning P.R.N. Provide pain relief Check vital signs Use humidifier Culture and sensitivity of sputum Emergency medical treatment—call physician immediately Check vital signs Administer antibiotic therapy Respiratory support Culture and sensitivity of sputum Perform nasotracheal suctioning P.R.N.

Examples of Surgical Treatment		
1. Pneumonectomy		
2. Lobectomy		
3. Head and neck surgery and tracheostomy		
Special Nursing Concern: Care of chest tubes		
3. Staphyloccal and other types of pneumonia	Fever Systemic toxicity Respiratory difficulty Consolidation and rales	Check pulmonary status. Encourage coughing and deep breathing Change positions Perform nasotracheal suctioning P.R.N. Administer antibiotic therapy Provide positive pressure ventilation Culture and sensitivity of sputum
4. Pulmonary embolism and pulmonary infarction	Usually occur 7–10 days after surgery Rising respiratory and pulse rate inconsistent with degree of fever Sudden onset of dyspnea and anxiety Hemoptysis Pleuritic pain Less severe dyspnea	Call physician immediately (medical emergency) Check vital signs Administer anticoagulation therapy Bedrest in Fowler's position Administer oxygen

TABLE 8.11
Peritoneal Assessment

High Risk Variables	Problems	Signs and Symptoms	General Nursing Intervention
Tissue damage and/or decreased tissue healing due to chemotherapy, radiation therapy, poor nutritional status, and/or tumor	1. Peritonitis secondary to breakdown of anastomotic suture line	Moderate to severe abdominal pain (unless masked by incisional pain and potent analgesic)	Check central venous pressure
			Check hourly urine output
		Burning ache aggravated by any motion, even respiration	Care for nasogastric tube
			Administer intravenous fliud replacement
		Anorexia, nausea, and vomiting	Administer antibiotics
Ischemia, hemorrhage, mucosal eversion, infection		Temperature, chills, thirst, and scanty urine	Check respiratory status
			Provide oxygen set-up
Bone marrow suppression due to chemotherapy and/or radiation therapy		Inability to pass feces or flatus, and abdominal distension (symptoms of adynamic ileus, which is secondary to the peritonitis)	Check vital signs
			Preoperative preparation
			Check laboratory tests
Tension of suture line		Tachycardia, with weak thready peripheral pulses	Administer analgesics
Excessive free peritoneal fluid		Rapid and shallow respirations	Provide wound isolation
		Decreased BP, subnormal temperature, and septic shock	Provide wound care
			Check amount and type of drainage
Examples of Surgical Treatment			
1. Esophagogastrectomy	2. Intraabdominal abscesses secondary to localized collection of leakage from the operative site	Frequently gradual onset after recovering from surgery	
2. Ileal conduit		Pale, weak, anorectic	
3. Colectomy		Abdominal distention, vomiting	
4. Gastrectomy		Increased temperature, blood and WBC count	
5. Colostomy			
6. Pancreaticoduodenectomy			

TABLE 8.12
Urinary Assessment

High Risk Variables	Problems	Signs and Symptoms	General Nursing Intervention
Surgery on urinary tract	1. Urinary retention	Bladder distention	Check amount of urine output
Bone marrow suppression due to chemo-		Low urine output	Check bladder distention
therapy and/or radiation therapy			Check abdominal pain
Tissue damage and/or poor tissue healing	2. Renal failure	Urine output less	Check amount of urine output
due to chemotherapy, radiation therapy,		than 30 cc/hr.	Monitor cardiovascular function;
and/or poor nutritional status			correct hypovolemia with ad-
Decreased bladder capacity secondary to			ministration of plasma or blood
radiation therapy and/or surgery			Check vital signs
			Check fluid and electrolyte im-
Examples of Surgical Treatment			balance
1. Segmental resection of the bladder			
2. Ileal conduit	3. Urinary tract infection	High fever	Check urine output—amount,
3. Nephrectomy		Flank tenderness	color, specific gravity, odor
		Pus or bacteria seen	Check vital signs
		in urine	Check abdominal pain
			Force fluids
			Administer antibiotics

255

TABLE 8.13
Gastrointestinal Assessment

High Risk Variables	Problems	Signs and Symptoms	General Nursing Interventions
Surgery on gastrointestinal tract with one or more anastomosis sites	1. Paralytic ileus	Quiet and distended abdomen (no flatus) Gastric aspiration: (a) green to yellow fluid at 1–2 liters every 24 hr. (paralytic ileus); (b) dark brown or black fluid (bowel obstruction)	Provide nasogastric care—suctioning and decompression Check abdominal distention Check bowel sounds Check bowel tenderness Administer fluid and electrolyte replacement Check for nausea, vomiting, and constipation Check vital signs
Sepsis			
Bone marrow suppression due to chemotherapy and/or radiation therapy			
Peritonitis			
Tissue damage and/or decreased tissue healing due to decreased nutrition, radiation therapy, chemotherapy, and/or disease process	2. Postoperative intestinal obstruction	Vomiting Abdominal cramps Constipation	See Problem 1 in Table 8.11
Adhesions due to radiation therapy			
Examples of Surgical Treatment	3. Peritonitis secondary to defects in anastomosis	See Problem 1 in Table 8.11	
1. Bowel resection			
2. Colostomies			
3. Ileostomy			

TABLE 8.14
Pain Assessment

High Risk Variables	Problems	Signs and Symptoms	General Nursing Interventions
Type, site(s), extent of surgical procedure Patient's perception of his pain, which may be influenced by certain variables: Anxiety Environment Social interaction patterns Meaning of the pain to the patient Knowledge of pain and pain-relief methods General body condition Availability and administration of analgesics Past pain experience Coping mechanisms Cultural orientation	1. Acute post-operative	Uncomfortable sensation, which may vary in *intensity*, from mild to excruciating, *type*, such as stabbing, throbbing, or spasmodic, and *duration*, such as intermittent or continuous *Physiological Responses:* Increased pulse and respiration rates Increased blood pressure Pallor Dilated pupils Increased muscle tension Possible nausea Decreased body movement *Facial Expressions:* Sober expression Facial tightness and contortions	Provide comprehensive pain assessment; manipulate variables that are increasing patient's perception of pain Be accountable for pain relief; medicate promptly, adequately, and with most effective drug; medicate before pain is acute Offer alternative pain relief measures in conjunction with analgesics; e.g., distraction, relaxation, guided imagery

TABLE 8.15
Nutritional Assessment

High Risk Variables	Problems	Signs and Symptoms	General Nursing Interventions

Poor preoperative nutritional status
Cancer surgeries that interfere with the mechanical process of eating
Cancer surgeries that interfere with absorption of essential salts and nutrients
Radiation therapy that results in taste alterations, decreased amount of saliva, dysphagia, nausea/vomiting
Chemotherapy that results in nausea and vomiting, anorexia
Depression
Anorexia, constipation
Nausea and vomiting causing fluid and electrolyte imbalance, sensory impairment, anemia and fatigue
 	
Examples of Surgical Treatment
1. Head and neck surgeries
2. Subtotal gastrectomy
3. Pancreatectomy
4. Extensive resection of the small bowel
	1. Malnutrition	*Physical Symptoms of protein–calorie malnutrition:*
		Edema
		Dyspigmentation of the hair
		Easy pluckability of the hair
		Muscle wasting
		Flaky-paint rash
		Dermatosis
			Check anthropometric tests
			Check biochemical analysis
			Check dietary analysis
			Check clinical examination
			Nutritional assessment:
			  Check problem area
			  Check food preferences
			  Check patterns and behavior related to food intake
			  Check intake and output
			  Check calorie count
			Provide relief from nausea and vomiting with use of antiemetics
			Encourage good mouth care
			Provide relaxed environment without pain
			Check presentation of food
			Encourage family to bring in favorite food
			Work with dietician to provide *diet* and and *supplements* that meet patient's needs
			Care for and monitor intravenous total parenteral nutrition
			Care for feeding tubes
			Provide nutrition teaching for patient and family before discharge

one holds about oneself at a given time, formed from perceptions particularly of others' reactions, and directing one's behavior" [6]. During the postoperative period, the ability of patients to adapt to the changes in their self-concept is influenced by : (1) the actual and perceived body changes; (2) feelings expressed in the grieving process; and (3) the perception of how others are reacting to the physical changes.

Physical changes in appearance and function due to cancer surgery can be quite extensive in an attempt to achieve cure. For the most part, wide excisions of the involved area, lymph node dissections, diversions, grafts, amputations, mastectomies, and resections continue to contribute to both the internal and external physical changes felt by patients following cancer surgery. Advancements in the surgical treatment of cancer attempt to find procedures that can achieve maximum effectiveness and minimal physical loss.

Patients react to these changes and often experience grief over losses that may be actual, imagined, or anticipated. Such losses include: (1) loss of significant others; (2) loss of self-image; (3) loss of a valued object; and (4) loss of function. The meaning of the losses experienced by patients will influence their grieving response and ultimately their adaptation to changes in self-concept.

For many families and friends, this will be their first experience with extensive cancer surgery. They, too, are frightened about the physical changes as well as their own reaction to these changes. Patients who are trying to adapt to a change in self-concept are very sensitive to the reactions of their families, friends, and even the health team. Sexual expressions of affection may be altered by the surgical procedure, the environment, and fears of the patient or significant other. It seems critical that patterns of sexual communication are initiated postoperatively as a means of comforting the patient who is experiencing such feelings as grieving, loss of control, shame, and helplessness. These feelings are caused by threats to one's body image and can lead to low self-esteem and maladaptive patterns of behavior.

A major nursing problem in the postoperative period can be described as acute grieving related to feelings of low self-esteem caused by physical or functional losses from cancer surgery resulting in the inability to perform necessary postoperative activity. Nursing interventions for this problem are aimed at manipulating, to the patient's advantage, those factors that influence self-concept such as perception of body change, ability to grieve, and reactions of others. See Table 8.16 for a description of selective nursing interventions.

TABLE 8.16
Postoperative Nursing: Self-Concept

Nursing Problem

Acute grieving related to feelings of low self-esteem caused by physical or functional losses from cancer surgery resulting in the inability to perform necessary postoperative activity.

Nursing Goal

Patient will demonstrate a more functional level of grieving and increased feelings of self-esteem as evidenced by performing necessary postoperative functions at a satisfactory level.

Nursing Interventions

1. Discuss with patients the meaning that the physical changes have for them including any fears (real or symbolic) about physical or personal losses.
2. Provide a supportive relationship to patients based on concern, trust, and acceptance.
3. Identify and reinforce effective coping behavior.
4. Accept and acknowledge the painfulness of the situation.
5. Allow patients to express and experience grieving in a safe environment.
6. Provide realistic yet hopeful education to patients regarding postoperative management, physical appearance, physical and sexual functioning, role changes, and alterations in interdependency.
7. Positively reinforce feelings of self-worth.
8. Positively reinforce and support open communication between patients and families.
9. Assist families in communicating their love, concern, support, and acceptance of patient.

Some patients experience significant role changes following extensive cancer surgery. Role can be defined as "the functioning unit of our society; it defines the expected behaviors that a person should perform to maintain a title" [13]. After cancer surgery, patients are faced with additional permanent or temporary expectations that may call for nursing interventions.

The threat of cancer and its surgical treatment can interrupt a patient's particular developmental stage. For example, Mr. L. is a 67-year-old who recently retired. One week ago he received a permanent colostomy as treatment with curative intent for a malignant tumor of the rectum. He had expected to spend his retirement traveling around the United States with his wife. Cancer and surgery changed his perception of his role as a "retired adult male."

For some patients, cancer surgery can alter roles within the family, among friends, and in a career. Questions asked in a nursing assessment may include: What changes do patients and their families perceive? What meaning do these changes have for patients and their families? Do patients and their families view the role changes congruently or accurately?

The "postoperative cancer patient" role must also be assessed. Are patients performing the necessary functions of this role (for example, deep breathing, coughing, learning self-care, and other required functions)? Are patients able to emotionally accept, at a functional degree, the diagnosis and the results of the surgical treatment? What are the new roles that patients must take on due to the surgical procedure?

Nursing problems occur following cancer surgery when patients: (1) find their patient role incompatible with their self-concept; (2) receive a conflicting message regarding appropriate role performance; and (3) do not perform the expected role behavior [22]. Cancer surgery can affect the multitudinous roles the patient holds at the time and nursing problems can occur. Three examples will illustrate these possible nursing problems.

1. Mrs. G., 32, views herself as a competent and loving mother who is actively and independently involved in the care of her three small children (3 months to 5 years of age). Mrs. G. underwent a hemipelvectomy for osteogenic sarcoma. Currently, Mrs. G. is very depressed because the role of mother that she has incorporated into her self-concept is incompatible with the physical limitations associated with a hemipelvectomy.

2. Mr. W., 60, is recovering from a sigmoid colostomy for localized cancer of the rectum. The nurses are trying to teach Mr. W., who is independent and agile, self-care of his colostomy. He does fairly well when his family is not around. Mr. W.'s family does not want him to touch his colostomy. "Let the nurses do the dirty work." They get very angry at the nurses who are teaching Mr. W. and criticize Mr. W. for performing his own colostomy care. Mr. W. is very confused regarding his expected role.

3. Ms. S., 62, is extremely depressed following a right modified radical mastectomy for breast cancer. She refuses to take deep breaths and cough; she will not keep her right arm elevated. Mrs. S. refuses to start beginning right arm exercises; and she will not ambulate.

The problem statements for the three examples discussed above are found in Table 8.17. Nursing goals and nursing interventions are also provided.

Dependent and independent needs change for patients following cancer surgery. Sutherland [25] points out: "There is considerable realistic dependency in the early postoperative period. If these emotional and physical dependency demands are inadequately met, a considerable amount of anxiety may be generated and the individ-

TABLE 8.17
Postoperative Nursing: Roles

Nursing Problems

1. Patients find their patient role incompatible with their self-concept.
2. Patients receive conflicting messages regarding appropriate role.
3. Patients do not perform the expected role behavior.

Nursing Goals

Patients will demonstrate ability to incorporate their new roles into their self-concept, demonstrate knowledge of expected behavior, and perform appropriate role behavior.

Nursing Interventions

1. Explore feelings regarding the loss or change in roles.
2. Clear up misinformation about role alterations with patient, families, and friends (in selective cases).
3. Provide comprehensive teaching to patients and their families (if appropriate) regarding functions of new roles.
4. Be sensitive to the difficulties that patients face in changing role behavior patterns and provide immediate and consistent positive reinforcement for their efforts.
5. Arrange for privacy and visitation by family, children, and friends since patients continue to function as members of their families. Encourage patients to use the phone for contact with their young children.
6. Allow patients off the floor for periods of time when they are physically and emotionally ready. A trip to the main lobby, cafeteria, or patio is often met with enthusiasm and provides some relief from the demanding role of "patient."
7. Obtain career counseling for patients who must seek a new role in their career.

ual convinced either that nobody can help him, or that he is not worthy of help."

During the immediate postoperative period, patients frequently may have an increased need for attention and affection by others such as family, friends, colleagues, and the health team in order to cope with the findings of surgery. This is considered an acceptable dependent behavior. Another realistic dependency need is seeking both physical help and psychological help during this period which is emotionally laden and physically limiting. The amount of physical help needed is partly due to the type, extent, and location of surgery. Physical dependency on devices such as ostomy bags, tracheostomy cannulas, crutches, or slings, is very necessary and appropriate following some types of cancer surgery. Dependency is considered a common grieving response following a significant loss. Emotional dependency on others is appropriate at this time. Frequently, patients need to seek recognition, approval, and praise in order to maintain self-esteem following cancer surgery.

As time moves on following cancer surgery, patients prepare for discharge and usually assume an increasing amount of independent behavior. Examples of independent type behavior would be: (1) taking the initiative to talk with the surgeon about further treatment plans (chemotherapy, immunotherapy, radiation therapy); (2) looking at the wound and learning wound care if necessary; (3) keeping intake and output records; (4) suctioning and cleaning a tracheostomy; (5) changing and emptying ostomy bags and keeping the skin clean and dry; and (6) learning to function without the presence or use of a particular limb or organ. These independent functions reflect the patient's ability to take initiative and to complete a simple or difficult task alone [2].

It is hoped that by the time of discharge the patient can achieve a state of interdependence. McIntier [15] defines interdependence as "the comfortable balance between dependence and independence in relationships with others." In other words, a patient who demonstrates independence in appropriate areas and accepts dependence in other appropriate areas achieves interdependence.

Nursing problems occur when patients exhibit independent, dependent or interdependent coping styles that are in conflict with the independent, dependent or interdependent demands following cancer surgery. These demands can change during the postoperative period. Dependent behavior that may be acceptable immediately after surgery may prove to be in conflict with the new demands of learning self-care for discharge. Table 8.18 describes an appropriate nursing goal and selective nursing interventions.

TABLE 8.18
Postoperative Nursing: Interdependency

Nursing Problem

Patients exhibit independent, dependent or interdependent coping styles that are in conflict with the independent, dependent or interdependent demands following cancer surgery.

Nursing Goal

Patients will demonstrate interdependent behavior that is appropriate to their physical and emotional capabilities and needs following cancer surgery.

Nursing Interventions

1. Observe for dependent behavior (for example, seeking help, seeking physical contact, seeking attention, seeking proximity), and independent behavior (for example, obstacle mastery, taking initiative, completing activities, trying to do tasks alone) [15].
2. Assess if these behaviors are adaptive to meet the independent or dependent demands at the current time.
3. Assess the importance of dependent and independent behavior. Has the cancer surgery significantly altered independent or dependent functioning?
4. Allow patients to utilize their normal independent or dependent coping styles whenever possible.
5. Create alternative methods to achieve interdependence.
6. Provide positive reinforcement for appropriate independence or dependent behavior.
7. Provide theoretical and clinical postoperative and predischarge teaching to the patient and family (when appropriate) so the patient can achieve an optimal level of interdependency prior to and after discharge. Topics that may be included in a teaching guide include: (a) wound care; (b) purpose, use, and care of needed devices; (c) signs and symptoms of high-risk problems with appropriate interventions if a problem occurs; (d) medicine administration and pertinent side effects; (e) nutritional guidance; (f) appropriate level of activity; (g) sexual counseling; (h) plans for future treatment regime; (i) the importance of medical follow-up; (j) psychological and social service availability; (k) other community resources. (This teaching guide will have to be made more specific for the particular needs of each individual patient.)

In summary, during the postoperative period, patients and their families face the surgical results associated with the malignancy of the tumor, the extent of spread, and the extent of surgery. Physical, psychological, and social adaptation is required. Nursing problems and nursing interventions have been explored with emphasis on the psychological and social adaptation of postoperative cancer patients.

POSTDISCHARGE AND FOLLOW-UP

The thought of going home after cancer surgery is often very pleasant and hopeful for most patients, their families, and the nursing staff. Yet, the postdischarge and follow-up period brings with it additional challenges for patients and their nurses. Patients confront with more reality the effect of the malignancy and surgical treatment on their everyday life. Patients often respond to the impact of this reality with acute emotional responses. The overall reported incidence of suicide in cancer patients is small. However, Jamison's [11] research shows that in a sample of 41 women with mastectomies, 25% of them had serious suicidal thoughts after discharge. These women attributed such thoughts to depression and other emotional reactions associated with their mastectomies. It is difficult to pinpoint a specific length of time before the acute impact is felt. However, Jamison [11] found that 15.8% of the mastectomy patients she interviewed thought that from an emotional and psychological standpoint, the second and third months after surgery were the worst.

What new stimuli do the patients face as they leave the hospital after cancer surgery? First of all, there is a change in environment. Patients leave the supportive care of the health team and face the challenge of caring for themselves in facilities different than those available in the hospital. Patients meet more neighbors, friends, relatives, and possibly other family members. Some patients change from sleeping alone in a hospital bed to sleeping with a spouse or roommate.

Patients also confront changes in roles. With the current use of adjuvant therapy and multimodality therapy, many patients have a long-term "outpatient cancer patient" role. Patients may be up and about and feeling fine, but continue with long-term medical treatment that often produces acute and chronic side effects. The effects of cancer surgery on the ability to return to work depends on the patient, the type of job, the surgical site, the complications of surgery, and the follow-up treatment regime. Patients must also adapt to the possible role changes in the family system. For example, a father may not be able to lift his child for a while after a midback wide excision of a melanoma with split thickness skin graft and bilateral auxiliary lymph node dissections. Or a husband may be impotent after an abdominal perineal resection for cancer of the colon. His role as lover is changed and alternative patterns of sexual activity must be explored. Or a wife who has always had a dependent role in the family system faces quite a change if her husband requires physical, emotional, and financial support following a surgery for cancer.

At home, patients continue to adapt to the changes in self-concept. Patients face the day to day living with: (1) physical and functional changes; (2) continuous emotional responses; (3) questions and discomfort of others in talking about the cancer or its treatment; and (4) continual need for affection and support.

The ability to maintain an optimal level of interdependence may be compromised by many factors. An optimal level of interdependence may be influenced by the following factors: side effects of chemotherapy, radiation therapy, or immunotherapy; fatigue of the patient or primary caregiver; depression; and the inability to problem solve caused by acute anxiety.

Patients who are at risk for developing physiological problems must be followed closely by the medical and nursing team. A few general physiological areas of concern include infection, obstruction, malnutrition, bleeding, fistula formation, lymphedema, and decreased mobility. Side effects of chemotherapy, radiation therapy, and immunotherapy can increase the risks for oncology patients who have undergone surgery.

Rehabilitation of patients with cancer will be discussed in Chapter 10. Nursing care in the home or clinic, from a surgical perspective, has two general goals:

1. Patients will continue with appropriate follow-up medical care (with or without additional treatment regimes).
2. Patients will achieve a rehabilitative status that is optimal for them.

Nursing interventions that can be implemented in the patient's home or in the surgical oncology clinic following discharge include:

1. Provide continual nursing assessment of the physiological, psychological, and social adaptation of the patient and family.
2. Provide continual patient and family education regarding self-

care, the importance of medical follow-up, symptoms related to high-risk problems and metastasis, significant medications, and side effects of surgery and other treatment modalities (if applicable). Giving positive reinforcement to the patient and family for appropriate behavior and care is critical.

3. Provide formal or informal family counseling that: (a) allows the family members to verbalize their feelings and concerns in a nonthreatening environment; (b) helps the family members interpret the felt change in the family system; (c) assists the family in solving problems related to the changes; (d) provides the family members with emotional support.

4. Provide continuity of nursing care. A concise discharge nursing summary by the patient's hospital nurse could be sent to the home care nurses or clinic nurses. A telephone call can supplement the report when special instructions or concerns arise.

5. Assist the patient and family in utilizing support groups, community resources, and other nursing agencies when appropriate.

In summary, during the postdischarge and follow-up period, patients come face to face with the everyday reality of their surgical loss and ongoing fight with cancer. Nursing interventions call for skill in education, counseling, communication, and locating available community resources. The nurse's hope is to assist the patient in achieving a high quality of life which is a realistic goal following cancer surgery.

This chapter has addressed concepts related to the physiological, psychological, and social adaptation of surgical oncology patients during four different time periods. Nursing care was discussed in relation to the unique and significant variables confronting patients, general behavioral responses, general nursing problems, appropriate nursing goals, and selective nursing interventions.

Nursing is tremendously rewarding in this field of surgical oncology because nurses frequently see positive results from their nursing interventions. They have the opportunity to work with many patients who are cured or live a high quality of life despite physical changes from cancer surgery.

REFERENCES

[1] AGUILERA, D. *Crisis Intervention Theory and Methodology.* St. Louis: C. V. Mosby, 1974.

[2] BELLER, E. Dependency and Independence in Young Children. *Journal of Genetic Psychology,* 87:25–35, 1955.

[3] CAPLAN, G. *An Approach to Community Mental Health.* New York: Grune & Stratton, 1961.

[4] de TORNYAY, R. *Strategies for Teaching Nursing.* New York: John Wiley, 1971.

[5] DONOVAN, M., and PIERCE, S. *Cancer Care Nursing.* Englewood Cliffs, N.J.: Prentice-Hall, Inc., 1976.

[6] DRIEVER, M. Theory of Self-Concept. In *Introduction to Nursing: An Adaptation Model,* ed. Sr. Callista Roy, pp. 169–179. Englewood Cliffs, N.J.: Prentice-Hall, Inc., 1976.

[7] DUNPHY, J.E., and WAY, L. *Current Surgical Diagnosis and Treatment.* Los Altos: Lange Medical Publications, 1975.

[8] GIACQUINTA, B. Helping Families Face the Crisis of Cancer. *American Journal of Nursing,* 77:1585–1588, 1977.

[9] GRUENDEMANN, B. Problems of Physical Self: Loss. In *Introduction to Nursing: An Adaptation Model,* ed. Sr. Callista Roy, pp. 192–201. Englewood Cliffs, N.J.: Prentice-Hall, Inc., 1976.

[10] HOLLAND, J.C. *Cancer Medicine.* Philadelphia: Lea & Febiger, 1973.

[11] JAMISON, K.; WELLISCH, D.; and PASNAU, R. Psychosocial Aspects of Mastectomy: The Woman's Perspective. Unpublished paper.

[12] KLEEMAN, K. Distortions in Body Image in Adulthood. In *Distortions in Body Image in Illness and Disability,* ed. F. Bower, pp. 73–96. New York: John Wiley, 1977.

[13] MALAZNIK, N. Theory of Role Function. In *Introduction to Nursing: An Adaptation Model,* ed. Sr. Callista Roy, pp. 245–255. Englewood Cliffs, N.J.: Prentice-Hall, Inc., 1976.

[14] McCAFFERY, M. *Nursing Management of the Patient with Pain.* Philadelphia: Lippincott, 1972.

[15] McINTIER, Sr. TERESA MARIE. Theory of Interdependence. In *Introduction to Nursing: An Adaptation Model,* ed. Sr. Callista Roy, pp. 291–302. Englewood Cliffs, N.J.: Prentice-Hall Inc., 1976.

[16] MURPHY, L. *The Widening World of Childhood: Paths Toward Mastery.* New York: Basic Books, 1962.

[17] PARKES, C. *Bereavement Studies of Grief in Adult Life.* New York: International Universities Press, Inc., 1974.

[18] PEPLAU, M. A Working Definition of Anxiety. In *Some Clinical Approaches to Psychiatric Nursing,* ed. S. Burd and M. Marshall, pp. 323–327. New York: Macmillan, 1963.

[19] PORTNOY, I. The Anxiety States. In *American Handbook of Psychiatry,* ed. A. Silvano, Vol. 1, 307–323. New York: Basic Books, 1959.

[20] ROBERTS, S. *Behavioral Concepts and the Critically Ill Patient.* Englewood Cliffs, N.J.: Prentice–Hall, Inc., 1976.

[21] ROY, Sr. CALLISTA. Adaptation as a Model of Nursing Practice. In *Intoduction to Nursing: An Adaptation Model,* ed. Sr. Callista Roy, pp. 3–39. Englewood Cliffs, N.J.: Prentice-Hall, Inc., 1976.

[22] SCHOFIELD, A. Problems of Role Function. In *Introduction to Nursing: An Adaptation Model,* ed. Sr. Callista Roy, pp. 265-297. Englewood Cliffs, N.J.: Prentice-Hall, Inc., 1976.

[23] SCHWARTZ, S. *Principles of Surgery.* New York: McGraw-Hill, 1974.

[24] SUTHERLAND, A., and ORBACH, C. Depressive Reactions Associated with Surgery for Cancer. In *The Psychological Impact of Cancer,* pp. 17-21. New York: American Cancer Society, 1974.

[25] SUTHERLAND, A. Psychological Impact of Cancer and Its Therapy. *Medical Clinics of North America,* May, pt. 3:705-720, May 1956.

[26] VETTESE, J. Problems of the Patient Confronting the Diagnosis of Cancer. In *Cancer the Behavioral Dimensions,* ed. J.W. Cullen, B.H. Fox, and R.N. Isom, pp. 275-282. New York: Raven Press, 1976.

[27] WELLISCH, D. Cancer and Families: Life on a Foundation of Quicksand. *UCLA Cancer Center Bulletin,* 5:8, 1978.

chapter nine

ANAYIS DERDIARIAN, R.N., M.N.
Assistant Clinical Professor
Teaching in Graduate Nursing
Oncology Program
School of Nursing, UCLA

Nursing in prevention of cancer

--- **INTRODUCTION: HISTORICAL PERSPECTIVES** ---

After 14 years of observation, experience, and thinking on the subject of bedside care of the sick, Florence Nightingale presented her conclusions in *Notes on Nursing* [32], written not "as a manual to teach nurses to nurse" but rather to help nurses to "think how to nurse." Thus the book was intended "to give hints for thought to women who have personal charge of the health of others . . . knowledge which everyone ought to have—distinct from medical knowledge, which only a profession can have." More specifically, the book was intended to help mothers or special groups of women to be known as nurses to nurse the sick and keep people well. One clearly can conclude in reading these notes that: (1) the fundamental needs of the sick and the principles of good care for the ill and the well are the same today as they were observed by Florence Nightingale over a century ago; (2) many of the modern concepts in the fields of nursing and public health have their origins in the publication of these notes in 1859; and (3) many of the improvements in those fields are due, in great part, to Miss Nightingale's efforts. In this respect she demonstrates an epidemiological approach to the study of the causes of illness and the care of the sick: "In Life Insurance and such like societies, were they instead of having the person examined by the medical man, to have the houses, conditions, ways of life of these persons examined, at how much truer results they would arrive!" In warning against the habit of observing conditions and making judgments on the basis of insufficient information, she suggests that "power of forming any correct opinion as to the result must entirely depend upon an inquiry into all the conditions in which the patient lives." This reflects her acknowledgment of the concept that disease is multicausal. Therefore, intervention must be multidimensional.

NURSING'S PHILOSOPHY IN REGARD TO HEALTH AND DISEASE

Florence Nightingale's notes [32] clearly express the philosophy of nursing. Prevention is envisioned as an integral part of care of nursing. Earlier in nursing's professional history, this vision was captured and related to more practically. With technological advancement, social and industrial changes, and control of many diseases, nursing has identified more closely with the acute care setting. Unfortunately, in this process, we not only have drifted away from the calling initially considered to be the nursing function, namely, care for maintenance and promotion of health and care after illness, we have at the same time drifted away from the clear vision of our professional goal as unique and different from that of medicine. Consequently the interpretation of our professional functions in terms of their nature, method, and outcome have been muddled and restricted to much narrower scopes. Rereading Nightingale's writings, one refreshingly finds the goal and direction for a unique nursing. The main concepts she presents for the understanding of nursing's place in health and control of disease, are that: (1) nursing has responsibility for the health of others; (2) individuals are capable of maintaining and promoting health; (3) knowledge about maintenance of health and prevention of disease is everyone's right; (4) prevention is fundamental to maintenance of health, effective cure of disease, and recovery from the effects of disease; (5) disease is multicausal and, therefore, promotion and maintenance of health as well as prevention and defeat of disease must accordingly be multidimensional; (6) systematization of observations in discerning the elements of prevention, cure of disease, and recovery from it is basic to the effective control of disease. Indeed those ideas are consistent with knowledge developed since their conception. The literature is rich in findings in support of these concepts.

Emphasis on prevention rather than cure in control of disease is compatible with the trends of prevalence of chronic rather than acute diseases plaguing mankind in most parts of the industrialized world. The virulence of agents of infectious disease has been replaced by noxious environmental stimuli of physical, environmental, social, psychological, and emotional nature. The concept of multicausality of disease, as in the traditional model of epidemiology, has been supported through research in the last decades. Strong inference can be made that the etiological complex resulting in disease involves three elements: (1) the resistance or the susceptibility of the host; (2) the disease producing agent; and (3) the nature of the environment in which the agent and the host interact. Further implied here is that disease or the disease-causing agent, as well as susceptibility or resistance of the host, must be understood in a psychosocial and biological sense. Cassel's findings [8], among several similar research outcomes, take the point a step further in proposing that the relationship between the psychosocial variables and disease outcome may be similar to the relationship between a microorganism and the disease outcome. Such a view of the health-disease continuum suggests that not only must the physical factors affecting the relationship between host, agent, and environment be understood, but also those psychosocial factors that are capable of changing human resistance in important ways in making groups of individuals more or less susceptible to those agents in the environment. This is particularly true and important in preventing, curing, or minimizing the effect of chronic disease. The particular relevance this has to cancer and its control will be discussed shortly. It is essential that the reader bear in mind that although general, the discussion is specific to cancer.

PREVENTION

Traditionally, prevention was defined as inhibiting the development of a disease before it occurs. The more current usage of the term is extended to include measures that interrupt or slow the progression of disease. Therefore, many levels of prevention, rather than one, exist: (1) *primary prevention* is effective, if applied in stage of susceptibility, by altering the susceptibility or reducing susceptible individuals' exposure to harmful agents; (2) *secondary prevention* is effective, if applied during preclinical and clinical phases, by early detection and treatment of disease; (3) *tertiary prevention* is effective, if applied in the advanced stage of disease by alleviating disorder or disability resulting from the disease or effects of treatment and restoring effective functioning [26].

In order to understand each of those levels of prevention, their relationship to control of disease, and implications for role and method of practice to professionals, particularly to nursing, it is necessary to have some knowledge of the natural history of disease and its relationship to prevention.

THE NATURAL HISTORY OF DISEASE

Many diseases, particularly chronic diseases, have a *natural life history*. Although each disease has its own life history, the natural history of disease in general, as well as different approaches to prevention and control of disease, may be understood within a general framework. Such a framework is illustrated by Mausner and Bahn [27].

Stage of Susceptibility

In the stage of susceptibility, although disease is not developed, the existence of factors that favor its occurrence make up a groundwork for its development. For example, chronic intake of large amounts of alcohol increases susceptibility to liver cirrhosis; smoking increases susceptibility to lung cancer; and chronic psychosocial stressors seem to increase the likelihood of emotional illness. Those factors whose presence is associated with increased likelihood that disease will develop at a later time are known as *risk factors*. The need to identify those factors is becoming more obvious as knowledge reveals that chronic diseases present the most major health challenge. It is known that some risk factors can be changed; for example, smoking can be given up, alcohol intake can be stopped; and help through and reduction in psychosocial stresses may be provided [27].

Stage of Presymptomatic Disease

In the presymptomatic stage, although there is no manifest disease, some changes have begun to take place through the interaction of factors. Those changes are, at this point, below the threshold of clinical manifestation through detectable signs or symptoms. Examples are atherosclerotic changes in coronary vessels before coronary disease signs or symptoms and premalignant changes in cells before onset of cancer [27].

Stage of Clinical Disease

In this stage, anatomic and/or functional alterations have begun and signs or symptoms are recognizable. It is important to subdivide this stage for better management of cases. Each disease has its own bases for subdivision. Cancer, for instance, is classified based on morphologic grounds, that is, histologic type and location of tumor. Categorization of disease by staging was discussed in detail previously [27].

Stage of Disability

Although many diseases run their course and then resolve either spontaneously or with therapy, some diseases give rise to residual defects of short or long duration, leaving the afflicted person disabled to a greater or lesser extent. Some diseases, usually self-limiting, may later give rise to chronic condition [27].

The National Health Survey [31] defines disability as "any temporary or long-term reduction of a person's activity as a result of an acute or chronic condition." In the broader sense, disability means any limitation of a person's activities including her psychosocial role. The implication here is loss of function and not necessarily loss of a body part. This distinction is important since loss of function is not solely related to loss of body part, as individuals afflicted with the same disease may suffer disability to the same extent, yet they may vary in their level of disability.

LEVELS OF PREVENTION

According to the natural history of disease, disease evolves over time during which pathologic changes may become irreversible. Therefore, the important thing is to prevent rather than cure disease, that is, to detect and intervene in the precursors and risk factors of the disease during the susceptibility and presymptomatic stages of disease. Thus prevention, rather than cure of disease, becomes the focus in control of disease and maintenance of health.

With prevention as a major focus, it may be well to refer to the definition of the term and elaborate on its meaning in various levels of prevention.

Primary Prevention

The prevention of disease consists of measures classified under two major categories: (1) general health promotion; and (2) specific protective measures. The first includes such things as good nutrition, safe work conditions, adequate rest, shelter, social, psychological comfort, and the like. A very important measure in this category is the broad area of health education, which includes anticipatory guidance of parents and children, counseling, teaching good health habits, and teaching with the intent of extinguishing habits hazardous to health such as smoking, overeating, and drinking. The second category includes environmental sanitation such as purification of water supplies or reduction of environmental pollutants, and protection against accidents and occupational hazards.

In developed countries, public health measures have been effective largely by primary preventive measures such as immunization and environmental manipulation. The current health problems yet awaiting solution are chronic diseases whose prevention requires modification of attitudes and behaviors. Those problems are complex in terms of their etiologies and treatments. Of such are use of alcohol, tobacco, and other drugs, dietary patterns, physical activity, lifestyle, socioeconomic status, and careless work or driving habits.

Secondary Prevention

The effectiveness of secondary prevention of disease is in early detection and prompt treatment of it. The aim is to either cure disease at the earliest stage possible or slow its progression, prevent complications, and limit disability. Examples of diseases most amenable to secondary prevention are hypertension, diabetes, in situ carcinoma of the cervix, and glaucoma. As much as it is the responsibility of health departments to conduct screening programs, it is the responsibility of all health professionals to help the public, through education, motivation, and community organization, to adopt measures for health maintenance on the individual, group, community, and societal level.

Tertiary Prevention

The aim of tertiary prevention is limitation of disability and rehabilitation where disease has occurred and left residual damage. Rehabilitation in the broader sense means to help an affected individual to return to a useful, functional, satisfying, and, where possible, self-sufficient role in society. The main theme is maximal utilization of the individual's residual capacities with emphasis on her remaining abilities rather than her losses.

Rehabilitation includes psychosocial, vocational, medical, and nursing components. As such it is an interdisciplinary enterprise. Its usefulness is effective until death in that, at each stage of the progression of disease process, appropriate interventive measures may be applied to prevent continued progression of the disease and deterioration of the patient's physical, mental, psychological, and emotional condition.

The different levels of prevention can be fully understood only in relation to the natural progression or natural history of a disease. The clearer our understanding of the natural history of disease, the greater will be the chances for developing effective points and methods of intervention. The interrelationship between natural history of cancer and levels of its prevention will be illustrated next.

THE NATURE OF CANCER AND ITS RELATIONSHIP TO PREVENTION

The Nature of Cancer

In view of the discussion related to the nature, etiology, classification, and treatment of cancer that was given previously, a brief overview is presented here of the way in which the natural history of cancer relates to the three levels of prevention. This understanding provides a framework within which nursing's functions may be envisioned.

Cancer can be thought of as a variety of nearly 200 different diseases, with one general characteristic—the multiplication of a disorganized and diseased group of cells in any tissue of the body which grow and spread locally or by transportation to the other areas of the body. Cancer cells undergo changes in their size, shape, and in the pattern of their nucleus, presumably over a period of many years. Knowledge as to the causes or the nature of the changes is not well established. Chapter 3 refers to several theories about the etiology and natural history of cancer, all of which have lead scientists in this field to vast and productive research. Three main categories are usually used to classify cancers: (1) carcinoma, (2) sarcoma, (3) lymphoma and leukemia. The first two groups are unicentric, that is, they originate in tissue cells in a local area and metastasize to other localities in the body. The third group usually first appears in already generalized form, although these are also unicentric forms of both lymphoma and Hodgkin's disease.

Incidence and Distribution of Cancer

Although there are several different forms of cancer, there is greater incidence in some sites of origins than in others. In women, the current principal primary sites of cancer are the breast (23%), the uterus (13%), the intestines (13%), the skin (13%), the ovaries (4.5%), the lungs (4%), and lymphomas (3.5%). In men, the primary sites are the skin (23%), the lung (18%), the intestines (10.9%), the prostate (10.6%), the bladder (4.5%), and lymphomas (4%). The present annual incidence of new cancer in the United States is 635,000. The new cases added to those being treated brings the estimated count of 975,000 Americans under treatment for cancer during a given year. It is projected that more than 52 million Americans now living will have cancer. The cure rate for cancer is four out of every ten cases [10].

The incidence of cancer varies in different geographic areas of the world from the standpoint of sites of origin in the body. According to several demographic and geographical studies done during the past decade, changes in civilization and advances in industrialization seem to be related to the incidence of cancer. For example, in Africa, as in Indonesia, primary liver cancer is common, whereas it is rare in other parts of the world. In Ireland, Scandinavia, and Japan the rate of cancer of the stomach is higher than in the United States. In Western Europe, as in the United States, breast cancer is more frequent than it is in Japan [33,23]. Observations reveal that the incidence of cancer in general varies according to differences in socioeconomic status, ethnic, or even religious differences.

Research uncovering various factors that promote or inhibit the advance of cancer, as well as some of those internal and external factors that predispose to the development of cancer, has increased our knowledge about the disease. Among such factors some of the better understood are hereditary elements, internal and external irritants and chemicals, cellular reaction and transformation, immunity factors, and viral agent effects. Among the better-established external predisposing factors are exposure to the sun, which results in more frequent skin cancer incidence; constant irritation of a mole, which may cause malignant melanoma; certain dyes, particularly those containing anyline which can cause cancer of the bladder; and cigarette smoking, which is strongly associated with development of cancer of the lungs and the larynx. Many cancers develop without known external predisposing causes. It is believed that factors that ultimately cause the change to malignancy are those that are internal or endogenous to the individual. Of such factors, some of the better known are the hormones upon which cancer of the breast and prostate are considered to be dependent. Conditions that may undergo malignant change include polyps in the colon, rectum, or cervix; senile keratosis; and leukoplakia of the mucous membranes of the mouth [19].

Diagnosis and Treatment of Cancer

Diagnosis and treatment depends on the patient's history, on a careful physical examination, and on the outcome of special diagnostic procedures. Establishment of the evidence of malignancy in a specific site or sites leads to further diagnostic tests and procedures. Treatment modalities are selected after consideration of all available data. Treatment of cancer follows three major directions: chemotherapy, surgery, radiation therapy. These may be used alone or in combination and all have consequences needing careful and extensive preventive, interventive, and rehabilitative nursing considerations.

According to National Cancer Plan, 1972 [29], accelerated efforts are currently directed toward identification of the problems and the approaches for a concerted effort to control cancer. This is a major concept; in fact, it is pivotal to understanding not only the nature and the approaches to cancer control, but more importantly to understanding the main focus of each profession on the interdisciplinary team involved in total cancer management. The two major means along which meaningful cancer control efforts must be directed are: (1) physical-biological; and (2) psychosocial. According to this plan, present principal research objectives are:

1. To reduce the effectiveness of external agents that may increase the probability of cancer development in existing or future populations
2. To increase individuals' resistance—for example, by vaccination—which would decrease the likelihood of their developing cancer
3. To prevent the transformation of the normal cell to one capable of developing a cancer by means of blocking or interfering with the steps involved in the transformation of the potentially cancer forming cells
4. To prevent tumor establishment in those cells already capable of forming cancer
5. To achieve accurate assessment of the presence, the extent, and the probable cause of cancer risks in individuals, groups of individuals or populations, so that helpful means be developed in prevention, cure, or prognosis of cancer

6. To cure as many patients as possible and maintain optimal control of cancer in patients who are not cured
7. To restore patients suffering from the sequelae of the disease or treatment to an optimal functioning state.

It seems obvious that the second of the major means mentioned above, the psychosocial, is not addressed separately and specifically in this plan. Yet given the extent of the existing knowledge in the physical-biological realm of cancer control, the psychosocial is and will continue to be equally important in the control of cancer. It must be borne in mind that control of cancer implies prevention in the primary, secondary, and tertiary stages of the health-illness continuum of cancer.

THE NATURE, SCOPE, AND METHODS OF PREVENTION OF CANCER

It is obvious, through a short overview of the natural history of cancer, that there is no substantially strong evidence that causal relationships exist between external or internal factors and the onset of cancer. Research in this area in the biological, physical, environmental, and demographic fields has been vast and fruitful; however, much remains to be explored. Advances in the therapeutic approaches to treatment of cancer have been impressive, yet here, too, much remains to be understood. Therefore, emphasis must be directed to the important counterpart, namely, the psychosocial realm of cancer control in the primary, secondary, and tertiary preventive phases of the disease. Tertiary prevention is such a vast area, since presently most treatments focus on this phase, that a separate chapter is devoted to it.

Since the determination of the nature, the scope, and the method of prevention of a disease depends on the available knowledge about all phases of the natural history of that disease, at some point in time it may be inferred that the nature of prevention of cancer would be psychosocial as much as it would be physical-biological or medical. For example, to stop smoking, or to take precautions in sunbathing, or to seek medical attention soon after a detected physical change, or even to adjust to postdiagnosis, medical, and psychosocial requirements would depend on: (1) what the patient or the caregiver knows; and (2) what they do or do not do. This point will be elaborated as all levels of prevention are dealt with separately.

Professor Pierre Denoix [10], the president of the Eleventh International Cancer Congress in Florence, Italy, in his opening speech, directed a plea to authors and journalists throughout the world to "bid them to abandon 'cancer' as a dramatic motif and a term that denotes terror and tragic inevitability. Eliminate the false connotations from your writing and you will have made an incalculable contribution to the campaign we are waging, together, against this disease—since you will have helped to reduce the unjustified terror that the inept use of this word tends to perpetuate."

These words perhaps speak to one aspect of why the term *cancer* spreads fear. Another aspect that needs analysis can be understood by asking: (1) why fear of cancer prevails; and (2) why behaviors conducive to prevention or early detection do not exist. For example, why do the chronic cigarette smokers continue to smoke while reading abundant warnings of the dangers of developing lung cancer, or why do individuals delay in seeking medical attention after noticing a change in a mole or a lump in the breast.

Some of the reasons for such behaviors may be rooted in partial knowledge relative to the natural history of cancer, and the behaviors can be set straight with proper education. Such knowledge includes the following [9]:

1. Cancer can occur silently, without warning, until the skills of the physician are no longer adequate to save the life.
2. Cancer is not confined to the original site but spreads silently to any body tissue if not checked.
3. For centuries, nothing could be done to arrest the course of cancer after an early period of growth, particularly for those cancers that were not evident externally.
4. Cancer deprives the rest of the body tissue nutrients, causing wasting of these tissues while it thrives.
5. Advanced cancer often causes intractable pain, often not responsive to available narcotics and analgesics.
6. Cancer causes an attitude of hopelessness in many people, including many physicians, leading to abandonment of cancer patients by those who should be supportive.
7. Often the diagnosis of cancer and the type is unsure, and inadequate therapy may be administrated until metastasis has occurred.
8. Therapy is often mutilative and deprives the patient of familiar self-image, independence, and perhaps of a means of livelihood.
9. The etiologies of many types of cancer are not known.
10. The patient has little or no personal control over the disease process, in that even if she fully cooperates with her physician, there can be no guarantee that the therapy will be successful.

A close examination of this knowledge reveals the mixture of some truth about cancer and what is made of it in the mind of the public. It is this truth that the scientist and the practitioner must confront and understand if they are to wage war against cancer with the aid of whatever tools are available. What is in the mind of the public is often not very different from what is in the minds of some physicians, nurses, psychologists, social workers, health educators, or volunteer helpers. Those who know little about the truth related to cancer and its treatment, and who harbor the same fears and confusion as does the patient or the public, are not only nonfunctional in helping the patient or the family, but more unfortunately, actually become reinforcers of fear, confusion, and uncertainty in the mind of the public. William Boyd, the noted Canadian pathologist and bacteriologist, in his book, *The Spontaneous Regression of Cancer* [5], sums up the general attitude: "When we think of cancer in general terms we are apt to conjure up a process characterized by a steady, remorseless, and inexorable progress in which the disease is all conquering, and none of the immunological and other defensive forces which help us survive the onslaught of bacterial and viral infections can serve to halt the faltering footsteps to the grave." Although there has been more progress in acquiring knowledge about cancer and its treatment in the past few decades than in the previous history of medicine, very little of this knowledge is included in the core of curriculae of medical and nursing schools. The psychiatrist, the psychologist, the social worker, or the health educator are trained for and concerned with the patient's and her family's psychological and social adjustment to the sequellae of the disease. Seldom do all of those individuals realize that the crux of the problem of the proper physical, psychological, emotional, and social adjustment of the patient and her family is effective and efficient communication. Communication based on knowledge about the disease and the treatment, delivered with honesty, empathy, and understanding, is of paramount importance not only to the psychosocial adjustment of the patient, but also the healing process of her body. For medical history attested, long before Freud's contribution to behavioral science, that a patient's emotional status can directly affect both the course of the disease and the effectiveness of the treatment.

Clearly implied in the preceding paragraphs are the elements of the nature of prevention as well as the configuration of the scope and methods of prevention of cancer at all levels. Inherent in and underlying all of those levels of prevention are two central elements that will play pivotal roles in the control of cancer. The first is teaching to inform and to invoke behavior change. The second is research to identify: (1) behaviors deterrent to primary, secondary, and tertiary prevention; (2) factors causal to or associated with those behaviors; and (3) interventions specific to changing those behaviors and the evaluation of their effectiveness.

The Nature of Prevention of Cancer

The term *nature* is defined here as "the essential character of a thing; quality or qualities that make something what it is; essence . . . the vital functions, forces, and activities of organs" [43]. Given the present knowledge about cancer and what this term means to the masses, the nature of prevention of cancer can at least presently be understood in terms of teaching to inform and to invoke behavior change. The available knowledge must be disseminated to the public in such a way that individuals will take responsibility and initiative to act on their own health and that of others. Becker's model [2] of Health Belief has been used as a conceptual guide for a number of studies of health behavior and is based on the thesis that under conditions of general motivation and in the presence of appropriate cues an individual will undertake a specific health related act. The major components of the model are as follows:

1. Individuals perceive a certain threat of a disease.
2. They perceive themselves to be susceptible to the disease.
3. They perceive the consequences of the disease to be serious for them.
4. They perceive the actions to be taken to be effective in dealing with the disease.
5. They do not perceive an unsurmountable barrier to taking the action.

Translated into operational terms, the model implies that the individual's *perceptions* of the disease, its treatment, and her action in relation to those determines her *behavior* with respect to the disease, the treatment, and her action. Although an individual's perceptions vary according to several complex variables, such as cultural background, past experience with respect to disease or treatment, educational background, socioeconomic status, and the like, inherent in the model is the assumption that teaching to inform and invoke behavior change will affect perception. Knowledge can affect perception by configuring disease as a threat, and help as attainable. Perception based on knowledge would energize and maintain behavior aimed at promoting and maintaining health. Threat of cancer based on an individual's misconceptions about cancer and its treatment may immobilize them to the extent of denial of apparent signals, or cancer phobia. Threat, as used in this model, does not imply this sort of stimulus. Rather, that threat of cancer means a realistic probability of an individual's vulnerability to the disease. More importantly, through proper education, the individual perceives her actions as determinant forces in dealing with the threat. Thus, in a way, the locus of control would shift from the disease to her health-related behavior. Motivation to initiate and continue to act will depend heavily on the availability of the necessary cues and means conducive to appropriate health behavior regarding primary, secondary, and tertiary prevention in cancer.

It must be noted that this model does not culminate in placing the entire responsibility of seeking and maintaining health on the individual. It does portion out responsibility to the environment of the individual. Knowledge about primary, secondary, tertiary prevention of cancer must be available. This is consistent with the concept that disease is multicausal, and so is its treatment.

Like its counterparts, this model may have its imperfections, and yet it provides guidelines for assessment, diagnosis, and interventions in dealing with health behavior of individuals or groups of individuals with respect to cancer prevention. Furthermore, it provides a basis for research in identifying factors deterrent or conducive to health behavior in relation to cancer control. Thus the nature of prevention of cancer is determined by the nature of the disease, available medical and psychosocial technology capable of dealing with it, and interdisciplinary research for generating knowledge in a concerted and collaborative manner in understanding the disease and its treatment including the psychosocial determinants affecting the control of cancer.

The Scope of Prevention of Cancer

The term *scope* is being used here as ". . . the range of view; . . . the area or field within which any activity goes on; range or extent of action; . . . room for outlook or liberty of action" [43].

The National Committee on Cancer, headed by the distinguished pathologist James Ewing [17], concluded in 1925 that "early diagnosis is so important that cancer detection clinics must be established in the United States." The Presidential Committee [40], investigating the problem of cancer in the United States in 1965 stated "Each premature death from cancer is a personal tragedy. Each preventable death is a national reproach. Each year more and more such deaths are occurring, for the pace of science is bringing them more within our reach, but the pace of application allows them to slip through our grasp." It is implicit in those statements that: (1) not only is necessary knowledge lacking, but what we do know is not being utilized adequately in a variety of cancer control efforts; (2) desirable national goals for prevention and early detection have not yet been reached; and (3) the application of knowledge in prevention of cancer implies the involvement of the nurse, the health educator, the behavioral scientist, the social worker, the epidemiologist, the public health worker, the government, and the individual, in addition to the physician and the scientist. All play complementary roles in the arena of cancer prevention. The complementarity of the roles is in the way of application of available knowledge by the scientists and the provision of feedback for further research by the practitioner through interdisciplinary network of communication and collaboration.

Therefore the scope of prevention of cancer, on all levels, requires the active involvement of the professional, the public, and the governmental sectors. Because the involvement of those sectors is ultimately interdependent, collaboration between them would be fruitful and efficient. A recent example of such collaboration is the campaign against smoking, which has involved will power, people power, and money power on the part of all those sectors to succeed to the current extent. This is a classic example of primary prevention of cancer. A classic example in secondary prevention of cancer is the concerted effort to combat breast cancer through breast self-examination programs. Teaching to inform and to invoke behavior change needs to be aimed at every sector.

Educating and training the professionals in the health care system as well as increasing programs in the system of education of health professionals is the primary step of concerted efforts. Personnel knowledgeable in the primary and secondary preventive measures are needed to develop programs of education and practice in promoting cancer control at the primary and secondary levels.

Educating the public to utilize available health care facilities and demand more facilities requires educational and organizational programs which create a need for people power and money power. Community pressure made up of professional and consumer collaboration can result in social and legislative action. Such actions are needed not only to increase the means of application of available knowledge but also to increase research power in the area of cancer control.

The Methods of Prevention of Cancer

The methods of prevention of cancer are alluded to in the foregoing discussions. The nature of cancer prevention defines the scope of cancer prevention which in turn defines the methods of cancer prevention.

One high-priority step is to increase professional training in primary and secondary prevention of cancer. An immediate way of achieving this is to increase cancer-related content in the core curriculae in the generic training of the nurse, physician, dentist, and public health professional. Although cancer is the second major cause of death, there is at present relatively little content on cancer in the training process of those professionals. The effort to strengthen the core content of generic education can be complemented by simultaneously increasing continuing education programs for those individuals. Both of these educational media should include content relating to beginning skills in community organization. Education and service in health can certainly use the expertise of health educators in this area.

Another necessary step related to the increase in professional training in cancer control is to increase training for specialists in cancer prevention. From the academic and training standpoint, nursing is the profession naturally best situated to mobilize its forces and contribute to cancer control. Therefore, specialty programs, both those on the formal graduate level as well as those on the continuing education level, can be efficient, effective, and cost containing.

Another high-priority step in cancer control efforts is that of increasing the primary and secondary prevention programs in communities through better utilization of existing knowledge and people power. This can be achieved by making money available to develop such programs and to develop coordinative and collaborative systems among the existing agencies concerned with the control of cancer. The community, including both professional and lay sectors, can exert efforts for the utilization of existing facilities such as the public education system as media for the education of the public in the primary and secondary prevention of cancer. Both the public and the private sector can be motivated to support, through financial and social means, the education of the professional and the lay communities as well as utilization of the professional skills in the primary and secondary prevention of cancer.

Another high-priority step, and an outgrowth of the preceding two, is to increase governmental support, through financial and legislative means, of the primary and secondary prevention of cancer. Cost-free education as well as screening and early detecting services need to be available and accessible to the communities, particularly to those at high risk for certain cancers. One practical way is to encourage the life and health insurance industries to promote and maintain primary and secondary cancer preventive behavior on the part of their clients, through reward mechanisms.

PRIMARY PREVENTION OF CANCER: SPECIFIC ISSUES

The measures specific to the primary preventive phase can be classified under two major categories: (1) technological; and (2) psychosocial.

Technological Measures

Presently, there are no known specific technological measures which, when applied to individuals, would prevent the onset of cancer in those individuals. Research in this area is active, particularly in the field of immunology, and it is hoped that like techniques will be developed.

Psychosocial Measures

Psychosocial measures specific to this phase comprise teaching to inform and to invoke behavior change. The health professionals and the public can be taught about: (1) the better-known factors or those suspected to be etiologically linked with incidence of cancer; and (2) the ways and means of minimizing or avoiding exposure to those factors.

Social-Environmental Factors. Etiological factors in carcinogenesis were discussed in Chapter 2. Some of the factors most pertinent to patient education and intervention will be highlighted here.

Tobacco use and its association with cancer of the lungs, larynx, throat, mouth, esophagus, and bladder, has been documented based on prospective and retrospective studies. Since 1950, with reports by Doll and Hill [12] and Wynder et al. [43], there has been evidence strengthening such associations. Chronic use of alcohol is associated with the development of squamous cell carcinomas of the oral cavity, pharynx, larynx, and esophagus. Continuous exposure to the ultraviolet rays of sun is associated with cancer of the skin.

In females, douching and Trichimonas infections are associated with cervical cancer [43]. Intercourse begun early, and with several partners, is also associated with cervical cancer[43]. In males, those not circumcised have more risk of developing cancer of the penis and pose more risk of cervical cancer in their partners than those who are circumcised [43].

In experimental animals, increased amount of animal fat in the diet is associated with an increased incidence of breast cancer; particularly when the subject is exposed to chemical carcinogens. In human populations, a strong positive correlation has been shown between fat consumption of a given country and the incidence of breast cancer in that country [7]. A similar correlation between animal fat and protein intake and increased incidence of breast cancer can be demonstrated in several countries [7]. However, whether a single carcinogenic pathway is involved in a relationship, such as that suggested between fat and protein intake and cancer of the colon, is not well known. Burdette [6] suggests that both adducts and proximal carcinogens are probably involved. Weisburger [41] adds that the intestinal microflora participates in and are required for the activation of carcinogens by liberating the reactive intermediates from a conjugate.

Physical-Chemical Factors. Urban living appears to increase the incidence of lung cancer [1]. This increase seems to be more significant among smoking males, although there is also an increase among smoking urban females in recent years. Whether air pollution is linked with lung cancer is not conclusively evident. It is believed that some other variables such as infectious agents or immunological state related to overcrowding in urban living may be linked to increase in lung cancer. The carcinogenic effects of exposure to asbestos is well documented [1]. Exposure to asbestos and cigarette smoking heightens the risk of mesothelioma more than that produced by either risk factor alone [35].

The potential hazards of nitrosamines in certain foods and halogenated hydrocarbons in drinking water have received particular attention in recent years. Nitrates are found in small amounts as additives in meats and water supplies. Under certain circumstances these nitrates can be reduced to nitrite, which can react with some classes of amines to produce nitrosamines which in turn, under certain circumstances, act as carcinogen precursors [42].

Occupational Factors. The carcinogenic effects of exposure to asbestos in mining and to chrysotile in industry are well known. Exposure to other industrial factors such as arsenic, chromium, nickel, tar fumes, and vinyl chloride are associated with angiosarcoma of the liver [3]. The effects of suspected airborne carcinogens such as pesticides or insecticides are still not well known. Ionizing radiation associated with leukemia and exposure to uranium, sun, and benzo-a-pyrene associated with nonspecific forms of cancer are among occupational hazards.

Iatrogenic Factors.   Some drugs are suspected to be associated with development of cancer. Three studies in 1974 reported the use of rauwolfia (reserpine-containing drugs) having almost a doubling effect on the risk of neoplasms in users compared to the control nonusers [15]. The possible carcinogenic effects of estrogen, which is widely used as a contraceptive and as an additive in raising meat-producing animals, are still under investigation. Black and Leis [3] reported a prior history of estrogen intake to be three times as frequent among young nulliparas with breast cancer as in their age-matched control counterparts.

Biological Factors.   Although four different groups of viruses are known to cause cancer in animals, evidence for human cancer-causing viruses is limited to a few examples discussed in Chapter 2. Research in this area is ongoing. Among infections suspected to be carcinogenic is schistosomiasis, which acts as chronic irritant on the urinary bladder.

SECONDARY PREVENTION OF CANCER: SPECIFIC ISSUES

Most known effective interventions in cancer control presently center in this stage of prevention. This stage ordinarily encompasses the early detection to early treatment periods. From a cancer control standpoint, each of these periods is critical with respect to problems specific to each and thus worthy of separate treatment. Since the early treatment period of cancer management is dealt with elsewhere, the early detection period will be given particular attention here.

Early Detection of Cancer

Factors influencing early detection center around two major categories: (1) those related to individuals' internal environment; and (2) those related to their external environment. The former can be understood in terms of attitudes toward and knowledge about health and disease, the latter in terms of availability and accessibility of health care services. Several relationships must be considered in understanding the interplay of those categorical variables. Such consideration is aided by a model presented by Green [21]. This model summarizes those variables under three major components: (1) the predisposing factors; (2) the enabling factors; and (3) the reinforcing factors.

Predisposing Factors. It is believed that certain common patterns of health behavior are established that, when understood, may be used as predictors of variations in personal health practices. Fink et al. [18] found such common patterns of health behavior in women participating in the Health Insurance Plan of Greater New York breast screening program, respective to four types of women. The conformist women seek or do not seek health based on rotelike pattern of behavior which is not derived from a direct, substantive connection with a specific need or cognition. The rational goal-directed women tended to be inner directed, goal oriented, relatively well educated, distinguishing cancer as more catastrophic than other chronic diseases, not denying susceptibility to it, and goal oriented in terms of physical check-ups. The complacent-stoic women were similar to the goal-oriented type, but they differed in that, although knowing their susceptibility to cancer, did not initiate check-ups until clear evidence of symptoms interfered with function or death from cancer of loved ones occurred. The ambivalent-anxious women were characterized by a high level of anxiety in general but specifically with reference to cancer. They perceived themselves as less susceptible and prevention as pointless. Green [21] found the common variance among a set of nine preventive health practices in a statewide sample of young mothers was attributable to socioeconomic status—more specifically to the "maximum status identity" of the nuclear family. Thus a woman tended to behave in accordance with preventive health norms of the highest socioeconomic stratum to which she belonged by her own or her husband's educational level, occupation, and income.

Lack of knowledge concerning the symptoms of cancer is related to many factors. Simmons and Daland [37] reported that delay after onset of symptoms was due to lack of pain. Smith [38] found the reason of delay to be lack of severity of symptoms and disability. Pack and Gallo [34] and MacDonald [26] reported that ignorance and subsequent negligence accounted for delay in seeking medical attention. Hacket, Cassem, and Raker [22] concluded that those who labeled their conditions as "cancer" were significantly earlier in seeking medical care than those who referred to their condition as "tumor." Eardley [14] showed that the significant reductions in delay for breast symptoms in Britain were largely attributable to the increased reassurances of curability of cancer.

Enabling Factors. Enabling factors refer to the availability and accessibility of cancer detection and screening services. A classic example of this is the Pap smear programs which proved to be successful [11]. Another such example is breast cancer screening programs described in Shapiro [36]. Kodlin [25] and Dowdy et al. [13] concluded that such screening programs in addition to saving lives did prove cost effective in saving vast amounts of monies through early detection. This category includes teaching programs for professionals and the community aimed at preparing individuals to teach early detective techniques. It is hoped that such services will be available in screening for cancers of the colon, prostate, lung, skin, lymphatic system, and oral cavity.

The Reinforcer Factors. Patient and public education can reinforce early attention-seeking behavior even for other symptoms. Cancer screening of site-specific cancer can be done while detection is conducted for other less threatening diseases such as diabetes, hypertension, and the like. Health education on the part of health professionals must be encouraged and must be institutionally mandated. Through community organization and social and legislative action, the governmental sector can be made to act as a major enabler and reinforcer of cancer prevention through implementation of early detection programs free of charge.

It is apparent that it is not yet known whether generalization from primary preventive health behavior to secondary preventive health behavior can be made. It may be inferred, however, that each has its own unique problems and determinants. Common determinants of both are some predisposing and enabling factors such as availablity and accessibility of cancer preventive health care services, and public education about distinguishing suspicious changes in body parts or functions, or about the curability of cancer.

IMPLICATIONS FOR NURSING

Nursing Practice

As introduced by Florence Nightingale [32], nursing's functions included teaching prevention of disease and promotion of health. Driven by forces other than its own, nursing has moved away from these functions. It can and it must reexamine its roles in health—particularly in prevention of disease; including: (1) primary prevention; (2) early detection; (3) early treatment; and (4) optimum adaptation to the long-term illness and the preterminal phase.

In primary prevention nursing can be involved in teaching other nurses, health professionals, or the public about cancer preventive health practices and about cancer curability. If mobilized, nursing can be a tremendous force to further attitudinal and behavioral changes necessary for cancer control. In secondary prevention as well, nursing is a potent force for public contact. Nurses can aid in case finding, teaching recognition of cancer signals, teaching of breast self-examination, and developing and organizing community efforts for cancer control efforts. In tertiary prevention, which includes early treatment and continues until the preterminal stage, nursing's functions are collaborative with other disciplines. Earlier chapters have focused on these functions as they relate to specific cancer treatments. Chapter 10 will focus on rehabilitative functions in general.

Nursing Education

Given this orientation to the calling of nursing, it is natural that the educational content of the curriculae for neophytes as well as the advanced graduates be revised to include the necessary theory and practicum relative to skills in prevention of cancer. In this way education of the professional will become more consistent with the role of nursing in the broad management of cancer. Implications for such educational changes for continuing eduation for the practicing majority of nurses are also of paramount importance. Educational programs specific to all phases of the natural history of cancer are gravely needed.

Nursing Research

Again, referring to Nightingale's [32] vision of nursing, the need for acuity and scientific treatment of observations places nursing in an extremely responsible position. Due to its natural situation and therefore its contact with the public and the patients, nursing can and must contribute to research in cancer control. The problems, their descriptions, possible etiologic factors, and effective interventions specific to any or all of the phases of cancer need to be understood. Nursing can develop its own pure research and/or it can collaborate in interdisciplinary clinical research with all professionals allied in the management of cancer.

Finally, cancer nursing can and must create a model and set the pace in redefining its goals and functions according to those envisioned by Florence Nightingale.

REFERENCES

[1] ASHLEY, J.D.B. The Distribution of Lung Cancer and Bronchitis in England and Wales. *British Journal of Cancer*, 21:243-259, 1967.

[2] BECKER, M.H.; DRACHMAN, R.N.; and KIRSCHT, J.P. A New Approach to Explaining Sick-Role Behavior in Low-Income Populations. *American Journal of Public Health*, 64:205-216, 1974.

[3] BLACK, M.M., and LEIS, H.P. Mammary Carcinogenesis. *New York State Journal of Medicine*, 72:1601-1605, 1972.

[4] BLOCK, J.B. Angiosarcoma of the Liver Following Vinyl Chloride Exposure. *Journal of the American Medical Association*, 229:53-54, 1974.

[5] BOYDE, W. *The Spontaneous Regression of Cancer*. Springfield, Ill.: Chas. C Thomas, 1966.

[6] BURDETTE, W.J. Colorectal Carcinogenesis. *Cancer*, 34:872-877, 1974.

[7] CARROLL, E.K., GAMMEL, E.B.; and PLUNKETT, E.R. Dietary Fat and Mammary Cancer. *Canadian Medical Association Journal*, 98:590-593, 1968.

[8] CASSEL, J. The Contribution of the Social Environment to Host Resistance. *American Journal of Epidemiology*, 11:12-17, 1972.

[9] CLARK, R.L. Psychologic Reactions of Patients and Health Professionals to Cancer. In *Cancer: The Behavioral Dimensions*, ed. J.W. Cullen, B.H. Fox, and R.N. Isom, pp. 1-2. New York: Raven Press, 1976.

[10] DENOIX, P. Opening Address for Ninth International Cancer Congress, Florence, Italy, 1973.

[11] DICKENSON, L.; MUSSEY, M.E.; and KURLAND, L.T. Evaluation of the Effectiveness of Cytologic Screening for Cervical Cancer. 2. Survival Parameters Before and After Inception of Screening. *Mayo Clinic Proceedings*, 47:545-549, 1972.

[12] DOLL, R., and HILL, A.B. Smoking and Carcinoma of the Lung, Preliminary Report. *British Medical Journal*, 2:739-748, 1950.

[13] DOWDY, A.H.; BARKER, W.F.; LAGASSE, L.D.; SPERLING, L.; ZELDIS, L.J.; and LOGMIRE, W.P., Jr. Mammography as a Screening Method for the Large Populations. *Cancer*, 28:1558-1562, 1971.

[14] EARDLEY, A. Triggers to Action: A Study of What Makes Women Seek Advice for Breast Conditions. *International Journal of Health Education*, 17:256-265, 1974.

[15] Editorial. Rauwolfia Deviatives and Cancer. *Lancet*, 2:701-702, 1974.

[16] ENGEL, G. *Psychological Development in Health and Disease*. Philadelphia: Saunders, 1963.

[17] EWING, J. *Neoplastic Diseases,* 4th ed., Philadelphia: Saunders, 1961.

[18] FINK, R.; SHAPIRO, S.; and ROESTER, R. Impact of Efforts to Increase Participation in Repetitive Screenings for Early Breast Cancer Detection. *American Journal of Public Health,* 62:238-336, 1972.

[19] GARRETT, J.F., and LEVINE, E.S. *Rehabilitation Practices with the Physically Disabled,* p. 151. New York: Columbia University Press, 1973.

[20] GREEN, L.W. Site- and Symptom-Related Factors in Secondary Prevention of Cancer. In *Cancer: Behavioral Dimensions,* ed. J.W. Cullen, B.H. Fox, and R.N. Isom. New York: Raven Press, 1976.

[21] GREEN, L.W. *Status Identity and Preventive Health Behavior.* Berkeley: University of California, Pacific Health Education Reports, 1, 1970 (b).

[22] HACKETT, T.P.; CASSEM, N.H.; and RAKER, J.W. Patient Delay in Cancer. *New England Journal of Medicine,* 289:14-20, 1973.

[23] HEALEY, J., ed. *Ecology of the Cancer Patient,* Smithsonian Institution, p. 184. Washington, D.C.: Interdisciplinary Communications Program, 1970.

[24] KASL, S.V. The Health Belief Model and Behavior Related to Chronic Illness. *Health Education Monogram,* 2:433-454, 1974.

[25] KODLIN, D. A Note on the Cost-Benefit Problem in Screening for Breast Cancer. *Methods Inf. Med.,* 11:242-247, 1972.

[26] MacDONALD, E.J. Changing Reasons for Cancer Patient Delay. *Connecticut Health Bulletin,* 61:91-101, 1947.

[27] MAUSNER, J.S.; and BAHN, A.K. *Epidemiology,* pp. 9-12. Philadelphia: Saunders, 1974.

[28] MAUSNER, J.S., and BAHN, A.K. *Epidemiology,* pp. 6-9. Philadelphia: Saunders, 1974.

[29] *National Cancer Plan, 1972.* U.S. Department of Health, Education and Welfare, National Cancer Institute, 1972.

[30] *National Committee on Cancer, 1965.* Washington, D.C.: U.S. Department of Health, Education and Welfare, 1965.

[31] *National Health Survey: Concepts and definitions in the health-interview survey.* USPHS Pub. No. 584-A3. Washington, D.C.: U.S. Government Printing Office, 1958.

[32] Nightingale, F. *Notes on Nursing.* pp. 12-93. New York: Dover, 1969.

[33] PACK, G.T., and ARIEL, I.M. The History of Cancer Therapy. In *Cancer Management,* pp. 2-27, Philadelphia: Lippincott, 1968.

[34] PACK, G.T., and GALLO, J.S. The Culpability for Delay in the Treatment of Cancer. *American Journal of Cancer,* 33:443-463, 1938.

[35] SELIKOFF, J.J., and HAMMOND, E.C. Community Effects of Non-occupational Environmental Asbestos Exposure. *American Journal of Public Health,* 58:1658-1666, 1968.

[36] SHAPIRO, I.S. The Teaching Role of Health Professionals in a Formal Organization. *Health Education Monogram,* 1:40-48, 1973.

[37] SIMMONS, C.C., and DALAND, E.M. Cancer: Factors Entering into the Delay and Its Surgical Treatment. *Boston Medical Surgical Journal,* 183:298-308, 1920.

[38] SMITH, F.M. Factors Causing Delay in Operative Therapy of Carcinoma. *Surgical Gynecology and Obstetrics,* 60:45-53, 1935.

[39] U.S. DEPARTMENT OF HEALTH, EDUCATION AND WELFARE. *The Health Consequences of Smoking: A Report to the Surgeon General, 1971.* Washington, D.C.: U.S. Government Printing Office, 1973.

[40] *The Presidential Committee Investigation, 1965.* Washington, D.C.: Department of Health, Education and Welfare, 1965.

[41] WEISBURGER, J.H. Chemical Carcinogenesis in the Gastrointestinal Tract. In *Seventh National Cancer Conference Proceedings, American Cancer Society, Inc.,* pp. 465-473. Philadelphia: Lippincott, 1973.

[42] WOLFF, I.A., and WASSERMANN, A.E. Nitrates, Nitrites and Nitrosamines. *Science,* 1977:15-19, 1972.

[43] WYNDER, R.L.; ESCHER, G.C.; and MANTEL, N. An Epidemiological Investigation of Cancer of the Endometrium. *Cancer,* 19:489-520, 1966.

CAROL A. BRAINERD, R.N., M.N.
Oncology Program Director
Visiting Nurses Association
of Pasadena and San Gabriel Valley
Pasadena, California

chapter ten

Nursing concepts in rehabilitation of the cancer patient: The patient, the family, the community

THE CHALLENGE OF CANCER REHABILITATION

The challenge of cancer rehabilitation is a challenge based on several emerging factors. One such factor is the growing realization that for every cancer patient, regardless of stage, there are appropriate rehabilitative measures and goals that can enhance life. Statistics indicate that one out of four Americans or two out of three families are affected by cancer in their lifetime. One-third represent persons who will be cured. Half of the remaining two-thirds are estimated as curable with early detection and treatment. Whether cured, potentially curable, or incurable, each of these persons represents a potential for cancer rehabilitation. Those who are cured or whose cancer is potentially controllable may live with their cancer or the effects of the treatment for many years and can benefit from rehabilitation. Those whose cancer is incurable represent persons whose remaining life-span may have increased quality if appropriate rehabilitation measures are focused on supportive and palliative goals. There exists, therefore, a massive population, both with controllable and non-controllable cancer that can be positively affected by successful cancer rehabilitation.

A second factor that contributes to the tremendous challenge of cancer rehabilitation is the variety of diseases and the variety and extent of treatment that cancer represents. There is a myriad of basic kinds of cancers and many significant variations of these basic types [19]. Treatments include multiple modalities—surgery, chemotherapy, radiotherapy, immunotherapy—and of these major categories there are many, many types. Rehabilitation, then, if it were based simply on the type of treatment alone, would present a broad challenge in variety and extent.

A third factor is the expanding concept of rehabilitation. Rehabilitation has come to mean far more than the use of physical therapy. It now includes interventions by physicians, nurses, occupational therapists, physical therapists, speech therapists, nutritionists, social workers, psychologists, ministers, craftspeople, and lay persons. The concept has also expanded from a focus solely on the patient to a focus that includes the family and significant other persons as well as the patient in the rehabilitation process. This means that for every case of cancer, there may be several persons to be rehabilitated, and that for every case of cancer there may be many professional and nonprofessional persons involved in providing for that rehabilitation.

A fourth factor is that the time period considered to be appropriate for cancer rehabilitation is changing. It is no longer considered effective to wait for definitive treatment and then initiate rehabilitation. Rehabilitation in cancer now means predicting potential disability and assisting the patient early to develop skills and life-styles that may prevent the disability from occurring or at least limit its severity.

Rehabilitation nursing of the cancer patient, therefore, is now appropriate for nurses at all levels of expertise and in all settings—office, hospital, outpatient clinic, home, or community—wherever nurses find themselves relating to the cancer patient.

——— PERSPECTIVES ON CANCER REHABILITATION ———

Rehabilitation is closely linked with prevention, both practically and conceptually. An element of each is to be found in the other. Practically, rehabilitation can be a means of preventing further disability, while preventive efforts can be a means of rehabilitation. Perhaps the major difference between the two is that prevention focuses on inhibiting the disease, while rehabilitation focuses on restoring ability.

Stages of Disease

The concepts of stages and levels have been useful concepts in prevention [16]. Understanding these stages and levels also seems to be a useful concept in rehabilitation. The course of a disease generally follows a natural history of signs and events. This is true of cancer. Since cancer actually consists of many diseases, each kind of cancer has its own stages and course of events. Not every cancer goes through all stages and not every individual with the same kind of cancer goes through the same stages. Yet conceptualizing the disease process in general stages aids in focusing rehabilitation efforts appropriate to each stage.

Stage of Susceptibility. In this stage, factors are present that favor the occurrence of cancer even though the disease has not yet developed [16]. For some, the factors that favor the development of cancer are high. Smoking, exposure to industrial carcinogens, or a familial history of cancer are high-risk factors in the development of certain cancers. Persons exposed to these factors are in the stage of susceptibility. With the causative factors in many kinds of cancers still to be discovered, however, it is possible to say that to some degree we are all in the stage of susceptibility and at risk of developing cancer.

In this stage there may also be factors present that would inhibit the individual from dealing effectively with cancer should he develop cancer. Fear, poor health-seeking behaviors, lack of adequate health care, or lack of available health care are some of these factors. Each of these might make the individual more susceptible to potential disability. Rehabilitation efforts then might focus on rehabilitating the individual with excessive fear so as to prevent potential disability that results from delay in seeking treatment or noncompliance with treatment.

Stage of Presymptomatic Disease. In this stage there is no manifest disease, but pathogenetic changes have started to occur. These changes usually result from the interaction of multiple risk factors. At this stage, although the disease is not yet detectable by signs and symptoms, premalignant or even malignant changes are occurring [16]. Some cancers are believed to have a longer presymptomatic stage than others. It is possible that this stage will be shortened for some cancers as more sensitive measurements are developed for early detection.

Stage of Clinical Disease. Recognizable signs and symptoms of cancer are present in this stage [16]. Subdivisions of this stage, that is, staging by location, histologic type, and presence of metastasis, are used to further classify the stage of clinical disease and to make management and evaluation of treatment more effective. It is in this stage that active treatment to cure or prolong life is administered.

Since it is not necessarily true that persons move along the continuum from stage to stage, some persons who have been classified as having presymptomatic disease never do progress to the stage of clinical disease. This stage of clinical disease presents many opportunities for rehabilitation, particularly with acute disabilities.

Stage of Disability. It is in this stage that the cancer gives rise to residual loss of function of either short- or long-term duration [16]. The loss of function or body part and the subsequent disability may be a result of the disease or of the treatment. For example, the use of chemotherapy may have resulted in residual nerve damage or in cardiac problems. There may be loss of speech following laryngectomy, or loss of limb following amputation. This is the stage of more chronic disability, the stage most commonly believed to be the point of rehabilitation of the cancer patient.

End Stage. Not all cancer patients, of course, pass through the end stage of cancer, but for many the disease is indeed terminal. It is in this stage that active treatment to prolong life is no longer administered but treatment is instead focused on palliation. Approximately one-third of cancer patients are expected to reach the end stage of disease [2]. Rehabilitation efforts focus on palliation so that the individual can experience maximum quality of life.

Acute Versus Chronic Disabilities

A second perspective regarding cancer rehabilitation is the consideration of disability as either acute or chronic [20]. *Acute disability* is found frequently during the active treatment period. Postoperatively, for example, the patient may experience pain, fear, lack of mobility, eliminative problems, or the inability to eat. All of these acute disabilities prevent him from making maximum use of his resources. Preventative rehabilitation, such as good preoperative teaching, can help to reduce the degree of acute disability as well as the time needed for recovery from the disability.

Chronic disability is encountered when a long-lasting handicap is present. Many of the chronic disabilities presented by the cancer patient represent general categories of disabilities that are much the same as those arising from other conditions. Amputations are representative of such a disability. Some chronic disabilities, however, are particularly related to cancer and its treatment, such as changes related to a particular surgical procedure or long-lasting secondary effects of chemotherapy or radiation therapy. With this group, preventative rehabilitation may help to minimize predictable chronic disabilities and definitive rehabilitation may help restore the patient to maximum potential.

Levels of Rehabilitation

The concept of levels of rehabilitation provides another perspective helpful in understanding rehabilitation of the cancer patient. I have developed this perspective out of my experience and have utilized levels of rehabilitation that are similar to the levels of prevention discussed by epidemiologists [16]. These levels are primary, secondary, and tertiary rehabilitation. They differ according to goal or focus. These levels of rehabilitation may be used at any stage or point in the natural history of the cancer.

Primary Rehabilitation. The focus of *primary rehabilitation* is on restoration to a level of function that *prevents or inhibits* disability or the progression of the disability. Primary rehabilitation is preventative rehabilitation. Primary rehabilitation involves awareness of predictable disability, that is, disability that has not yet occurred but has the potential for occurring.

Predictable disabilities are present at any stage of cancer and therefore primary rehabilitation is possible at all stages. For example, in the stage of susceptibility, we can encourage individuals who have developed a life-style of stress to adopt stress-reducing behaviors, and perhaps, therefore, assist them in experiencing greater well-being should cancer develop.

Likewise, we can predict that the individual who has a high level of fear of cancer or who has inadequate health-seeking behaviors may delay in seeking regular checkups during the presymptomatic stage. That delay, therefore, is a predictable disability, keeping the person from optimal function. Rehabilitation efforts to reduce fear of cancer will, it is hoped, reduce the length of time between checkups and perhaps keep the patient from entering the stage of clinical disease.

In the stage of clinical disease, examples of primary rehabilitation are numerous. Predictable disability occurs, for instance, with the amputee. Training in crutch walking prior to surgery may greatly improve the patient's function and confidence postoperatively and therefore, reduce the predicted disability. Predictable disability may also occur in the patient receiving chemotherapy and radiation therapy. If nausea, for example, is an expected problem, consideration should be given to medication dosages and schedules, patient relaxation, and nutritional support during the course of the treatment. These measures may prevent or reduce the disability of nausea and enable the patient to make maximal use of resources during treatment.

Even in end-stage disease it is possible to predict disability and to take a rehabilitative approach that reduces the severity of the disability or prevents it from occurring altogether. For example, some cancers can be predicted to cause severe pain during end-stage disease. This pain is a debilitating symptom to the patient. The severity of pain can be reduced significantly if the patient can be taught early in end-stage disease how to take pain medications effectively and how to evaluate and reassess the pain regimen prescribed.

Secondary Rehabilitation. The secondary level of rehabilitation deals with actual disability situations in which the existing disability or its effects can be reduced significantly. The focus of the *secondary level of rehabilitation is prolongation of life and return to maximal functioning* with little residual handicap or, at the least, control of the problem.

Efforts with this level of rehabilitation may involve: (1) subtractive measures; (2) additive measures; or (3) measures that manipulate the existing environment or resources. Subtractive measures remove the source of the problem, such as the removal of disabling stress or fear, or the removal of the tumor that causes the pressure or pain. Additive measures include such rehabilitative measures as a prosthetic device, use of colostomy equipment, or institution of an adequate pain regime. Efforts involving manipulation of the patient's resources or environment might include rescheduling of medications or food intake or rearrangement of the patient's physical environment.

The secondary level of rehabilitation can include attention to both acute and chronic disabilities. Postoperative instruction, adequate medication, or range-of-motion exercises all might be definitive measures that reduce the acute disabilities of pain, immobility, and fear postoperatively. The secondary level of rehabilitation may also focus on chronic disabilities, such as loss of an extremity following amputation, facial disfiguration after radical head and neck surgery, or loss of voice following a laryngectomy. The common focus in all these examples of secondary level of rehabilitation is the reduction of disability and the restoration to maximal function in order to prolong life both in quality and in quantity.

Tertiary Rehabilitation. The tertiary level of rehabilitation occurs when disability is already present and the patient cannot be restored to predisability function. The focus of *tertiary rehabilitation* is primarily *palliative*; that is, the goal of rehabilitation is to make the patient more comfortable and thus improve his quality of life. Tertiary rehabilitation is generally thought of in connection with end-stage disease, for it is at this stage when symptom control of pain, anorexia, or eliminative problems can add immeasurably to a person's ability to function at maximum potential.

Tertiary rehabilitation may occur, however, even at earlier stages of disease. In the stage of susceptibility, a habitual smoker may be unwilling or unable to stop smoking. Using the level of tertiary rehabilitation, that person could be taught to incorporate such efforts as good nutrition, frequent checkups, or use of low-tar cigarettes to reduce the risk of moving from the stage of susceptibility into the stage of presymptomatic or clinical disease.

NURSING CONCEPTS OF CANCER REHABILITATION

Rehabilitation of the cancer patient is a complex problem requiring the skills and cooperation of all members of the health team. Because this is so, roles frequently overlap and health care givers ask who should do what, or who is responsible. In practice, overlapping roles do not need to be a problem. The health care giver who possesses the required skills and who has primary access to the patient, both in terms of time and relationship, is probably the most logical team member to do the job.

Use of a Nursing Model

It is appropriate, however, and extremely useful for nurses to possess an understanding of their unique roles, of their specific goals, and of their unique expertise in rehabilitation. In order to have a systematic way of understanding these focuses, nursing models have been developed. These nursing models, discussed in Chapter 13, provide some-what differing but systematic ways of understanding the patient.

The model chosen by the nurse as a guideline for nursing practice may fit into one of several categories: a systems model, which focuses on the patient as a functional unit with end boundaries; a developmental model, which focuses on the patient as having processes of growth and development; or an interactionist model, which focuses on nursing as a social act or a social relationship. Choice of a model will help the rehabilitation nurse in understanding what problems to focus on and what interventions to use.

My preference in working in the rehabilitation setting has been to use a systems model, the Johnson nursing model [11], for conceptualizing the patient and the patient's problems. In this model the patient is seen from the nursing viewpoint as a system of many behaviors, a system that attempts to maintain those behaviors in a stable and predictable balance. When the patient becomes ill, begins to have symptoms of cancer, is diagnosed, is treated, and subsequently lives with the effects of cancer and its treatment, many factors or variables upset the usual balanced way of behaving. The patient then tries to regain that balance or tries to "normalize" his life. This is the process of rehabilitation.

The nurse's unique function within such a framework is to facilitate the patient's return to stable, predictable, and effective behaviors, behaviors that meet the patient's own goals and facilitate health. The nurse can accomplish this by several means: by protecting from stresses; by stimulating and nurturing effective behaviors; or by inhibiting or restricting ineffective behaviors.

NURSING ASSESSMENT IN CANCER REHABILITATION

Broad categories of behaviors described by the Johnson model provide a basis for assessing the patient for rehabilitation needs. Figure 10.1 lists the broad categories that are to be observed and demonstrates a simple form for recording observations that might be noted [6].

Information needed to determine the type of rehabilitation suitable for the patient can come from many sources: charts, documents, health care givers, or the patient and his family. A preliminary look at the chart can often be a very satisfactory beginning showing age, sex, type of cancer, treatment, and payment source. Many of the important facts, however, need to be obtained directly from the patient and family.

NAME

MEDICAL DIAGNOSIS:

CHEMOTHERAPY:

RADIOTHERAPY:

SURGICAL PROCEDURES:

IMMUNOTHERAPY:

OBSERVATIONS DURING PATIENT/FAMILY EVALUATION:

Dependence for physical needs and/or emotional support:

Relationships with spouse, family, friends, and/or others:

Goals or plans/and efforts toward achieving these goals:

Threatening physical and/or emotional situations and ways of coping

Eating and drinking patterns including medication schedules:

Eliminative patterns including urine, bowels, discharges:

Sleeping, relaxation, and stress–reduction patterns:

Sexual functioning including roles and body image:

NURSING PROBLEMS AND DIAGNOSES:

FIGURE 10.1

When interviewing, it is important to sit with the patient, giving undivided attention and providing for no interruptions. Every effort must be made to ascertain the patient's and family's own values and goals since success in rehabilitation is dependent upon cooperation with these goals and values. During the interview special attention to the patient's first and last remarks may be of value. The first remarks made in introduction to the problem will reveal much about his attitude toward seeking help. Remarks at the end of the interview may indicate the patient's attitude toward the interview or the degree to which he will use his own efforts toward rehabilitation.

Questioning the patient and family can be done with one of two purposes: (1) to direct the patient's conversation into channels that will supply needed information; or (2) to obtain specific information. Table 10.1 includes a series of questions that are appropriate in eliciting the information that is needed to plan a suitable rehabilitation program [6]. These data can provide guidance in choosing the approach for rehabilitation and in helping to make plans for short- or long-range goals.

TABLE 10.1
Interview Schedule—Rehabilitation Assessment

Dependence

What kind of help will you need at home, and how will you manage?
What kind of equipment do you have available or need?
What responsibilities do you have to others?

Relationships

Who are your significant supportive persons?
How are they reacting to your illness?
What are your concerns about these persons?

Goals and Plans

What are your hopes and plans for activities for the future? for this week?
Do you have any immediate concerns about those activities?

Threatening Situations and Coping Mechanisms

What things are causing you problems now? the treatment? pain? medications? breathing difficulties? sensory problems? financial problems? family problems? ambulatory difficulties? other?
How do you usually cope? How are you coping now?
How do you feel about your illness?

Elimination

What is your usual pattern and way of handling bowels, urination, any other discharges?
What problems do you have now?

TABLE 10.1 (continued)

Intake—Eating, Drinking, Medicines

What is your usual eating and drinking pattern?
What medications do you usually take?
Any problems now?

Sleep, Relaxation, Stress Reduction

What is your usual sleeping and napping pattern?
How do you usually relax?
Any problems now?

Sexual Functioning, Roles, and Body Image

What is your usual role as wife/husband, mother/father, etc.?
Do you anticipate any problems with these roles?
Do you anticipate any change in your feelings about yourself
  or your body?
Any problems now?

Variables Affecting Rehabilitation

The major factors that seem to determine how the patient is affected by the illness and what success can be expected in subsequent rehabilitation are as follows [17]:

1. Developmental experience, both physical and psychological
2. Family, social, and cultural influences and their psychosocial effects
3. Symbolic meaning of experiences
4. Motivation, that is, level of aspiration and tolerance of frustration

Developmental Experiences. The patient's past experiences and relationships seem to have considerable effect on the prediction that successful rehabilitation will occur. A study of patients with head and neck cancer [17] indicated that a good postoperative course and successful rehabilitation were more likely to occur if the patient:

1. Was able to verbalize fears openly
2. Had adapted well in previous stressful situations
3. Had a successful work record
4. Had generally related well with family members
5. Had good relationships with previous doctors
6. Had good social relationships in general
7. Had positive past medical and surgical experiences

These factors seem to indicate the importance of understanding the patient's primary relationships and patterns of adjustment in predicting successful rehabilitation.

Family, Social, and Cultural Influences. Family members and family dynamics are important both as a focus of care and as a significant factor in promoting or inhibiting successful rehabilitation. Family may mean the traditional unit of husband, wife, and children or it may include one or more other persons who form a primary group and are significant in the patient's life.

When working with the patient and the family as the unit of rehabilitation, it is important to understand who the family members are, to understand the meaning of cancer and its treatment to each family member, and to understand role relationships between family members. Some questions to ask are: How are decisions made in the family group? What is the general feeling/tone of the family group? What are the family's priorities and who sets them?

It is also important to understand their concept of health, disease, and cancer. What are the family's health practices? When do they seek medical help? How does the patient's illness affect each family member? The nurse who demonstrates recognition and respect for the values and strengths of the particular family group is more likely to be successful in rehabilitation efforts.

The family's ability to respond to the stress of the diagnosis and treatment of cancer and subsequent rehabilitation efforts may depend upon the degree to which they can understand the problem, their capacity to tolerate stress, and their ability to organize effective coping mechanisms to deal with the illness and its affects. Poorly defined roles or poor communication may hamper their ability to work together effectively with rehabilitation efforts.

Cultural factors also seem to have an important impact on rehabilitation. The extent of this impact may be hard to determine, thus making it hard to avoid extremes—that is, developing stereotypes on the one hand, and ignoring its influence altogether on the other hand. Nurses susceptible to stereotypes are those who see a patient of a particular ethnic descent or subcultural group as "different from" other persons from other groups. Nurses who are susceptible to ignoring the influence of cultural factors are those who may feel that all patients should be treated alike and that it is prejudicial to consider the patient's race, creed, nationality, or even socioeconomic status.

In spite of the difficulty in determining just how cultural factors do affect the patient's response to illness and the chances for rehabil-

itation, there may still be some fruitful areas for consideration [24] :
How does the patient define illness? When should the patient seek
treatment in this subculture? What are common responses emo-
tionally, physically and behaviorally to cancer and its treatment?
How is a convalescing patient regarded by other family members?
How are health professionals regarded?

Sometimes attention to cultural attitudes toward the sick role,
toward compliance with medical instruction, or toward appropriate
time for a convalescent period may also uncover some important
variables affecting the patient's rehabilitation.

Symbolic Meaning of Experiences. An important variable to be
considered during the assessment is the unique meaning of cancer or
of the prescribed cancer treatment to the patient and family. Life-
styles, financial resources, or family attitudes are but a few of the
many factors that can be involved in what an individual's disease
means in his particular situation. The meaning of cancer will be discussed more comprehensively later in this chapter.

NURSING DIAGNOSIS
IN CANCER REHABILITATION

After assessing the patient's and family's needs for rehabilitation as
well as the variables involved, the nurse is ready to make a decision
regarding the underlying problem to be solved or the area that will be
the focus of rehabilitation. This decision is called nursing diagnosis.
Nursing diagnoses that accurately state the problem that must be
solved before rehabilitation occurs are not always clear-cut or easily
identified. Making the nursing diagnosis can be facilitated if several
perspectives are considered.

Perspectives in Rehabilitation Diagnoses

Some problems or diagnoses in rehabilitation seem common to the
general population of cancer patients rather than related to the particular cancer or the kind of treatment given. Other problems and
diagnoses are more directly related to the kind of cancer and to the
usual treatment for that kind of cancer. Whatever the problem
source, the problem itself will generally be manifested in one of the
behavioral categories in which assessment for rehabilitation needs
was made. When determining nursing diagnoses that are appropriate
for the rehabilitation process, use of one of the three perspectives
described below can be helpful.

Use of the Nursing Model
To Suggest Nursing Diagnoses

One helpful method for choosing a nursing diagnosis is to consider the areas that are designated as problem areas in whatever nursing model is used to approach the patient. With the Johnson nursing model, the nurse would focus on each of eight general categories and look for problems in these categories. If in any one of the categories the patient is not functioning in a manner compatible with the way he functioned before cancer or its treatment, that area would be a profitable focus for rehabilitation efforts.

The areas to be looked at are:

1. Dependence for physical needs and/or emotional support
2. Relationships with spouse, family, friends, and/or others
3. Goals and plans or efforts toward achieving these goals
4. Threatening physical and/or emotional situations and ways of coping
5. Eating and drinking patterns including medication schedules
6. Eliminative patterns including urine, bowels, discharges or drainage
7. Sleeping, relaxation, and stress-reduction patterns
8. Sexual functioning including roles and body image

To determine a nursing problem or diagnosis that requires nursing management, it is helpful to look for one of the following four major dysfunctional patterns in any of the eight behavioral categories:

1. The first dysfunctional pattern is inability to function effectively in a particular area due to insufficient environmental resources such as insufficient knowledge, insufficient or improper equipment, or insufficient or inappropriate external support. The problem of the patient who wishes to return to work but cannot due to job discrimination regarding his handicap can be classified in this category. This problem is broadly termed *insufficiency* [11].
2. The second dysfunctional pattern is inability to function effectively because the patient's own behaviors or actions cannot effectively achieve the desired goal; that is, a discrepancy exists between the actual behaviors and the desired goals. Inadequate nutrition due to anorexia, or leakage of an ileostomy appliance due to infrequent pouch changes are nursing problems that are classified in this category. This problem is broadly termed *discrepancy* [11].
3. The third dysfunctional pattern is dominance of one group of be-

haviors to the detriment of other behaviors. In this category would be the problem of uncontrolled pain which so dominates the patient's life that he is unable to eat or maintain his usual family roles. This problem is broadly termed *dominance* [11].

4. The fourth dysfunctional pattern occurs when the goals or behaviors of two different areas conflict with one another. The patient who desires to maintain a previous job that requires independent mobility but is now dependent on adaptive devices that require him to be dependent on others is an example. This problem is broadly termed *conflict* [11].

If one or more of these dysfunctional patterns are identified, rehabilitation efforts are indicated.

Use of Key Problem Areas for the Chronically Ill To Suggest Nursing Diagnoses

Another very helpful perspective in looking at the problems that cancer patients must face in rehabilitation is the consideration of key problem areas faced by chronically ill patients in "normalizing" their lives.

Some of these key problem areas are: (1) prevention and management of medical crises; (2) control of symptoms; (3) management of regimens; and (4) preparation for the trajectory, that is, the future course and prognosis of the disease [22].

In the area of *prevention and management of medical crises* or potential problems, all patients with disabilities from cancer must learn to read the signs of potential problems and know how to prepare for or organize for handling these potential problems. For example, patients with an amputation, loss of voice, chronic pain, or an ostomy all must know what problems to expect and how to manage if they should occur.

The patient with an ostomy will need to have an understanding of skin breakdown, what it looks like, what will cause it, and what will prevent it. That person would also need to know how to read the signs of good stomal circulation and stomal size and what to do if poor stomal circulation or constricting stomal size occurs. Likewise, management of potential problems of leakage, gas, constipation, odor, or infection, must all be a part of such a patient's repertoire.

Sometimes preparation for the potential problem includes teaching someone else in the family to manage the patient's care should the patient not be able to manage it independently. It also usually includes giving the patient referral phone numbers of appropriate people to call in an emergency—the physician, the Visiting Nurse Association, the enterstomal therapist, or others.

The problem of *symptom control* involves the need to learn about symptoms and their consequences. Pain, constipation, edema, discharges, night sweats, and odor are but a few possible symptoms. Each patient must learn what causes and controls each symptom. The patient with a colostomy, for example, must learn what happens if certain foods are eaten. The patient with amputation must learn what happens if perspiration of the stump occurs. The patient also learns the patterns of these symptoms, how long they last, when they occur, how they can be prevented, or how they can be diminished. The patient's attention to and awareness of the pattern of his symptoms will give him data for rehabilitation.

The patient also will consider, when attempting control of symptoms, what limits are present and how much can be done in spite of the symptoms. For example, how much communication can be achieved with and without esophageal speech? How much mobility is possible with and without the prostheses? All this data assists the patient in symptom control.

Along with recognizing the patterns, there is a lengthy task of trial and error, of testing out various means of control and evaluating them. The nurse has much to offer from experience in suggesting effective means of controlling symptoms. The major responsibility for control, however, rests with the patient.

The third key problem area includes *managing the regimen.* This involves the problem of learning how to manage diet, medicine regimens, and activity levels. It includes learning how to deal with the equipment used, learning how to use a new prosthesis, learning how to apply a colostomy pouch, or learning esophageal speech.

When considering what regimen it is that the patient will need to manage, it is essential to consider what the patient's choice of regimen is or will be. A regimen is not automatically accepted just because it is recommended by the physician or nurse. Regimens are evaluated on the basis of many factors such as:

1. The degree of difficulty in learning or in doing the regimen
2. The time involved
3. The amount of discomfort caused by the regimen
4. The amount of energy required to perform the regimen
5. The effectiveness of the regimen in relieving the troublesome symptoms
6. The expense of maintaining the regimen

7. The amount of social isolation caused by the regimen
8. Unpleasant side effects of the regimen

The patient's evaluation of these factors will determine his acceptance or rejection of the regimen [22].

If the regimen is easy to do, has minimal effect on the desired life-style, and greatly eases the bothersome symptom, the patient will probably accept the regimen. For example, the patient will be more apt to use a prosthesis if he finds it easy to apply, is able to walk satisfactorily with it, and can still maintain his usual life-style and investment of time and energy in his home, job, and relationships.

Acceptance or rejection of a regimen is also affected by the response of family members. If they are supportive, such as in giving the patient assistance when necessary, the patient is more apt to accept a particular regimen. Most patients also "shop around", that is, they get the advice of others—neighbors, friends, or even other professionals. This additional data greatly affects their evaluation of the regimen.

Sometimes the problem faced by the nurse is to find ways to minimize problems that are inhibiting acceptance of the regimen. In the final analysis, if the patient's choice is respected and his strengths recognized, he will choose a regimen that effectively fits in with his goals and life-style.

The fourth major problem area in which the cancer patient and family require rehabilitation is in *preparation for the expected outcome* and in dealing with the future course of the disease. Questions such as, "When can I resume sexual intercourse?" or "How do I buy a breast prosthesis?" are questions that deal with the future course. It is important to determine what the patient and family perceive as the potential outcome. Indeed, the patient's idea of his future and how to prepare for it may be very different from the idea held by the family or the health worker.

When facing the expected outcome and preparing for the future course of the disease, the meaning of cancer to the patient and family must be discussed, for the meaning of his cancer is an important determinant of how the patient sees the future. The meaning of cancer is unique to each individual. Age, socioeconomic status, culture, and profession are all variables that affect the meaning.

The meaning is also different for the same person at different times; for example, the meaning of a patient's cancer may change between the time he is first diagnosed and when he has completed his treatment. Because the meaning of cancer is different for different people at different times, the health care giver can only know the specific meaning to a specific patient if the patient is asked. The health care giver can make some intelligent guesses based on experience, research, or intuition, but in the end, the patient himself is the authority on what his particular cancer means for him.

To determine the person's view of cancer, that is, what it represents uniquely to that person, there are some key questions to ask:

1. What kind of cancer does the patient have?
2. What is the patient's knowledge and understanding of his cancer and where was that information obtained? Past experiences? Public media? Doctor? Family or friends?
3. How long has the patient known about his cancer? Because cancer represents a series of losses, perhaps ultimately ending in the loss of life itself, the individual goes through many stages. It becomes important, then, to know how long the patient has known about the illness because this will be a factor in what the meaning is for the patient at the present time.
4. Has the cancer metastasized? Is the patient facing palliative measures? Is he facing death?
5. Has the patient had radical treatment? Surgery, chemotherapy, radiation, immunotherapy, loss of a body part, or loss of a body function all radically affect how or what the cancer represents.
6. What are the patient's basic personality, life-style and life roles? What is his approach to life or ways of coping? Most persons remain fairly consistent in their approach to life. This basic life approach will be a fairly strong determinant in the meaning of his cancer.
7. How does the staff, family, and the surrounding environment react or act toward the patient's disease? Hopeful? Pessimistic? Realistic? Avoidant?

Among the common meanings or concepts that cancer represents to individuals are the following:

1. Guilt or punishment for some wrong action in the past
2. Fear of abandonment or social isolation
3. Debilitation, that is, loss of function, loss of energy, etc.
4. Disfigurement, such as in mastectomies, head and neck surgeries, and ostomies
5. Changes in livelihood with accompanying loss of self-esteem or financial difficulties
6. Contagion

7. Pain
8. Dependence on others and resulting loss of freedom.

These are some of the major meanings of cancer for the individual that affect his ability and effort in preparing for the future.

Use of Kinds of Cancer or Treatments
To Suggest Nursing Problems

A third major perspective for predicting the most common nursing problems and diagnoses to be found in the rehabilitation of the cancer patient is to consider the kind of cancer or treatment. The following is a list of the nine major areas in which rehabilitation needs are particularly evident:

1. Radical neck dissections
2. Cancer of the face and mouth
3. Laryngectomies
4. Ostomies
5. Mastectomies
6. Cancer of the lung
7. Nervous system tumor involvements
8. Bone and soft tissue involvements
9. Leukemias and lymphomas

The particular problems of each of these special groups of patients will be discussed in more detail.

Cancer of the Face and Mouth and/or Radical Neck Dissections. When caring for the patient who is being treated for cancer of the face and mouth or with radical neck dissection, the rehabilitation nurse faces several specific problems. Preoperatively, the patient usually experiences fears of death and mutilation, fears of loss of sight or of speech, or fears of loss of social relations. Postoperatively, these fears have become a reality. A period of depression usually begins. This depression is complicated by the fact of physical weakness postoperatively. The rehabilitation nurse must be prepared for severe emotional reactions with paranoid, hostile, or aggressive behaviors [17].

Patients who are treated with radical neck dissection experience cosmetic defects and disability in the shoulder on the operated side due to dissection of the accessory or eleventh cranial nerve. Muscle paralysis, dropped painful shoulder, and rotated scapula all may occur in varying degrees. Initial support to the arm and shoulder with sling, exercise programs, and surgical interventions attempting to use nerve grafts may all be required for this disability [9].

Some of the specific disabilities encountered after treatment of cancers of the face and mouth may involve the following [17]:

1. Severe cosmetic problems and changes in body image
2. Speech defects and communication problems
3. Difficulties with chewing
4. Swallowing difficulties
5. Problems with salivary control
6. Attitudes towards prostheses
7. Family and social relations
8. Problems associated with return to work

For cancers of the eye requiring enucleation of the eye, the cosmetic problem will be complicated by changes in perception and reductions of the total visual field.

Because the areas of disfigurement around the face, mouth, and neck are difficult to hide, the patient experiences severe psychological responses to the treatment. Rehabilitation care ideally should be started in the preoperative period and should include psychological support.

The fact that surgical treatment in head and neck cancers is usually carried out in a series of stages is also a source of potential problems. At each stage temporary prostheses and rehabilitative efforts can help lessen disfigurement and restore as much functional ability as possible while the patient is waiting for the next stage of treatment [9].

Many services will be needed to cooperate before final rehabilitation of these patients is accomplished. Speech therapy, social services, surgeons, dentists, and nurses will all be required in helping the patient toward maximal restoration of his potential.

Laryngectomies. Patients having laryngectomies, although experiencing the general problems just mentioned for the patient with head and neck cancer, have other particular problems. They must learn a new way of verbal communication and must learn to live with a permanent opening in their lower neck. Difficulties of handling secretions from the tracheostomy, and coughing and wheezing may also affect intimate contact with others.

Learning esophageal speech is a particular challenge to the laryngectomy patient. He will need to learn to deal with the complications of esophageal speech, that is, with belching, rectal gas, abdominal distention, stomach troubles, or even ulcers. These problems can be very discouraging. If the patient is older or has no work or outside interests that require effective communication, it will be even harder to motivate him in the use of a new way of verbal communication. Usually success in esophageal speech is proportional to the amount of outside effort and incentive used to motivate the patient.

To complicate these inevitable problems of a patient with a laryngectomy is the fact that many of these patients have had a problem with alcoholism before treatment of their cancer [17]. For those with problems of alcoholism, there must be an understanding early in the patient's treatment of how this will affect the patient's rehabilitation, and of what plans will be made to assist the patient with this problem.

Problems of the Patient with an Ostomy. Rehabilitative needs of patients with ostomies occur at three principle times: (1)initial efforts preoperatively and postoperatively for the patient with a new stoma; (2) general rehabilitation with training adjustment and reassurance; and (3) crisis points or special situations where intervention is needed.

Rehabilitation begins with some important preoperative considerations. Preoperatively the placement of the stoma is essential for maximal rehabilitation [14]. The stoma must be at a functional site, that is, a place where an appliance can easily adhere, a place that will not interfere with wearing of clothes for work or recreation, and a place that will not interfere with belts or adhesives of other appliances should the patient need two stomas, such as the patient with both an ileal conduit and a colostomy.

General rehabilitation includes both practical problems and dealing with fears. Since the responsibility for his stoma becomes a lifelong task, the patient must understand the stoma and his own functional and physical signs. With this knowledge the patient will know when to seek professional advice and will know how to use the advice that is given to him. From my experience, insufficient instruction regarding practical problems seems to be a frequent deficiency in current rehabilitation of colostomy patients. Problems centering around appliances, skin difficulties, changes in the stoma; problems of odor, gas, or noise; and problems regarding the effect of foods on colostomy performance are some of the major problems of the ostomy patient. In 50% of males, impotence is experienced following abdominal-perineal resection usually performed with colostomies [9]. Potential sexual difficulties, then, also need to be discussed with the patient and his family.

Fears of the patient with an ostomy may revolve around: (1) fear of loss of self-esteem, especially if "normal" bowel or bladder function is believed to be a prerequisite to being accepted; (2) frustration with the interference or loss of the body function such as loss of bowel control after a colostomy or loss of bladder control after an ileal conduit; and (3) possible alterations in interpersonal relationships such as withdrawal from usual social events or withdrawal from a spouse.

Problems of the Mastectomy Patient. Special problems for the mastectomy patient after treatment are based on both psychological and physical factors. Some of the physical disabilities occasionally experienced are lymphedema, brachial plexus palsy, and shoulder dysfunction. Approximately 50% of mastectomy patients do experience some postoperative arm edema on the operative side with its resulting pain, restriction of shoulder motion, and swelling [9,13]. The swelling that appears early in the postoperative period and is slight most frequently subsides. The swelling is more likely to be persistent or progressive if it occurs weeks or months after the surgery [9]. Early efforts at rehabilitation, including positioning, exercises, and psychological support, will result in the best restoration of physical function and the control of edema.

There may also be brachial plexus palsy in the postoperative phase requiring the use of physical therapy or orthotic devices designed to restore function. Shoulder dysfunction can usually be prevented by immediately instituting full range-of-motion shoulder exercises postoperatively [9,13].

Specific psychological concerns of mastectomy patients are: (1) the patient's self-image, that is, dealing with the loss of a breast as well as the loss of a body part that is sexually significant; (2) the patient's desire to develop a healthy denial of the mastectomy but fear that telling others will prevent this from occurring; (3) the patient's fear of and worry over possible removal of the remaining breast; (4) the patient's choice of a breast prosthesis; and (5) the patient's plans for return to work or former life-style [23,12].

Group methods of psychological support of the mastectomy patient have been frequently and successfully used [23]. In these groups patients can help and be helped by each other. Since all mastectomy patients must make some adjustments, the group approach is especially helpful to patients in coping, for assistance is available without waiting for a crisis or physical disability to occur.

Cancer of the Lung. The effects of thoracotomy and associated procedures are the primary focus of disability in the patient with cancer of the lung. The effects of the surgery may include restriction of pulmonary function, decreased respiratory reserve depending on the amount of lung tissue removed, or difficulty with the mechanics of breathing if the chest wall has been resected [9]. Preoperative teaching of breathing and coughing exercises and encouragement of these exercises postoperatively can assist in maintaining full range of motion and strength on the operated side.

Problems of Patients with Tumor Involvements of the Central and Peripheral Nervous System. Any malignancy that involves the brain and spinal cord or peripheral nerves, whether primary or metastatic, may result in disabilities that affect coordination or sensory abilities [8]. If sensory abilities are lost, other sensory modalities must be trained to substitute for the loss. If motor coordination is impaired, special training exercises may improve function.

Persistent pain is another disability that often occurs with nervous system involvement. Pain requires many approaches. Steroids, radiation therapy, surgical procedures, hypnosis, medications, the application of hot packs and cold packs, and gentle massage in certain cases are all various methods employed to reduce a variety of kinds of pain [9,18].

Problems of Patients with Amputations. Cancer patients with prostheses due to amputation of extremities experience much the same problems as patients requiring amputation from other diseases. The major difference between the cancer and the noncancer patient requiring amputation is the degree of fear. This fear involves a fear of the unknown, an uncertainty of the future, and a fear of reoccurrence of disease.

In the opinion of some, the most important elements in successful rehabilitation are the patient's desire and stamina. If the patient needs an excuse to be helpless and dependent, the amputation can serve this purpose well. The degree of dependence experienced is seemingly more related to the motivation to become self-sufficient than to the amputation itself [3].

Problems of self-image can be similar to those problems of self-image that accompany the loss of any body part. These problems include the patient's frustration over the loss of function of that extremity, and fear that he will not be loved or accepted. The patient with amputation may have difficulty with certain social events such as dancing and therefore may fear living a less active or socially isolated life.

Patients with amputations often have problems of adjusting to activities of daily living. Restrictions requiring adjustment are based on the type and severity of amputation experienced and may include problems of bending, bathing, fitting of clothes, riding escalators, or simply the fear of falling on such things as wet pavement.

There are also problems related to the prosthesis itself. Difficulty in maintaining an adequate fit due to weight gain or loss may occur. Perspiration of the stump may cause discomfort and breakdown of tissue. There may also be physical pain in the remaining portion of the limb resulting from exposed nerve ends or broken down tissue.

Other problems experienced by the amputee include problems of finding employment and problems of transportation. Expense is also a consideration because of special devices and equipment that are required.

Rehabilitation Problems of Leukemia and Lymphoma Patients. Rehabilitation with leukemia and lymphoma patients is primarily involved with long- and short-term side effects from chemotherapy and radiation therapy. With these patients there is also a fear of recurrence and fear of death from cancer, as well as the need to deal with the weakness and other effects of the disease itself.

For the young patient with leukemia, there may be particular problems associated with growth and development, or problems associated with adolescence. As the patient becomes an adult, he may experience problems with infertility, difficulty in obtaining health insurance, or job discrimination, all areas requiring rehabilitative efforts.

NURSING INTERVENTIONS IN CANCER REHABILITATION

Effective rehabilitation is primarily the process or philosophy of setting realistic goals. How realistic a goal is depends on: (1) what the patient and family unit are capable of achieving; (2) what the patient and family unit desire to achieve; and (3) what resources are available to them either from within themselves or from the outside. Such outside resources include friends, community facilities and services, available health care givers and specialists, available equipment, and financial resources. It is not a realistic goal, for example, for an elderly patient who lives alone and has end-stage cancer to expect to spend the final days of his illness at home if there are no friends, attendants, or other persons such as volunteers from the community, available to provide primary care as his condition weakens. It is a reasonable goal for that patient, however, to spend his final days at home if there is someone willing and able to give primary care when it is needed.

Realistic expectations or goals for the patient can be classified into four broad categories: preventative goals, restorative goals, supportive goals, and palliative goals [20,10]. These varying approaches serve to emphasize that rehabilitation can take place at many levels. If the appropriate approach and goal is chosen the potential for successful rehabilitation is high.

After realistic and appropriate goals are set, evaluation criteria should be defined so that it will be evident to the patient, family, and nurse when rehabilitation is achieved. For example, if a palliative goal such as pain control is chosen, the evaluation criteria of successful pain control can have a broad range of possibilities. The patient may consider his pain controlled when he is able to be awake, alert, and conversing coherently and pleasantly with other family members. For other patients, the preferred criteria for pain control might be the ability to sleep through the night without pain or restlessness.

A more precise way of designating behaviors that measure successful rehabilitation would be to specify certain behavioral targets that could be counted and then to specify the direction of desired change as to the increase, decrease, or maintenance of frequency. These behavioral targets might include such things as social behaviors, that is, number of persons visited, number of personal contacts, number of telephone calls, or number of minutes of family interaction. Other activities to measure might include such things as the number of minutes of work in the house, number of minutes spent watching TV, number of minutes spent resting, and so on [21]. The goal for each of the specific criteria must be set realistically, that is, it must be something that is possible for the patient to achieve.

After the goal is set and the evaluation criteria are determined, nursing interventions can be planned. Four major types of nursing interventions emerge in the field of cancer rehabilitation: (1) patient and family education; (2) patient and family assessment; (3) patient and family advocacy and referrals; and (4) patient and family counseling.

Patient Education

Patient education seems to be particularly appropriate in terms of rehabilitation efforts. Particularly when patients make the transition from the hospital to the home setting, they are ready to ask questions, ready for teaching, and motivated to learn such things as how to manage symptoms, equipment, or activities of daily living. Patients at this point are also ready to hear what the effects of their particular treatment might be [6].

Teaching Preparation for Medical Crisis. First let us look at how to teach the patient and family how to prevent and prepare for potential medical crisis. These types of teaching efforts can be seen as primary or preventative rehabilitation. Here the family and the patient are prepared for potential problems that might occur, are assisted in developing organizational efforts to prevent potential crises from occurring, and are taught to manage them should they occur. The patient and family prepared with these skills can prevent serious results from a potential crisis.

The patient and family are first taught how to properly read the signs that indicate impending crisis. The ileostomy patient is taught not only how to prevent skin breakdown but how to recognize the signs of beginning skin breakdown. He is also taught what to do if skin breakdown actually occurs. Likewise, the family of the bed-bound patient in end-stage cancer is taught how to prevent decubiti by frequent turning, as well as what to do if beginning signs such as redness occur.

Not only is the patient and family taught how to read the signs of crisis but how to organize for the crisis. For example, in end-stage disease there is considerable organization required of family members in order to provide care for the patient. Some family members may need to take time off from work and rearrange schedules, or attendants may need to be hired. If the patient then becomes comatose or severely weakened the family has already organized available resources to meet the crises satisfactorily.

Teaching the Patient How To Manage a Regimen. Rehabilitation frequently involves the learning of a new regimen, whether it be to add something such as taking a drug or learning a new activity, or whether it involves eliminating something such as eliminating a certain food. The regimens that must be learned can be very complex or simple. A complex regimen—the learning of esophageal speech—is required of the patient with a laryngectomy. Some regimens are complex at first, such as learning to irrigate a colostomy, but become rather simple with practice.

To a great degree learning the regimen requires "learning through experience." This suggests that the nurse can help the patient become aware of what the patient's own unique reactions are to various aspects of the regimen and then assist him in learning how to handle these reactions.

Teaching the Patient Symptom Control. Teaching the patient symptom control requires that the patient learn in detail about symptoms and their consequences. He must discover his limits, what he can do in spite of the symptoms, and how he can plan activities around the symptoms.

Learning symptom control also means the patient must learn to acquire an awareness of his own body, what it can and cannot do now as opposed to what it could do before the illness or treatment. The patient who learns energy conservation, how to make the most of the energy that remains, is learning how to manage symptom control.

Many people are very inventive about arranging things or working out special devices that permit them to do the activities they wish to with minimal discomfort, pain, or drain of energy. The experienced nurse who has met a great number of patients with virtually identical symptom problems has much to offer. She or he can be alert to how those individuals inventively manage their symptoms and pass useful information along to other patients.

Teaching the Patient How To Plan for the Future Course. The future course refers to the anticipated sequence of phases. The predictability of these sequences may be relatively uncertain or fairly certain. When it is uncertain, the patient and family may have a difficult time making arrangements and knowing how to plan and prepare. If the sequence of phases is relatively predictable, such as knowing that a new stoma will reach maximum shrinkage in about 6 weeks postoperatively, plans can be made to prepare for the expected event, such as waiting to decide on the size of the permanent appliance until the stoma has reached maximum shrinkage. The nurse's knowledge of predictable phases can be helpful data for the patient and family in planning ahead.

At every step or phase the patient must reassess where he is and determine anew what arrangements are necessary in order for him to effectively manage his symptoms, daily life, and preparations for the future. At each phase he becomes a new person. Teaching the patient and the family how to deal with this new person at a new phase becomes an important part of the rehabilitation process.

Patient and Family Assessment

Another major intervention of the nurse in rehabilitation of the cancer patient is intervening by giving feedback through the process of patient and family assessment. Many patients in the rehabilitative phase will state that they are "doing okay" and yet when the nurse shows interest and time in assessing the problems, are eager to have feedback on problems that are bothering them. Often they have been trying to assess their own problems, have made certain evaluations, and yet are uncertain as to whether their symptoms or evaluations are normal or abnormal and whether or not they are "doing the right thing." Patient and family assessment is valuable to the nurse in providing a basis for nursing interventions but is also valuable to the patient and family in gaining feedback on their own assessments and interventions.

Patient Advocacy and Referrals

During the rehabilitation process the nurse has frequent opportunities for teaching the patient his rights, communicating with other services on behalf of the patient and in making patient referrals to appropriate sources. Rehabilitation is a cooperative effort involving many team members—physical therapist, occupational therapist, speech therapist, physician, nurse, family members, and the patient himself. This team effort requires communication and a willingness to refer.

Frequently it is the nurse who becomes the appropriate person to suggest other team members who might be of assistance in the rehabilitation process. Spiritual support, financial counseling, learning new skills—all may be needs of the patient for which the patient would like assistance from persons other than the nurse. To have an extensive knowledge of the community and its available resources becomes a particular asset when referring patients to appropriate resources.

Communicating with other services on behalf of the patient helps to coordinate the team effort in rehabilitation and provides for continuity of care. Through these efforts the patient can be taught how the health care system works and how to make the transition from one phase to another.

Patient and Family Counseling

In this section we will deal with the interventions needed in rehabilitation that require patient counseling. Dealing with the diagnosis and mobilizing the life force are two significant areas of discussion.

Dealing with the Diagnosis. Counseling is seen as talking with the patient in a way that assists him in recognizing and utilizing his own resources. Teaching is seen as giving the patient new information. Since we are discussing counseling the patient in this section, we will not discuss the question of what to tell the patient so much as the question of how to assist the patient in coping with what he already knows. Dealing with the diagnosis may require such counseling techniques as crisis intervention and empathic listening.

Crisis Intervention. If the patient's emotional response to the diagnosis or the treatment causes a temporary inability to use his usual coping mechanisms, we consider the patient to be "in crisis." The steps in crisis intervention are: (1) assessing the patient's usual support systems; (2) clarifying the patient's perception of the crisis; (3) assessing the patient's usual coping mechanisms; and (4) helping the patient determine a plan of action [1]. This may include using a previous coping mechanism or developing a new coping mechanism. Sometimes simply helping the patient clarify how he perceives the diagnosis assists him in being able to resume his normally effective coping mechanisms.

Empathic Listening. An important counseling technique that can be used effectively in helping the patient respond constructively in the face of a threatening diagnosis and treatment is to use empathic listening. Active listening, empathic listening, and creative listening are all terms used to describe a similar approach to listening to the patient so that he feels understood. When a person feels understood, that person may then be able to move on to creatively dealing with the situation.

The first skill of empathic listening is using attending behavior. This means sitting wth the patient, using good eye contact, nodding the head at appropriate times, that is, using body language that shows one's full attention is directed towards the patient.

The second skill of empathic listening is for the listener to be able to "feed back" or restate what he or she hears or senses the patient is saying. A phrase such as, "Let me see if I understand what you are saying . . ." followed by a paraphrase of what the patient has described about the situation and his feelings may help the patient feel understood. This restatement of key phrases that the patient has used in conversation will indicate that the listener has heard what has been said and that nothing has been "missed" in what was important to the patient.

Checking out implications, if done in a tentative way that does not assume that the nurse knows more about the patient's feelings than the patient does, may also help the patient to feel understood. For example, the sentence might be started by "It seems as though ...." The patient then is free to respond to this tentativeness of the implication with agreement or disagreement. This author believes the patient is always the final authority on how he perceives the situation and that the patient should never be talked into a feeling, either positive or negative, that he does not express.

Another skill that helps the patient feel understood is agreeing with him or affirming whatever can be agreed with or affirmed in the conversation. For example, to say, "It would seem frightening to me too in that situation," is an affirmation to the patient that the expressed feelings are okay and might be experienced by someone else in the same circumstances. To help the patient know that he is believed or that his feelings might be experienced by others in similar circumstances often helps the patient feel understood and can then give the patient the basis to move on to creatively solving his problems.

Mobilizing the Life Force.   It is common to hear talk about helping the patient to maintain the hope that there is always something more that can be done, a hope based on the security that the patient knows he will never be abandoned. This author believes, however, that quality of life is based on something in addition to maintaining hope. The exhilirating feeling of watching someone who has cancer and fully lives life or who may be in end-stage cancer and yet has an unmistakable quality of life comes from seeing a person who has the characteristic often called the "will to live." LeShan [15] calls this will to live "the life force." His interesting paper on "Mobilizing the Life Force" reveals that there are two problems: the fear of death and the fear of life. The fear of death is actually the minor problem while fearing to live life or fearing to face life "head on," whatever that may be, is the major problem.

LeShan believes that patients may fight to live for two different reasons: (1) the wish to live; and (2) the fear of death. The wish to live is a much stronger force in binding together the resources of the person.

The counseling person who wishes to assist the patient in his fight to live is working to increase the "person," the "being," or the "soul" in whatever aspect it exists. This will to live is connected with the freedom to be oneself fully without fear, to develop in one's own special way. This involves giving up concerns about the opinions of others, about "success," or even about one's own fears. It means becoming concerned about inner development. The nurse can approach the patient by such questions as, "What do you really want in life?" Exploring this can help the patient find his own strengths and perhaps discover what blocks the use of these strengths. In the final analysis, the patient must look into his inner resources and listen to those internal messages that say "I enjoy this," "I like doing this," "I do not like this."

The patient can experience reduction of fear of death when these creative internal impulses are rearoused. The nurse's function is to help the patient find these creative impulses and then assist in stimulating them. Use of these impulses gives the individual goals in life that are meaningful to him.

THE COMMUNITY AND REHABILITATION

Understanding the Mechanisms of the Community

Due to the variety and extent of diseases and treatments which cancer represents, and due to the sequential nature of the many stages, rehabilitation depends on the involvement of and the utilization of many community resources. The first step in utilizing community resources in rehabilitation is knowing what resources are available and understanding the mechanisms involved in utilizing them.

Categories of Available Facilities

Available services and facilities within a community may be many and varied, and may function differently depending on the community in which they are located. Some community facilities that can be assessed as potential resources in rehabilitating the cancer patient are described below [5].

Hospitals. Hospitals may be public or private, teaching or nonteaching. The facility may be set up to handle most situations, from diagnosis to rehabilitation, or it may be equipped to provide only simple services with comprehensive treatment provided elsewhere. It is important to know if the hospital has a staff of well-qualified specialists, what social services are provided, where special consultation can be obtained, and how persons can be transported to the facility.

Extended Care Facilities. Extended care facilities may have beds available only for continued treatment and rehabilitation after acute hospitalization, or they may also have beds available for persons who can no longer be maintained in their own homes because of increasing disability. Some facilities have an understanding of the special needs for cancer rehabilitation.

Clinics and Outpatient Facilities. Assessment of clinics and outpatient facilities includes knowledge of ambulatory facilities available for cancer patients, transportation available to these facilities and the qualifications of staff in these facilities. Type of rehabilitative services provided, manner of funding, and communications with existing inpatient services are other important areas of assessment.

Emergency Services. Emergency services refer to ambulances, paramedics, and 24-hour services. The service may be limited to a specific geographical area and, in the case of ambulance service, may be willing to take patients in an emergency only to specific facilities. Investigation will reveal the kind of emergency care for which the rescue personnel are trained. If they are trained only in heroic measures, they may not be the appropriate persons to call for a person in end-stage disease who does not want heroic measures.

Personnel. Specialists may be available in the community, such as oncologists, internists, radiotherapists, enterostomal therapists, clinical nurse specialists, nurse practitioners, psychologists, psychiatrists, and social workers. Useful knowledge includes where these people are located, the agencies with which they are associated, and the specialists' specific qualifications and abilities. It is important to know who is eligible to receive their services, how their services may be purchased, and how their services are coordinated with others in the community.

Voluntary Agencies. Voluntary agencies may exist in the community specifically to aid cancer patients, such as American Cancer Society, Cancervive, Cancer Line. They may offer equipment, counseling, funds for home care, drugs, homemakers, transportation, or volunteer help. Eligibility and the process for obtaining assistance must be assessed. Other agencies existing in the community, although not designed especially for cancer patients, can also be of assistance in cancer rehabilitation. Meals-on-Wheels, Homemakers Associations, and Seniors-on-the-Move are some of these agencies.

State Agencies. Each state has its own funded programs designed to assist disabled persons. Many of these programs are appropriate for the cancer patient. State agencies may work toward such goals as eliminating job discrimination, providing social services, or operating rehabilitation programs. In-Home Supportive Services is an example of such a program.

Self-Help Groups. Groups of persons sharing a common disability and a common goal of helping one another cope with the disability are available and effective in many communities. Reach to Recovery is an organization of women with mastectomies who assist other women in learning to cope with a mastectomy. The Lost Chord Club, for those with laryngectomies, and the Ostomy Association for those with ostomies are similar self-help groups.

Home Health Agencies. Home care programs have two purposes: (1) to provide hospital type services for patients who are inappropriately hospitalized and can be cared for at home; and (2) to provide preventative and rehabilitative services in the home when this is the most appropriate setting. The range of services offered by the home care program may include acute care, chronic care, or hospice care. Nurses, physicians, homemakers, home health aides, physical therapists, occupational therapists, social workers, and speech therapists may be available. Investigation of the population which they serve, how referrals are made, and who pays for the services may also reveal their relationship with the other health facilities in the community.

Consumer Services. Although not specifically designed for cancer patients and perhaps not designed specifically for the ill at all, the availability of consumer services affects the plan of rehabilitation. Assessment should include what grocery stores are available, what special products they carry, and whether delivery and competitive prices are available. Significant to cancer rehabilitation are pharmacies or stores that carry the products needed such as drugs, ostomy supplies, breast prostheses, and dressings. The manner in which billing is done, the accessibility to various geographical areas, home delivery of products, and the availability of sales personnel who are well-trained and sensitive to rehabilitation problems of the cancer patient will determine their usefulness.

Hospices. A type of care focusing on symptom control and supportive services for the dying patient and family is called hospice care. Such care usually includes: (1) emphasis on symptom control; (2) treatment of the patient and family as a unit; (3) use of an interdisciplinary team; (4) involvement of volunteers especially for supportive assistance; (5) 24-hour availability of the team for consultation or assistance; and (6) bereavement care. Such care may be provided by a specially designed in-patient facility and/or home care service called a hospice or may be part of the care given by professionals and volunteers in in-patient and home care services who understand supportive and palliative care.

Categories of Funding for Rehabilitation Services

Ways of financing rehabilitative services are many and varied. The general classifications of financial resources are discussed below [4].

Personal Payment.   The individual's own financial resources are utilized, including those resources that are borrowed or received from someone else such as a relative, friend, or loan company. The individual privately purchases the service.

Charity.   Charity funds come from voluntary sources who are not direct beneficiaries of the services. United Way, the Leukemia Foundation, American Cancer Society, and hospital auxiliary funds all collect and distribute funds to appropriate persons or organizations who are in need of resources.

Voluntary Insurance.   Financing of health care services by voluntary insurance is supported by periodic contributions or payments by groups of persons. The benefits are available only to those persons or their dependents who have contributed. Blue Cross, Blue Shield, and various other insurances are widely used in our population. Group-sponsored plans, such as Kaiser-Permante, that provide comprehensive services through group medical practice and health maintenance organizations, also can be classified as voluntary insurance. Although many people in our population use such payment for health care needs, large segments of the population—the poor, the elderly, people in rural areas—frequently are not covered by this kind of insurance.

Social Insurance.   Social insurance is insurance required by law to pay for certain services to designated persons. Medicare, which covers hospital and home care for the elderly, is an example of this kind of insurance. People who may benefit from Medicare are those who are 65 and older and those under 65 who have been disabled and who qualified for Social Security cash disability benefits for at least two years.

General Revenues. Money that comes from local, county, state, or national governments through taxation on income, property, and the like is often used to support health services. These services are generally not limited only to taxpayers, but are available to needy or low-income people who are eligible. Medicaid is an example of this source of financing.

A plan for rehabilitation of the cancer patient at any stage is not viable unless there is a source of financing available. Becoming familiar with these resources and with the patient's current and potential eligibility for these resources is an important task of the nurse who assists in designing the rehabilitation plan.

Mobilizing and Using the Community Resources

Once the nurse understands what resources are available in the community in which the patient functions and understands what the mechanisms are for utilizing these resources, how does she or he then mobilize these resources for the patient and family? The key roles for the nurse in this part of rehabilitation are "patient advocate" and "change agent." Both of these terms, advocate and agent, indicate one who acts "for" or "in the place of" the originator of the idea or plan. These concepts recognize that personal responsibility of the patient and the family is a basic premise and that their needs and their rights can never be bypassed. They also recognize that effective rehabilitation only occurs when those who have the power and the responsibility, that is, the patient and the family, support the plan and support the referral to a community resource.

I have also found that whenever feasible, that is, when the mechanism for referral allows for it and when the patient and family have the capability to do it, it is more effective for the patient or family to contract with the referral sources themselves. This does not mean that the nurse or other health care giver's efforts are not needed, but that these efforts usually take the form of education regarding available resources, supervision and support during utilization of resources, and coordination of these multiple resources.

Potential conflict between the patient/family unit and the caregiver may occur. This conflict may follow the introduction of a new idea or new resource. Such conflict is a natural phenomenon as the individual patient will be overcoming resistances that naturally occur before a new idea can be accepted. The flexibility of the nurse to allow modification will do much toward effectively utilizing this conflict.

The conflict may also focus on the issue of the best action to implement to achieve the desired goal. This too is healthy conflict, conflict that can be constructively utilized toward change. For example, if the mutual goal of both patient in end-stage disease and the nurse caring for the patient is for the patient to have a comfortable peaceful death, but they have conflicting ideas about whether this death is to take place at home or in the hospital, the goal of a peaceful death can still be achieved if flexibility toward implementation is maintained.

Community resources must be introduced with sensitivity towards appropriate timing. The patient's and the family's situation itself will be in a state of change, so that plans thought to be appropriate earlier may no longer be so. Keeping an eye toward alternatives at each step in the rehabilitation process will prevent the patient and family from involvement in obsolete or inappropriate resources.

In the matter of timing, it also becomes apparent that the implementation of community resources will be most effective if the patient himself feels a need for assistance. In rehabilitation of the ostomy patient, for example, introduction of a visitor from the Ostomy Association to help support the patient is usually not accepted unless the patient is beginning to feel the need to compare his situation to that of others outside himself.

Coordinating the Community Resources

Particularly in the multiproblem situations represented by most cancer patients who are working toward rehabilitation, a frequent problem is duplication of services or an inundation of persons and pressures from multiple agencies. This inundation of persons can cause the patient to retreat from or resist efforts made in his behalf. Acting as a mediator or advocate, the nurse can, by suggesting an interagency conference or by communicating individually with involved people, help to identify the agency or personnel with the best rapport with the patient and recommend that those persons be the ones primarily responsible for carrying out the plan. In this way the nurse continues to act as facilitator and coordinator but the patient is not further inundated with the nurse's presence as well.

The way in which nurses go about using the community resources effectively for rehabilitation of the patient will depend on the kinds of relationships they establish with other agencies. It will also depend on how they interpret their own nursing role to the patients, families, and other agencies, and on how they interpret the role of other agencies to the patients.

Providing Leadership Toward Desired Change in the Community

When providing leadership toward desired change and toward establishing and improving needed services, four major phases emerge: (1) identifying goals and priorities; (2) surveying and analyzing needs and resources; (3) getting community action; and (4) evaluating and adapting the program [7].

Identification of Goals and Priorities. In cancer rehabilitation, the nurse in the community must be involved in identifying existing need and in helping to set goals and priorities to meet that need. Suppose the nurse involved in cancer rehabilitation becomes involved with patients in end-stage disease. That nurse may observe that these patients seem to experience impersonalized care during the final stages, have inadequate symptom control, or have families who experience severe disorganization and distress during this time. The nurse may believe that a form of hospice care is needed, care which from the viewpoint of the nurse does not seem to exist in the community at present. It is important at that time to voice these perceptions to the health facility or agency with which the nurse is involved. With the nurse's knowledge about the power structure of that facility and of the community in which it functions, it is possible to begin the process in which many persons can express their perceptions and priorities about care of the dying patient and family. The goal of this process would be that a priority for care of the terminally ill be set and that all groups represented would have their perceptions incorporated into the final plan.

Survey and Analysis of Needs and Resources. Once the priority has been set, then there must be a thorough study of the needs that led to selection of that goal and of available or potentially available resources to meet that goal. For example, if the priority of hospice-home care was set, then it would be important to survey the community involved to determine the persons who would utilize services, what their specific needs for service are, what kinds of gaps in service exist, who might be utilized to provide such services, and a cost analysis of such services. This kind of survey and analysis takes some specific knowledge and skill in epidemiological and demographic study. Such persons with these skills should be utilized to make an effective study.

Community Action. Even as the survey and analysis is being done, community action will begin. This action includes all the activities that are utilized toward achieving the goal. In the example of the hospice need, hospital discharge planners may begin to include the option of home care, physicians may encourage the patient to receive care at home, courses in death and dying may be established in community education programs, and interest groups may spring up.

The agency or facility working toward the planned change must be prepared to offer some possible plans or approaches as community action begins, but must also remember that it is the community itself which must plan for and implement the plan whenever possible.

The nurse's role in the community action phase would depend on that nurse's specific skills. Participation in the treatment programs designed to give home care to the dying patient is appropriate for the nurse who is a clinician. Involvement in training and supervising others who will provide hospice-home care is appropriate for the nurse whose skills are educational or consultant based. The nurse might also be a member or leader of a team, either of professionals or of nonprofessionals who are planning to provide some of the necessary aspects of that hospice care.

Evaluation and Adaptation. From the beginning of the planned service, ways of evaluating the results must be considered. Both the desirable and the undesirable outcomes must be measured. For example, patients and families' judgments regarding the effectiveness of the hospice service as well as the professional judgments of the effectiveness of these services would be valuable in determining the effectiveness of the community action. Even if this evaluation shows that the planned action was not successful, it is one step toward a new cycle of adapting the plan and again progressing toward the desired goal of rehabilitative care.

REFERENCES

[1] AGUILERA, D.C., and MESSICK, J.M. *Crisis Intervention: Theory and Methodology.* St. Louis: C. V. Mosby, 1974.

[2] AMERICAN CANCER SOCIETY. *1977 Cancer Facts and Figures,* p. 3. New York: American Cancer Society, 1976.

[3] ANDERSON, B.R. Problems of the Amputee. In *Rehabilitation of the Cancer Patient, Annual Clinical Conf. on Cancer 1970 at the Univ. of Texas M. D. Anderson Hospital,* pp. 75-78. Chicago: Year Book Med. Pub., Inc., 1972.

[4] BENSON, E.R. and McDEVITT, J.Q. *Community Health and Nursing Practice,* pp. 183-200. Englewood Cliffs, N.J.: Prentice-Hall, Inc., 1976.

[5] BENSON, E.R., and McDEVITT, J.Q. *Community Health and Nursing Practice,* pp. 246-266. Englewood Cliffs, N.J.: Prentice-Hall, Inc., 1976.

[6] BRAINERD, C.A. The Cancer Patient and Continuing Care. Unpublished paper, UCLA Graduate School of Nursing, June 1977.

[7] DeLOUGHERY, G.W., GEBBIE, K., and NEWMAN, B. *Consultation and Community Organization in Community Mental Health Nursing,* pp. 168-192. Baltimore: Williams and Wilkins, 1971.

[8] DIETZ, J.H., Jr. Neurological Problems of the Cancer Patient. In *Rehabilitation of the Cancer Patient, Annual Clinical Conference on Cancer 1970 at the Univ. of Texas M. D. Anderson Hospital,* pp. 95-99. Chicago: Year Book Med. Pub., Inc., 1972.

[9] DIETZ, J.H., Jr. Rehabilitation of the Cancer Patient. *Medical Clinics of North America,* 53 (3):607-624, May 1969.

[10] DIETZ, J.H., Jr. Rehabilitation of the Cancer Patient: Its Role in the Scheme of Comprehensive Care. *Clinical Bulletin,* 4(3):104-107, 1974.

[11] GRUBBS, J. An Interpretation of the Johnson Behavioral System Model for Nursing Practice. In *Conceptual Models for Nursing Practice,* ed. J.P. Riehl and C. Roy, pp. 161-197. Englewood Cliffs, N.J.: Prentice-Hall, Inc., 1974.

[12] HEALEY, J., Jr. Role of Rehabilitation Medicine in the Care of the Patient with Breast Cancer. *Cancer,* 28(6):1666-1671, December, 1971.

[13] HEALEY, J.E., Jr., and VILLANUEVA, R. Cancer of the Breast: Role of Rehabilitation Medicine. In *Rehabilitation of the Cancer Patient, Annual Clinical Conference on Cancer 1970 at the Univ. of Texas M. D. Anderson Hospital,* pp. 181-190. Chicago: Year Book Med. Pub., Inc., 1972.

[14] LENNEBERG, E.S. Continuing Needs of Patients with an Abdominal Stoma. In *Rehabilitation of the Cancer Patient, Annual Clinical Conference on Cancer 1970 at the Univ. of Texas M. D. Anderson Hospital,* pp. 225-235. Chicago: Year Book Med. Pub., Inc., 1972.

[15] LeSHAN, L. Mobilizing the Life Force. *Annals of the New York Academy of Science,* 164(3):847-861, 1969.

[16] MAUSNER, J.S., and BAHN, A.K. *Epidemiology: An Introductory Text,* pp. 1-20. Philadelphia: Saunders, 1974.

[17] MILLER, R.N. Psychological Problems of Patients with Head and Neck Cancer. In *Rehabilitation of the Cancer Patient, Annual Clinical Conference on Cancer 1970 at the Univ. of Texas M. D. Anderson Hospital*, pp. 19–31. Chicago: Year Book Med. Pub., Inc., 1972.

[18] MILLER, R.N. The Control of Pain in the Cancer Patient. In *Rehabilitation of the Cancer Patient, Annual Clinical Conference on Cancer 1970 at the Univ. of Texas M. D. Anderson Hospital*, pp. 129–139. Chicago: Year Book Med. Pub., Inc., 1972.

[19] MOORE, G.E. Cancer: 100 Different Diseases. *American Journal of Nursing*, 66(4):749–756, April, 1966.

[20] RUSK, H. Rusk on Rehabilitation. *Medical Times*, 105(1):64–75, January 1977.

[21] STEIN, G.H., GOLDSTEIN, M.K., and SMOLIN, D.M. Remote Medical-Behavioral Monitoring: An Alternative for Ambulatory Health Assessment. In *Cancer: The Behavioral Dimension*, ed. J.W. Cullen, B.H. Fox, and R.N. Isom, pp. 361–367. New York: Raven Press, 1976.

[22] STRAUSS, A.L. *Chronic Illness and the Quality of Life*, pp. 13–67. St. Louis: C. V. Mosby, 1975.

[23] TRACHTENBERG, J.M. Team Involvement and the Problems Incurred. In *Rehabilitation of the Cancer Patient, Annual Clinical Conference on Cancer 1970 at the Univ. of Texas M. D. Anderson Hospital*, pp. 181–190. Chicago: Year Book Med. Pub., Inc. 1972.

[24] WILLIAMS, M. A. Ethnocultural Responses to Hysterectomy: Implications for Nursing. In *Transcultural Nursing: A Book of Readings*, ed. P.J. Brink, pp. 219–223. Englewood Cliffs, N.J.: Prentice-Hall, Inc., 1976.

chapter eleven

JOSEPHINE A. GATAN SHIPLACOFF,
R.N., M.N.
Clinical Research Nurse Coordinator
Division of Surgical Oncology
Department of Surgery, UCLA

The oncology nurse: Clinical oncology team research

INTRODUCTION

The evolving nature of therapy for cancer provides frequent opportunities for the nurse practitioner in oncology to participate in clinical investigations. Most cancer patients under medical care undergo experimental procedures or therapies at some point in their management or become subjects in research studies designed to elucidate aspects of the disease process.

Oncology nurses are involved in human research in three ways:

1. As practitioners giving care to cancer patients who are undergoing experimental treatments or procedures or who are subjects in research studies designed to increase knowledge about the biology of cancer
2. As members of a research team involved in such studies
3. As principal investigators directing research studies which may include patients and nonpatients

Ellis delineates (1) and (3) above as the two major roles of nurses in human research [4]. Most oncology nurses, however, are involved in research as an integral part of their role as oncology nurses or as members of a research team.

This chapter delineates the research aspects of the role of the oncology nurse, who is a member of an oncology team. It also presents those general concepts of clinical research that have bearing on the practice of oncology nursing. This chapter does not focus on the oncology nurse whose primary concern is the care of patients who are subjects in clinical studies. It also does not delineate the research functions of the oncology nurse who has transcended the participatory and collaborative roles and is herself an independent nursing investigator. This chapter is primarily directed to the oncology nurse who needs to become familiar with all aspects of research protocols.

Job descriptions for oncology nursing positions with varying labels such as oncology nurse clinician, oncology nurse specialist, nurse coordinator, or research nurse invariably include several statements related to their roles in the implementation of a clinical investigation protocol. Other nurses without such labels, who take care of cancer patients, are frequently involved in human research simply by virtue of their ordinary nursing care activities in the course of their daily work. In this instance, the nurses may not even be aware that they are participants and very likely their consent to be involved in research is not sought.

The role of principal investigator is a relatively new one for nurses. It is a role not frequently encountered, especially in clinical nursing. Oncology nurses in general seem to be very research oriented, and more oncology nurses are assuming this role [10,15]. A quick survey of abstracts submitted to the Oncology Nursing Society's 1979 annual meeting bears out this observation [20]. In 1979, 202 abstracts were submitted, compared to 45 abstracts submitted in 1977—more than a fourfold increase in 2 years [19]! Despite this heartening trend for greater involvement in designing and directing research studies relevant to the practice of oncology nursing, nursing involvement in research for the most part is limited to participation and at best to collaboration.

PARTICIPATION VERSUS COLLABORATION

In the hospital setting nurses as practitioners are frequently involved in research because they care for patients receiving investigational drugs or other experimental therapy as part of medical treatment. As part of their regular nursing responsibilities nurses must make observations and assess such patients. Nursing care often may involve actual administration of the experimental drug or treatment procedure; however, the individual nurse's participation may be unintentional, as mentioned earlier.

Participation means taking part in the implementation of a research study. Active involvement by the nurse is specified by the protocol and directed by the investigator. This may include data collection, performance of skin tests, and other actions prescribed by the methodology of the investigation. Collaboration, on the other hand, implies more than just contribution in a quantitative sense of work performed [22]. It denotes a creative or qualitative contribution, that is, sharing in the identification of a research problem, in the formulation of a research question, and in designing the study. Thus, the responsibilities for and the fruits of the joint effort are shared. In actual practice, however, what is frequently regarded as collaboration is in fact participation confined to sharing in the implementation of the investigation. This probably stems in part from the historical and functional relationships between medicine and nursing.

THE NURSE'S UNIQUE CONTRIBUTION TO THE RESEARCH TEAM

Regardless of the extent of the research participation of nurses, their contributions derive for the most part from nursing functions and because they are nurses [4]. However, a unique opportunity for such collaboration between medicine and nursing exists more often in oncology than in other areas of practice [10]. The special contributions of nurses are recognized by most clinical investigators as essential in the implementation of a clinical trial or any research study where the subjects are patients. Indeed, the integrity of investigational regimens may be highly dependent on the oncology nurse. Contributions of the oncology nurse may affect not only the conduct of research but also, of great importance, the patient's attitude toward it. The nurse's usefulness to patients as they perceive and experience the nurse's ministrations, supportive care, and attitude toward the investigative treatment can influence patient compliance to the protocol. The unique role of the oncology nurse in clinical research lies in the nurse's ability to translate and implement required treatment regimens in a manner that is both acceptable to the patient and her family and least disruptive to their life-styles without compromising the scientific integrity of the investigation. The nurse must strive to maintain a balance between two sets of goals: the needs of the patients and the requirements of the study. The nurse's value rests in the inherent differences in orientation between medicine, which is primarily concerned with the diagnosis, treatment and cure of the disease, and nursing, which is primarily concerned with the care, comfort, and psychosocial adaptation of patients.

GENERAL ELEMENTS OF THE ONCOLOGY NURSE'S ROLE

The role of oncology nurses as members of the research team cannot be separated from their general clinical role as oncology nurse specialists. In fact, it is precisely this participation in clinical research that contributes to and distinguishes the oncology nurse's expanded role. Despite myriad ways of assigning or attaching a title to the oncology nurse, that is, specialist, clinician, practitioner, and research coordinator, there are roles and responsibilities common to all oncology nurses in various settings by virtue of their oncology practice. To be sure there is a wide range of degrees of autonomy and accountability. However, the oncology nurse's role in general includes the following:

1. Collaboration with physicians and other health professionals in the management of patients in various settings
2. Coordination of health services needed by the patients
3. Primary nursing care responsibility for a group of patients
4. Administration of chemotherapy, immunotherapy, and/or other treatment procedures
5. Evaluation of patient's clinical status and observation of responses to therapy
6. Data collection and maintenance of records
7. Consultation, liaison, and educational activities with other members of the profession, other health professionals, and the community
8. Involvement in clinical trials, which includes aspects of the above

In addition, specific research activities may include the following:

1. Screening and selection of patients eligible for a particular protocol
2. Collaboration with the physician-investigator in the preparation

of informed consents, research protocols, and publications arising from the research.

3. Primary responsibility for the initiation and conduct of research

A collaborative climate is essential for the oncology nurse to be able to function effectively as a member of the clinical research team. The oncology nurse's participation or contribution may be an uncontrolled factor affecting the conduct of research or the patient's attitude toward it. Clinical investigators frequently rely on the oncology nurse to interpret aspects of the protocol requirements to the patient, to administer investigational agents and to make and record observations and measurements required by the protocol. One aspect of the oncology nurse's participation that is often overlooked is the impact of the nurse's attitude toward investigative procedures as a factor in determining the cancer patient's attitude or responses to the investigation. When the oncology nurse is well informed about a protocol and is encouraged by the physician to become actively involved in a collaborative sense, the nurse's deliberate or unintentional actions, conveyance of information, or attitude is bound to have a positive influence on the study and its implementation.

CONCEPTS IN CLINICAL RESEARCH

Randomized clinical trials have become an integral part of the practice of oncology. The controlled clinical trial has become the definitive approach to evaluating new treatment. An informed and effective participation in clinical trials requires a knowledge of the research design of "controlled, prospective clinical trials." A clinical trial is any clinical research effort designed to answer questions of significance regarding the safety and effectiveness of treatment procedures or investigational drugs used in the management of diseases. In the management of cancer it is an organized inquiry into clinical problems of significant concern in the care of the cancer patient. A controlled experiment is the scientific ideal [11]. This is an experiment in which all the factors or variables, known or unknown, not themselves the object of study but which are likely to affect the experimental outcome are controlled. A proper research design has two functions: (1) to help the investigator obtain answers to the clinical research questions; and (2) to provide control.

There are several ways to control extraneous variables but only randomization will be discussed as it is the most relevant for the oncology nurse. The best way to provide control is to randomize whenever possible. Subjects should be selected at random and assigned to groups at random. In clinical trials often it may not be possible to select subjects or assign them into groups at random. However, it is frequently possible to assign experimental treatments to experimental groups at random and every effort should be made to do so.

With randomization the extraneous variables can be assumed to be present equally (depending on sample size) in both the group receiving the experimental treatment and in the control group. This serves to neutralize the effects of these unwanted variables, because the main difference between the two groups, then, is that the experimental treatment is applied to one group and not applied to the control group. Therefore, any experimental outcome different in the two groups is probably due to the experimental treatment.

RANDOMIZATION

As defined by Kerlinger [5], "Randomization is the assignment of objects (subjects, treatments, groups) of a universe to subsets of the universe in such a way that, for any given assignment to a subset, every member of the universe has an equal probability of being chosen for that assignment." Thus, whenever random procedures are applied, every member of a population has an equal chance of being selected or an equal chance of being assigned to the experimental treatment. Randomization applied to clinical trials is based on the premise that it is possible to identify a large group of patients all having the same disease in the same stages, the same subsets, so that the disease can be predictable in such a large group. Then by random assignment, eligible patients are assigned to the different treatment arms of the clinical study. This procedure gives each patient an equal chance of receiving any of the treatments under study. The essence of randomization is that chance and chance alone must determine which treatment is assigned to each patient.

Since controlled trials are feasible only when similar groups of patients can be compared, it has wider applicability to Phase III or comparative clinical trials usually conducted with a homogeneous patient population to compare the effectiveness or results of new treatments with other treatments of noneffectiveness. Randomization of patients is also employed in some Phase II trials when two dose regimens or routes of administration of an agent are under investigation.

Having comparable groups of patients is necessary for the internal validity of any scientific inquiry. It is the sine qua non of a controlled clinical trial [5].

Pseudo-approaches to randomization have been employed in clinical research. They include such techniques as assigning treatments or procedures to patients by their hospital number, birth dates, date of entry into the study, or even by tossing a coin. The best procedure is based on a table of random numbers. Clinical trials frequently require that an equal number of patients be randomized to each treatment to facilitate comparison. This procedure is called restricted randomization [9]. In a truly random procedure the ratio of patients assigned to each treatment is random, that is, treatment A might be assigned to only three out of ten consecutively randomized patients. In a restricted randomization, the selection of subjects may be set up so that an equal number of patients is assigned in each treatment group after a fixed number of consecutively randomized patients. For example, in a study comparing two treatment drugs, BCG (B) and Levamisole (L), it is possible to assign each drug to two out of every four patients so that each of the two treatments is equally represented. In sequence 1 below, the first and fourth patients seen can receive BCG, while the second and third receive Levamisole:

1. BLLB   3. BLBL   5. LLBB
2. LBBL   4. LBLB   6. BBLL

To apply the random process, random numbers are then assigned to each of the six possible sequences of treatment. If the number 2 was arbitrarily assigned in advance to the treatment order BLLB, each time the number 2 is drawn from a table of random numbers, the next four treatment assignments would be in the sequence of BCG, Levamisole, Levamisole, BCG. An example of a restricted randomization treatment order that is actually predetermined before patients are randomized might be BLLBBBLLLLBB . . . and so on. In this example the first eligible patient seen receives BCG, the next two get Levamisole, BCG is then assigned to three consecutively seen patients, and the next four are all assigned Levamisole. However, of the 12 treatment assignments, BCG and Levamisole are equally represented.

Age, weight loss, histologic type of tumor, and stage of the disease are some of the possible variables influencing prognosis, and therefore comparability, of patients in a randomized study. When patients are grouped into categories ("strata" or subsets) based on these variables, randomization is said to be stratified. A potential disadvantage of having too many categories of patients is the difficulty of achieving a large enough patient accrual to allow comparability.

Frequently in clinical trials randomization is restricted to a predetermined system or arrangement of ensuring that there will be a balanced assignment of treatments to patients or to each stratum in a stratified grouping of patients. In a pure randomization, randomly selected subjects are randomly assigned to groups which, in turn, are randomly assigned the treatments or control conditions. In this instance, however, subjects are selected and assigned to groups according to predetermined criteria. This procedure also requires that an equal number of patients be assigned to each treatment. The order in which the treatments are arranged is random within the restriction of eventually having equal numbers of patients after a given number is accrued.

RANDOMIZED DESIGNS

When the study requires only one category of patients or when there is no way of grouping patients into prognostic subsets, a simple randomized design is employed. Patients are randomized to two or more treatment groups. One drawback is that there is no assurance, even with randomization, that the treatment groups are indeed comparable.

DOUBLE-BLIND STUDY

In a double-blind study, neither the patient nor the doctor should know the nature of the treatment. The purpose of keeping both the patient and investigator "blind" is to obtain unbiased subjective impressions and judgments of the course of the illness and the response to the new treatment being investigated. The crucial element is that the physician who manages and evaluates the patients on the study should have no knowledge of the actual treatment being used. This is to ensure that patients on each treatment regime are managed in identical ways. The treatment may be administered by a second physician who may know what he or she is giving the patient but who will not be involved in the management and evaluation of the patient. The code, of course, can be broken at any moment if the physician thinks it is in the best interests of the patient. When complications occur in the course of treatment, it may become necessary to know what drugs the patient is receiving to help establish a diagnosis and determine further treatments.

CROSSOVER DESIGN

A crossover design uses each patient as her own control. There are two ways of utilizing this design. First, half of the patients receive the treatment sequence of treatment A followed by B and the other half receive treatment B followed by A. This allows two comparisons between treatments A and B: (1) between different patients in the first phase; and (2) between different patients in the second phase. The second method of accomplishing crossover is to assign a patient to one of the two treatment sequences by random. Thus, a patient might receive treatment A for a specified length of time followed by another treatment, B.

There are several objections to this design. Knowing that tumor growth is not likely to remain stable, the patient's condition may not be comparable over time. This makes impossible the comparison of both treatments. The long-term effects, if any, of the first treatment cannot be evaluated nor is it possible to eliminate lasting effects of the first treatment in evaluating the response to the second treatment. A crossover study therefore, may be best conducted when a patient's condition is expected to remain stable for some time as in remission state at successive times.

FACTORIAL DESIGNS

Factorial research designs are frequently employed in Phase III clinical trials. In this design, two or more treatments are studied for their independent effects and for the effects of their interactions. Patients are randomly assigned to receive one of two treatments, or both, or no further treatment. In a surgical adjuvant study of melanoma, patients were randomized to receive BCB alone, or BCG with tumor cell vaccine, or no further treatment following regional node dissection. This study hopes to establish whether either of the adjuvant treatment arms (BCG alone or BCG in combination with tumor cell vaccine) is more effective than no further treatment following surgery. In addition, the design also allows for the study of a possible interaction effect between BCG and tumor cell vaccine.

This design can be extended to a study of more than two treatments which would require a large number of patients in order to have a sufficient number of subjects for each treatment arm.

PROSPECTIVE VERSUS RETROSPECTIVE STUDIES

A prospective study is one in which patients are randomized to a treatment arm at the time of entry into the study. The most important difference between prospective and retrospective studies is *control*. In a prospective study the investigator can exercise direct control by randomization and experimental manipulation. In the retrospective studies these kinds of controls are not possible. However, sample selection techniques offer some control. Historical controls may be of some value but the usefulness of retrospective controls in general is limited because of the difficulty of demonstrating the comparability of patients on the new treatment with those already treated.

ELEMENTS OF A PROTOCOL

A protocol is a detailed written plan of the proposed clinical research investigation. It is the blueprint for a clinical trial. The standard parts of a protocol are dictated by an agency's grant proposal application form. A protocol begins with a statement of the goal of the study. The significance of the questions asked or the answers sought is based on a scientific rationale. The evolving nature of clinical trials is such that previous trials frequently provide the background and impetus for further new trials. Answers to earlier questions generate subsequent questions and the process proceeds into a continuum. Before any intervention is put on a clinical trial there must be enough information about it, such as from a pilot study, to warrant a full research investigation. Sometimes a clinician may become so convinced of the efficacy of treatment based on his or her preliminary knowledge that further participation in a controlled trial may be precluded.

A protocol delineates the criteria for eligibility and specifies contraindications to participation. It also includes the procedure to be followed for randomization. Once a patient has been randomized she must be followed up and be included in the final analysis of the study whether the allocated treatment was given or not. How the treatments are to be administered is specified as to preparation, dose, and technique of administration. It is particularly important that the treatment regimen be implemented in a uniform way by all those participating, especially in collaborative multiinstitutional studies. The protocol should include a statement of anticipated toxicity and side effects with appropriate measures to be employed for dosage adjustment or terminating treatment. Study parameters and frequency of patient follow-up is indicated in the protocol.

A protocol should also indicate which tests are required and which ones are optional. Regular evaluation of patients provides data for the measurement of the effect of treatment. Measures of responses may include disease-free interval, recurrence, and survival defined by the protocol. The statistical plan of the analysis of results includes the required patient accrual to provide statistically significant information and the anticipated length of time necessary to accrue these patients into the study. The protocol also specifies how prescribed forms are to be completed and provides a schedule for regular submission of data forms to the study coordinating office. Any information relevant to the implementation of the study is included in a protocol. Therefore, a well-written protocol that provides precise definitions and specifies procedures and actions can guarantee a well-implemented study.

Oncology nurses or anyone assuming the care of cancer patients should make a point of becoming familiar with all aspects of the protocols under which their patients are being treated.

The care of cancer patients who are research subjects requires more of oncology nurses than an understanding of research designs and procedures. Nurses must also be informed and cognizant of the legal and ethical aspects of research affecting the patients under their care and of their own professional responsibilities. Participation in research activities under a physician's direction does not relieve professional nurses of responsibility for their own acts and judgments [4]. It is imperative for oncology nurses to understand the doctrine of informed consent and to have a clear understanding of their role in obtaining informed consent [1,6,7,8,13,18]. Oncology nurses must be aware of federal and local governmental regulations governing the conduct of research.

The protection of human subjects for experimentation is embodied in the Nuremberg Code [14], the Helsinki Declaration [3], and in governmental policies issued by the Department of Health, Education and Welfare (DHEW) [23]. Because the federal government has taken increasing responsibility for the ethical aspects of human research, some concern has been raised regarding the extent to which the government can and should regulate clinical research. However, these government regulations reflect technical standards, professional experience, and communities' attitudes.

In recent years, publicized accounts of abuses in human experimentation have drawn attention to the need for ensuring the protection of human subjects in the conduct of research. The DHEW through its two major branches—the Food and Drug Administration (FDA) and the National Institutes of Health (NIH)—have issued guidelines dealing with the protection of human subjects. The ethical issues involved in protecting the rights of research subjects are complex and difficult. This chapter will not focus on these.

A National Commission for the Protection of Human Subjects of Biomedical and Behavioral Research was established by the National Research Act enacted in July 1974. One of the most important problems that must be dealt with is that of providing for the education of those who are to conduct and to participate in future medical research. The DHEW requires that any organization receiving grant or contract support for research in which human subjects are at risk, must submit detailed assurances to indicate that "It has an ethical review committee to review and approve the ethical aspects of initial grant or contract applications and to monitor projects on a continuing basis to assure protection of subjects" [23]. Under DHEW guidelines/regulations an institutional review committee must be established wherever federally funded studies are being conducted. This practice has become so widespread in recent years that other nonfunded institutions voluntarily comply. The membership of such a committee should be multidisciplinary and should include, for example, theologians and philosophers as well as scientists from assorted disciplines. Before any clinical trial can be implemented, approval must be obtained from the review committee.

All proposals and protocols are reviewed by the committee under three specific criteria:

1. The risks to subjects must be so outweighed by the sum of the benefits to the subjects and the importance of the knowledge to be gained as to warrant a decision to allow the subjects to accept these risks.
2. Informed consent must be legally effective and obtained by methods that are adequate and appropriate.
3. The rights and welfare of the subjects must be adequately protected.

The institutional guide to DHEW policy on protection of human subjects considers an individual to be "at risk" if she may be exposed to the possibility of harm, be it physical, psychological, sociological, or any other harm resulting from any activity beyond those required by established and accepted methods necessary to meet her needs. The DHEW policy on protection of human subjects applies to all grants and contracts that support activities in which subjects may be at risk.

The concept of informed consent is the most problematic aspect of human experimentation. There is a great deal of legal and ethical controversy surrounding the process of informed consent [2,5,6,7,8,16,17,18,21,24]. Several questions have been raised to which there are no easy answers, including: How may an individual be best informed and under what conditions? Is it possible to obtain truly informed consent? Will the use of informed consent destroy the scientific design of some experiments? What are the responsibilities of paramedical personnel in the informed consent process? What is an informed consent?

BASIC ELEMENTS OF AN INFORMED CONSENT

Federal regulations define the basic elements of information that constitute an informed consent. Stated in clear, simple lay terms, consent forms must include the following:

1. A fair explanation of the procedures to be followed, including an identification of those that are experimental
2. An identification of the individuals performing the procedures and their degrees (i.e., M.D., PH.D., etc.; the word "Doctor" should not be used exclusively)
3. A description of the possible immediate and long-term discomforts, hazards, and risks, and their potential consequences (if none, so state); patients as subjects should be advised that their condition may become worse despite participation and that they may derive no specific benefit
4. A description of the benefits to be expected
5. A disclosure of appropriate alternative procedures that would be advantageous for the subject and that would include their risks and benefits

6. An offer to answer any inquiries concerning the study at any time
7. An instruction that the subject is free to withdraw his consent and to discontinue participation in the project of activity at any time without prejudice
8. An assurance that any information derived from the research project that personally identifies the subject will not be voluntarily released or disclosed without the subject's separate consent, except as specifically required by law
9. An assurance to subjects that if the study design or the use of the collected information is to be changed, they will be so informed and their consent reobtained (new consent forms must be approved by the review committee)
10. A statement that medical care and hospital treatment will be provided in the event of injury directly resulting from the subject's participation in the research study
11. A statement that questions, comments, concerns, and/or complaints about the study or the informed consent process may be addressed to the institutional officer responsible for overseeing the conduct of research

Additional information may be included as required by special circumstances—as when the subject is to be remunerated, is disabled, or is a minor—and by local state health and safety codes. In California, inclusion of a statement acknowledging receipt of a copy of the consent form as well as a copy of the Subject's Bill of Rights is required for research classified as "medical experimentation."

The extent of the oncology nurse's participation in obtaining informed consent is surrounded by some controversy. There are those who think, "Nurses must not get involved in the type of communications that are necessary for informed consent" [13]. There is, however, growing support for collaborative efforts among the health professionals involved in the care of the cancer patient in providing information. Carpenter and Langsner [1] recommended the development of a systematic and major role for the nurse in informed consent. Traditionally the nurse's role was limited to obtaining the patient's signature and acting as witness. Traditionally, nurses also were taught and expected to respond to the patient's questions about contemplated treatments and procedures with, "Ask your doctor." However, many of the same policy considerations that underly the physician's "duty to disclose" also govern the nurse's own duty.

The nurse's primary commitment is patient care and safety. It is obvious from the list of information that is contained in an informed consent that nurses cannot avoid the responsibility of being involved in the consent process. Nurses' typical nursing activities and their concern for patients will apply and continue despite clinical investigations. Because of their characteristic circumstance, nurses have the greatest opportunity for direct contact with patients. Being more readily available than other members of the multidisciplinary team, nurses are drawn more into the daily concerns of patients over problems and issues. Few patients will voice their doubts or raise questions when face-to-face with physicians, but many will to a nurse. The nurse-patient relationship imposes fewer constraints on the patients and their families when more information is needed. The nurse can provide and supplement information over time. Thus, frequently the nurse is asked to clarify and reinforce information given by the physician. Whether intentionally or not, the nurse is often in the position of having to interpret to the patient and the family what is involved in the research study.

For the oncology nurse to be able to assume an active role in helping patients acquire sufficient information on which to base their decision to participate in clinical trials, the nurse requires knowledge and self-confidence. This is possible only through a close collaboration and continuous exchange of information with the investigator. The physician enhances the nurse's knowledge and understanding of the protocol, and the nurse enhances the physician's awareness and understanding of the patient's ideas and concerns about proposed treatments and procedures. The role of oncology nurses is often expanded beyond the usual domain of nursing. However, it is exactly this aspect of their practice that many oncology nurses find most satisfying [12]. The overlap of medical and nursing functions that characterizes the practice of oncology nursing facilitates preparation of the oncology nurse to step into the role of primary researcher.

REFERENCES

[1] CARPENTER, W.T., Jr., and LANGSNER, C.A. The Nurse's Role in Informed Consent. *Nursing Times*, 71:1049–1051, 1975.

[2] CURRAN, W.J. Reasonableness and Randomization in Clinical Trials: Fundamental Law and Governmental Regulation. *The New England Journal of Medicine*, 300:1273–1274, 1979.

[3] *Declaration of Helsinki: Recommendations Guiding Doctors in Clinical Research*. Adopted by the 18th World Medical Assembly, Helsinki, 1964.

[4] ELLIS, R. The Nurse as Investigator and Member of the Research Team. *Annals of the New York Academy of Science*, 169:435–441, 1970.

[5] FOST, N. Consent as a Barrier to Research. *The New England Journal of Medicine*, 300:1272-1273, 1979.

[6] GARGARO, W.J. Informed Consent, Part I. A Good thing for Patients; a Better Thing for Doctors and Nurses. *Cancer Nursing*, 1:81-82, 1978.

[7] GARGARO, W.J. Informed Consent, Part II. How Much to Tell the Patient. *Cancer Nursing*, 1:167-168, 1978.

[8] GARGARO, W.J. Informed Consent, Part III. The Nurse's Right to Inform. *Cancer Nursing*, 1:249-250, 1978.

[9] GEHAN, E.A., and SCHNEIDERMAN, M.A. Experimental Design of Clinical Trials. In *Cancer Medicine*, ed. J.F. Holland and E. Frei, III. Philadelphia: Lea & Febiger, 1973.

[10] HUBBARD, S.M. Editorial. The Foreign Exchange Nurse Visitor Program: An International Program for Cancer Nurses. *Cancer Nursing*, 2:351-352, 1979.

[11] KERLINGER, F.N. *Foundations of Behavioral Research*. New York: Holt, Rinehart & Winston, 1973.

[12] MAXWELL, M.B. Nurse Practitioner Chemotherapy Clinic. *Cancer Nursing*, 2:211-218, 1979.

[13] MILLS, D.H. Whither Informed Consent? *JAMA*, 229:305-310, 1974.

[14] The Nuremberg Code. *In Trials of War Criminals Before the Nuremberg Military Tribunals Under Control Law No. 10*, Vol. 2, pp. 181-182. Washington, D.C.: U.S. Government Printing Office, 1949.

[15] McCORKLE, R. First Conference on Cancer Nursing Research. *Cancer Nursing*, 2:226-230, 1979.

[16] OBERST, M.T. Research Ethics. Part 1: Randomized Clinical Trials. *Cancer Nursing*, 2:385-386, 1979.

[17] OBERST, M.T. Research Ethics. Part 2: The Concept of Risk in Clinical Studies. *Cancer Nursing*, 2:481-482, 1979.

[18] OBERST, M.T. Research Ethics. Part 3: Risk Associated with Researcher Access to Clinical Records. *Cancer Nursing*, 3:57-58, 1980.

[19] ONCOLOGY NURSING SOCIETY. *Proceedings of the Second Annual Congress*, Washington, D.C., 1977.

[20] ONCOLOGY NURSING SOCIETY. *Proceedings of the Fourth Annual Congress*, New Orleans, 1979.

[21] RELMAN, A.S. The Ethics of Randomized Clinical Trials: Two Perspectives. *The New England Journal of Medicine*, 300:1272, 1979.

[22] THIGPEN, L. *Guidelines for Research in Clinical Nursing*. New York: National League of Nursing, 1967.

[23] U.S. DEPARTMENT OF HEALTH, EDUCATION, AND WELFARE. The Institutional Guide to DHEW Policy on Protection of Human Subjects. In *Federal Regulation of Human Experimentation, 1975*. Washington, D.C.: U.S. Government Printing Office, No. 48-2730, 1975.

[24] ZELEN, M. A New Design for Randomized Clinical Trials. *The New England Journal of Medicine*, 300:1242-1245, 1979.

chapter twelve

DONNA L. VREDEVOE, Ph.D.
Professor
Teaching in Graduate Nursing
Oncology Program and Nursing Research
School of Nursing, UCLA

The oncology nurse: Research designs for the future

INTRODUCTION

The oncology nurse will face a clinical area that abounds with researchable problems. There will be those who may identify researchable problems, but choose not to pursue the research study itself. There will be others who will participate in oncology research designed by principal investigators with whom they are associated. This chapter, however, is designed primarily for the oncology nurse who wishes to pursue research to its conclusion of providing an answer to a research question. Although this chapter cannot cover all of the important aspects of research it is intended to chart the path of research, to highlight the elements of the process, and to suggest ways to approach research so that the reader will be stimulated to seek more knowledge about the research process.

For those who are already deeply involved in research, this chapter may provide a few new twists to the basic ideas of research. It may be a source material that the researcher would use for orientation of assistants in studies.

ONCOLOGY NURSING RESEARCH PROBLEMS
OF THE FUTURE

In identifying those designs or research problems that are particularly pertinent to the oncology nurse, one can only reflect one's own biases and experiences. Thus, the design approaches or research problems relating to oncologic nursing discussed in this chapter stand out in this author's mind as particularly significant. The reader will soon form his or her own priorities. The significant point is that in approaching an area such as research it is important for each person to cull out those things that demand the greatest attention.

Methodological research is basic to the research process. Valid, reliable, and sensitive data collection instruments are developed by this research approach. The literature abounds with studies in which the researcher plunged ahead with data collection utilizing instruments that did not meet criteria for acceptable validity, reliability, and sensitivity. The result has been many studies in which the results could not be interpreted in a significant manner and the body of knowledge could not be increased by information from the research.

Methodological research designs are multifaceted. Separate designs, each with its own hypothesis or purpose, are created to deal with testing of a selected method of measuring either the validity, reliability or sensitivity of the instrument.

Validity is the ability of a measurement technique to measure the variable under study. Since questionnaires or interviews are frequently used data collection instruments in nursing research, these will be used as examples here. Validity can be established in a number of ways:

1. *Face validity* may be developed by simply stating that logically the questions measure the variable under test. This is a weak source of validity and relies only on logical analysis of the questions.
2. *Content validity* utilizes reference sources to establish validity. Literature or judge panels of experts can be used as reference sources. This is a practical way of developing a new tool in areas in which data collection instruments are nonexistent.
3. *Concurrent validity* utilizes an existing instrument as a criterion against which the new instrument is tested to see if similar results are obtained. In this type of validity there must be a rationale for development of the new instrument that indicates clearly why the existing instrument could not measure that variable

in the new setting or in the new sample as well as the new instrument.

4. *Construct validity* utilizes hypotheses that are created to define relationships about the interplay of variables to be tested. As the hypotheses are supported, the validity of the measurement technique for the variable about which the measurement technique has been developed is established.

5. *Predictive validity* utilizes a prediction about how a variable under study will behave at some future point in time. This prediction is made in the form of a hypothesis. When the hypothesis is supported the validity of the measurement technique is supported.

Reliability of a measurement technique may be assessed in a number of ways also:

1. *Test-retest reliability* is used to establish that the same sample, tested at two different points of time, gives similar results to the same questions. In this technique the time interval, care in minimizing intervening variables and equivalency of the two settings for administration of the questionnaire are important.

2. *Alternate form reliability* is a technique in which two equivalent forms of a questionnaire are developed to show that they measure the variable under study in equivalent or highly correlated manners. In this type of reliability the two forms of the instrument are administered at the same time.

3. *Split-half reliability* is a technique in which a set of homogeneous questions about a well-defined topic or variable are analyzed by comparing responses to the odd- and even-numbered questions. Again the entire questionnaire is administered at a single time.

Sophisticated computerized reliability systems are also available (Kuder-Richardson) which provide estimates of the reliability of questionnaires.

Sensitivity is a measurement of the degree of change in the variable which the instrument is capable of measuring. Here the measurement of change is critical. With variables such as temperature or biochemical tests this is more readily achieved than with the behavioral variables. In testing reliability a sample must be selected that has those characteristics of the population for which the instrument is intended for use. In testing or establishing validity one would use a sample for testing construct, concurrent, or predictive validity and a reference source for establishing content validity. Judge panels may be the only available reference source for establishing the validity of a new interview tool or questionnaire dealing with problems in nursing oncology. Until more research is published in nursing, judge panels will continue to be one of the best resources for establishing that: (1) questions measure what they are supposed to measure (validity); (2) that the style of the question is appropriate for the sample, setting, and measurement; (3) that similar questions are equivalent in their ability to measure the same variable (alternate form reliability); and (4) that the language used in the question is appropriate to the sample for which it is to be used.

The intricate process of methodological research is well worth the result of a measurement technique which is valid, reliable, and sensitive for measurement of the variable(s) under study. It provides a firm building block for subsequent survey or experimental research.

A second area of special concern to the nurse oncologist is measurement of the psychosocial responses of patients to the impact of the diagnosis, treatment, and long-term consequences of cancer. Since the psychosocial responses cannot be isolated from the physiological responses, the entire spectrum of variables must be analyzed. This poses an almost overwhelming problem to the researcher. How, then, is it possible to design research approaches to these multifaceted research problems? The key to this is a culling of ideas, designs, measurement techniques, and data analysis techniques so that new information can be gained about a problem area. This process goes on in all research, but it is particularly important in nursing oncology because of the great array of relevant variables that interplay.

Since research begins with a question, it may be appropriate to follow the process from the question to results to see the many facets of the narrowing down process. The ability to use this process is perhaps the most important characteristic of a successful researcher. Persistence, stamina, and ability to see the whole and the parts simultaneously are other important characteristics.

THE RESEARCH QUESTION

Research begins with a question. The findings should contribute something new to the body of scientific knowledge. Some questions are very different from previous questions. They ask about entirely new concepts or utilize a new way of thinking. Other research questions are only slightly different from previous questions, for example, those that ask "Can the assay utilized for subjects A in study A give similar results on subjects B in study B?" You must be able to defend that your research question if answered will contribute *new* knowledge. Thus, if you ask whether results of study A can be replicated by study B you must defend the need for study B and reasons why results of study B will yield new knowledge.

Research studies usually begin with one or more primary questions. These primary questions pertain to the problem to be solved. The nature of the question determines the type of research design. There then follow many secondary questions that determine the nature of the sample, the setting for collection of data, the methodology for data collection, and the plan for analysis.

Some questions asked as a preliminary step in the development of research are not researchable questions. For example, "Does immunosuppression cause cancer?" is not a researchable question. Descriptive or evaluative studies usually have a statement of purpose. Comparative or correlational studies usually have hypotheses. The differences in these types of studies will be discussed in subsequent sections. A researchable question can be defined as a question that:

1. Is different from previous research questions in that it has the potential, if answered, to generate new knowledge
2. Expresses (a) a relationship between variables, or (b) a question about a variable or variables
3. Expresses (a) the degree or direction of relationship between the variables or (b) the type of information required

In this list, (a) applies to studies with hypotheses and (b) applies to studies with purpose.

For example, "Does immunosuppression affect the incidence of cancer?" is a vague general question which does not specify the population involved, the type of cancer, the type of immunosuppression or duration, or the time relationship of immunosuppression to the development of cancer. The question "Does immunosuppression by agent X prior to the injection of lymphoma virus Y in animal species Z result in a statistically significantly higher incidence of lymphoma as compared to similar animals of species Z receiving lymphoma virus Y and no agent X?" is researchable. Here the nature of the variables of immunosuppression, oncogenic virus, and animal species is specified. It is also noted that a significant difference between control and experimental groups is expected. This question is similar to the hypothesis that would be stated, "There will be a statistically significantly higher incidence of lymphoma when immunosuppression by agent X is administered prior to the injection of lymphoma virus Y in animal species Z as compared to similar animals of species Z receiving lymphoma virus Y and no agent X."

This final researchable question was derived only after asking several preliminary questions.

1. What is immunosuppression?
2. What sample population will be involved?
3. What is the incidence of spontaneous lymphoma in the animal species?
4. How will immunosuppression be induced in the population selected?
5. When will the immunosuppression be introduced relative to the introduction of the cancer virus?
6. Will immunosuppression increase or decrease the incidence of lymphoma?
7. What comparison or control group will be used?

The research question now determines the design. If one creates a new situation, then an experimental design, with a control group for comparison, is used. Since agent X and lymphoma virus Y are introduced in this study, and a control group is used, this requires an experimental design. Basically there are two groups—that is, the one receiving agent X and lymphoma virus Y, and the other control group receiving only virus—but other groups to control the effects of these two agents must also be used. For example, the final design would include a group that received only agent X and no virus Y to control for spontaneous neoplasms. A group that received no injections of agent X or virus Y would also be included as a control for spontaneous neoplasms. Basically, however, the study involves two groups receiving lymphoma virus. The animal species chosen would likely be one that developed a low incidence of virus-induced lymphoma after injections of virus alone. In such a case the difference between immunosuppression and no treatment could be evaluated. However, if the incidence of spontaneous or virus-induced lymphomas after injection of lymphoma virus Y were high the high incidence would obscure the difference between the two groups since both groups would develop lymphoma regardless of immunosuppression.

There are six basic types of research approaches, each designed to answer different types of research questions:

Conceptual Models and Theory: The development of conceptual models and theory is particularly important in professions such as nursing where the body of knowledge is developing. Such studies ask questions about the nature of phenomena with which the practitioner deals. They define the parameters of the profession and its research. They pose research questions.

Historical Research: Historical research asks research questions about events that have occurred, why they occurred, the consequences, the persons invloved, and the issues involved. This type of research involves tracing events through time in an attempt to answer these questions. It may lead to the discovery of new documents, letters, or manuscripts, or it may involve examination of documents now available.

Methodological Research: Measurement tools for many of the variables of primary interest in nursing research are lacking. Frequently as research studies are developed it becomes apparent that the variables of interest can be conceptualized, but not measured accurately. For the study to progress, it is necessary to develop measurement techniques for the variables. Thus, studies that were originally to be survey or experimental approaches become methodological as the need for measurement becomes critical.

Survey Research: Surveys ask questions about things that are. They do not create new situations, as does the experimental approach, but they ask questions about things, people, phenomena, issues, and programs that already exist. Surveys are important approaches in nursing research since they provide comprehensive characterization of the variables and phenomena of importance in nursing research. For example, prior to an experimental study on the effects of intervention to teach mothers in techniques of mothering, careful study of mothering patterns in various cultural, economic, and other groups is required. One cannot intervene to change behavior until the "normal" patterns of behavior are known and appropriate interventions and time and need for intervention are determined.

Experimental Research: Experimental research asks questions about new situations created by the researcher. Experimental groups receive new treatments, teaching techniques, interventions, or other new variables and the effects of the introduction of the new variables are determined on the group. The effects can only be determined by comparing the experimental group to the control group which does not receive the new variable. It is left to the ingenuity of the researcher to control extraneous variables in the two groups so as to minimize the effects of these extraneous variables on the independent variable introduced. The independent variable then is the new variable introduced by the researcher. The dependent variable is the variable that is affected by the introduction of the independent variable. The independent variable has been termed the causal variable, the dependent the effect variable. Independent and dependent variables are also part of the design of survey research. However, in survey research the researcher does not introduce the independent variable, but studies a selected independent variable that already exists and notes its effect on dependent variables.

Applied Research: The result of survey and experimental research usually has implications for nursing practice. This knowledge frequently can be applied to the clinical setting, but often this application requires another research approach, that of application of previous findings to the clinical population and setting.

STEPS IN THE RESEARCH PROCESS

Defining the Research Problem

The research problem is that situation or phenomenon which the investigator seeks to: (1) clarify; (2) change; or (3) eliminate. The problem is basically the result of a question that is unanswered. It may stem from lack of measurement techniques, a need for improved techniques by modification of existing techniques, poorly defined clinical observations, lack of adequate description of phenomena, or inability to measure variables or to predict relationships between variables. The problem presents itself frequently as a deviation from expected behaviors or phenomena. For example, neoplasms are aberrant types of tissue growth distinguishable by their interference with normal metabolism, function, and anatomy as they progress in size. The research problem becomes that of developing a way to eliminate or control this aberrant tissue growth.

These deviations from expected norms can affect small or large percentages of given populations. For example, smog is a deviation from the pure air that one would hope would exist in urban areas. Smog can be a cause or effect depending upon the definition of the problem. For example, an environmental engineer may ask what combinations of atmospheric conditions, airborne particles, and emissions result in smog and so see smog as an effect variable. A biologist may observe the effect of smog on organisms and so see smog as a causal variable.

There is little doubt that a large portion of nursing research in oncology will involve patients or clients in clinical settings. However, nursing research may also involve animal experimentation, analysis of written documents, and other approaches that may not directly involve the patient or client. Researchable nursing problems can arise from one or two general sources: (1) basic science theory and findings of relevance to nursing; or (2) the clinical settings of nursing practice. Clinical setting is defined as the environment in which the nursing role is practiced.

Basic science research and theory may allow one to predict certain relationships between variables that might exist in clinical nursing settings and then to set up designs to see whether these relationships do indeed exist. Clinical settings can also be used to derive nursing research problems. Here one would observe a problem, then research the literature for related theories, studies, and design approaches. It should be noted that in the basic science approach, a wider variety of clinical applications and approaches may be possible since one is not bound to any one clinical problem. The important difference between problem solving and research has been discussed by Wandelt [9] and should be considered carefully in selection of a problem, particularly in the clinical setting.

Regardless of the approach used, flexibility of approach is critical. When one approaches a research problem by applying theory or findings from basic science, one must be certain not to preconceive the solution to the problem. Careful examination of theory and related research should allow one to approach the clinical setting with a number of possible applications in mind and the rationale for selection of a particular setting should relate directly to the theory being tested.

In approaching the definition of the research problem from the clinical settings, the approach may be narrower since it will be confined to the problem selected and related factors. Here again the researcher must be flexible enough to see the relevance of the specific problem being tested to other problems in nursing and must understand the underlying phenomena and theory with which he or she is dealing.

Search of the Literature

A thorough search of the literature is of primary importance in the development of the research study. In approaching this review, the researcher should first make a list of all relevant terms that pertain to the study. At this point, it is wise to project the possible types of design methodology and analysis that could apply to the research problem. These topics can then be researched in the literature so that the experience of other investigators will be available when the critical final choice of the research design, methodology, and analysis is made. In reviewing literature the following categories of topics may be covered:

I. THE PROBLEM
   A. *Has this problem been researched previously? If so, what research approaches, theoretical frameworks were used?*
   B. *Has this problem been recognized but not researched previously?* Frequently the problem has been recognized, but it has not been researched. In that case, there may be reference to the problem in the literature with suggested research approaches, variables involved or cause-and-effect relationships. Such observations and suggestions can be helpful in formulating your own research approach.

II. THEORETICAL FRAMEWORK
   A. *Which theories might be useful in explaining or analyzing this situation or phenomenon?* For example, if one is investigating behavioral responses of hospitalized pediatric preschool patients to specific nursing interventions, theories such as that of the child's cognitive processes response to separation from the mother, separation anxiety, developmental patterns, and physiological capacities should be investigated.
   B. *What are the findings of previous investigators studying this problem? Can these findings be woven together into a theoretical framework useful for predicting relationships between variables in your study?*

III. DESIGN
   A. *What previous studies have been done utilizing designs that may be appropriate?* For example, if you contemplate use of a two-group experimental design, how has this design been used in previous studies? What are its strengths and weaknesses?
   B. *In analyzing the literature pertaining to previous studies on the same or similar problems, what types of designs did previous investigators use? Which designs yielded the best results?*

IV. METHODOLOGY
   You may already know exactly what methodological techniques you will use or you may want to first survey the experience of other investigators with methodological approaches. Regardless of the approach, search the literature for information regarding the technique you select. For example, if you plan to do behavioral observations, ask

questions such as: What are suitable units of behavior for observation? What are reasonable time intervals for observation? Should all presenting behaviors be recorded at each observation time or should only certain types of behavior be recorded? Who will record the behaviors? What techniques of recording will be used?

V. ANALYSIS OF RESULTS

What types of data analysis are appropriate for this problem? How are the data presented in the final research report? Is all of the collected data reported?

VI. REPORTING RESULTS

What types of journals or books report research findings such as you anticipate reporting? What are the styles of these journals? If you are interested in a particular journal, read the section of the journal that pertains to format for contributors. If such a section is not in any of the issues of the journal for one calendar year, write to the editor for specific directions as to formats for presentation of manuscripts.

Such a detailed review of the literature may seem premature when you have just selected a research problem. You may want to approach it by doing certain sections at one time, summarizing your thoughts and then proceeding. However, eventually all of the above topics are covered in search of the literature. With a carefully defined research problem, it is frequently easier to approach the review considering all of the above questions in the initial review.

Analysis of Variables

A *phenomenon* is an observable event, situation, mechanism, reaction, relationship, response, or experience that is the focus of a research design. *Variables* are aspects of the phenomenon that have the capacity to change, move, evolve, exist in different forms, or be altered. Phenomena are thus clusters of variables and hence change themselves. This cluster of variables, or certain of the variables within the cluster, may be variables relating to other phenomena as well. Ideally a variable is as much as possible a single factor. However, such single-factor analysis is rarely possible in the real world and hence any variable should be regarded also as a cluster of subvariables or subfactors. These moving clusters of variables can be a source of challenge and interest or of frustration to the researcher.

There are many types of variables, some of which are of primary importance in the formulation of the design and some of which are necessary for control of the design.

An *independent variable* is the variable that you manipulate or that you view as the cause of some effect. You manipulate a variable when you change it. For example, if you develop a new way of teaching specific types of patients preoperatively, you may want to test this teaching technique in an experimental design. In this case, you have changed the existing technique of instructing patients preoperatively since your teaching technique is new. Your teaching technique is *an* independent variable in the broadest sense. Actually it is a cluster of many variables relating to information given, manner of presentation of information, nurse-patient relationship, and relevance of information to the patient's needs. For simplification in communication, the new technique, in the manner in which it is utilized for your study, is frequently referred to as *the* independent variable.

A *dependent variable* is the variable, or cluster of variables, that you do not manipulate. It is the effect variable, the variable that you hope to change when you introduce the independent variable. In the example of the introduction of a new technique for teaching preoperative patients, the dependent variable might be a variable such as the incidence of vomiting, sleep disturbance, or need for medication postoperatively, or it might be the level of the patient's anxiety measured in some specific way. In hypotheses you state the expected relationship between the independent and dependent variables. For example, you might hypothesize that use of your teaching technique preoperatively—which carefully explains the hospital and operative procedures, possible feelings preoperatively, and help that is available—might decrease the incidence of requests for pain medication postoperatively. Actually, the teaching technique is affecting the patient's cognitive response to his operation and the teaching might in turn decrease his anxiety, modify his physiological responses and perception of pain, and then result in a decrease of requests for pain medication. However, the variable that you are measuring as the effect is that of decrease of requests for pain medication and hence that is the dependent variable for your study. Your theoretical framework should allow you to project that such a response is possible and how it might occur.

Intervening variables are variables exclusive of the independent and dependent variables. They are particularly important in research designs that test hypotheses. These are the variables that can affect either the independent or dependent variables, and thus are necessary for definition of the sample, setting, and research approach.

For example, if one is studying the effect of a new medication on allergic conditions then the previous history of the patient's response to therapy, the type of allergen(s), the family history, age, and general physiological condition of the patient will be variables that could influence the patient's response to the drug therapy.

Intervening variables are of two types: (1) those that can mimic or distort the effect of the dependent variable; and (2) those that can mimic or distort the effect of the independent variable. The effect of the variables could be controlled by selection of a population either all presenting, all lacking, or matched for the variables, by techniques such as balancing or pairing. In this situation, the potentially intervening variable becomes a sample selection variable. For example, in a study of the effect of nursing intervention or separation anxiety of hospitalized children, one would want to control for the child's previous experience with separation from the mother. The study might be limited to subjects experiencing their first separation overnight from their mother. It could also be limited to subjects who had been hospitalized alone previously. Both control and experimental subjects, or both groups of a comparative survey, might include some children who had been separated previously from their mother and other children who had not been separated previously. If potentially intervening variables are not controlled through making them sample selection variables, they are handled by noting their presence through data collection techniques such as observations or interview questions about them. Effects of intervening variables may or may not be analyzed depending on the precision of the measurement and research design.

Extraneous variables are variables that are not the main focus of the study but that could be of interest for future studies. For example, in studying infection rates among preschool children, the occupation of the father might be a variable that would not be of direct concern for control of the primary study but about which data could be collected for future studies.

Selection of the Research Design

Selection of the research design is frequently governed by such practical considerations as patients, facilities, and funds available. For example, it is unrealistic to expect to construct a new type of unit to test the effect of varying the environment on behavioral responses of intensive care patients. Such construction would only be warranted after careful surveying of factors involved in the selected types of behavioral responses studied. A more realistic approach might be to first analyze responses of patients in two different settings, one in which noise of machines and personnel, patients' interruptions, and intense lighting were kept to a minimum and another in which these conditions existed most of the time. Was there really a difference in the behavioral responses such as hallucinations, sleeplessness, and irritability in the patients in the first environment? If so, you would have some basis for recommending that new hospitals utilize the first type of environment.

Second, survey the availability of the sample population. If you intend to study human rabies cases, do not expect to collect a sample of 100 in a 2-month period of data collection in the United States.

TABLE 12.1
Research Design

Question	Design
What are the specific characteristics of a single case or small number of cases of bone marrow transplant patients?	Case study
What are the expressed concerns of mastectomy patients during hospitalization immediately prior to surgery?	Descriptive survey
What is the level of powerlessness in baccalaureate nursing graduates tested by a powerless scale at the end of their first year of clinical practice after graduation?	Evaluative survey
What is the incidence of upper respiratory infections in premature as compared to full-term infants during their first year of life?	Comparative survey
Is there a positive correlation between scores on scale X and clinical expertise as measured by scale Y?	Correlational survey
What is the history of United States nursing care of patients with terminal illnesses?	Historical research
Will explanation and doll play of the technique prior to venipuncture result in more cooperative behavior as measured by X in 3-year-old children receiving venipuncture withdrawal of blood as compared to a similar group of children receiving no explanation or opportunity for doll play?	Experimental research
Will induced immunosuppression of inbred mice increase susceptibility to virus-induced leukemia as compared to mice receiving no immunosuppressive treatment?	Experimental research

On the other hand, if you are studying skin cancer patients, a sample of 100 patients, limited to some age category of even a 2- to 3- year time span, is not unrealistic in a large metropolitan area. Are the data going to be available during the time period when you are planning to collect data? For example, studies of curriculae of nursing educational institutions would be best conducted during the academic year.

Having ascertained that the setting, sample, and personnel that you might utilize for data collection will be available, determine whether it is realistic for you to carry out your design. For example, if you plan to do an experimental design that involves manipulation of the environment, will the hospital or agency allow such changes? Can necessary approvals of agencies, personnel, and subjects be gained for your design?

When the available facilities and personnel have been determined, one can determine the best design for the research problem. In a few ideal situations it is possible to first determine the design and then, regardless of the complexity of the requirements for the facilities and subjects, meet these requirements. However, a more realistic approach is to consider the practical aspects of securing the research environment simultaneously with development of the research design.

In selecting the research design consider the research question that you are asking. Table 12.1 illustrates how the question leads to choice of the design.

Selection of the appropriate design for the research question is important for the design determines the need for control groups, nature of the sample, and analysis techniques.

Selection of the Methodological Techniques

What do you want to know about your research subjects or environment? Are you describing something in quantitative terms only or will you measure something in quantitative terms. Consider first the type of data you wish to collect. Do you want to know whether or not a subject has a characteristic or how much of a characteristic he has? For example, do you want to know whether patients have antibodies to a specific pathogen or do you want to know how much antibody a patient has? Further, do you want to fractionate the antibody, or characterize its in vitro or in vivo activity? In another example, do you want to know whether a patient feels pain after a specific procedure or do you want to measure physiological variables that may correlate with perception of pain? In another example, do you want to know whether or not patients have infections after surgery (considering "infections" to include all types) or do you want to know specific types of infections, their etiology, time of onset, duration, treatment, immune response in the host, complications, and so on?

It is very important to decide just how simple or complex your entire research question is. For example, you may initially ask, What is the rate of postoperative infections in oncology patients receiving a specific type of nursing care postoperatively as compared to patients receiving routine nursing care? However, after examination of the question, you may find that "infection" is too broad a category and that you are really interested in a complete analysis of each infection encountered. First of all, a medical definition must be developed of the presenting symptoms that lead you to conclude that the patient has an infection. Then you may wish to run follow-up laboratory tests to determine the etiology of the infection. Further you may follow treatment, secondary complications, duration of the infection, and immune reactions of the host. Thus, as the question is developed it becomes more complex and more and more variables are important in analysis. The question should be explored exhaustively and all subquestions developed. For example, the above general question on infection rate developed into five subquestions involving: (1) etiological agent; (2) medical treatment; (3) secondary complications; (4) duration of infection; and (5) immune reactions of the host. Other variables could be added.

When all of the questions and subquestions have been asked, appropriate methods must be developed for collection of each of the types of data.

Data Collection

Prior to any data collection, permission of the agencies and subjects to be used must be secured. In some specific types of studies, permission of agency officials rather than the subjects is adequate, but such procedures are subject to careful review. Consult the administrator of the facility that you plan to use for your study regarding procedures for obtaining consent of subjects and supervisory personnel.

Second, determine how you will collect the data mechanically. Will you record all of the interview responses by longhand? Will you use a tape recorder? Will you use a shorthand or code for recording of responses during the interview.

Third, consider the possibility of recording your data in a manner that will facilitate keypunching for eventual computer analysis. Other references outline ways of coding data for this type of analysis [6,10].

Analysis of Findings

The type of data to be collected will determine the type of statistical tests. Several excellent texts and articles deal with this topic in depth [1-8].

Reporting Results

As the research problem, design, and methodology are developed, consider also the manner in which you plan to report your results. If you are planning on publishing in a professional journal, you may have already obtained a copy of the format for manuscript presentation. Follow this format as you write your report and list your references in the manner suggested by the journal. Tables should present data that cannot reasonably be presented in the text.

TEAM RESEARCH VERSUS INDIVIDUAL RESEARCH

The foregoing process of research is one which can be done alone or as a team with other colleagues. Sometimes there are no options. The research is so designed that it is only possible for it to be done by a team of researchers. However, for those situations in which there is a choice, several questions are posed here for thought.

1. What advantages and disadvantages will result if the research is done as a team effort?
2. How will individual contributions to a team effort be identified and rewarded?
3. What are the time restraints on the researchers involved? Is the design such that it is dependent upon certain people? What will happen if those people cannot complete their contributions?
4. When future research evolves, who is likely to lead that effort? Will funding be sought by individuals or the team as a whole for future studies?
5. Are the research abilities of the members of the team complementary in such a way that the loads can be carried in anticipated ways? Arc intrateam member dependencies recognized if they exist?
6. Will access to the sample group be jeopardized in any way by a team effort? If several individuals collect data in the same manner, will their abilities be equivalent? What will be the consequences in differences in data collection styles among team members if such differences exist?

7. If different interpretations of the data result, how will these be handled by the team members?
8. Who will report the results? How will credit be given to the team members?

Each of the above questions would be weighted versus the consequences of attempting the research alone. Most research today is done by teams. Sometimes these are teams of colleagues of equivalent status and responsibility. In other situations the team is headed by a principal investigator who hires assistants for specific tasks in the research process and who utilizes consultants for areas such as data analysis, instrument development, and sample selection.

Basically research is intended to add new knowledge. If it is based upon sound methods, designs, and analysis, new information emerges. Research results usually generate new questions; new questions generate new research, and hence the body of knowledge grows.

REFERENCES

[1] ABDELLAH, F.G., and LEVINE, E. *Better Patient Care Through Nursing Research.* New York: Macmillan, 1979.

[2] BABBIE, E.P. *Survey Research Methods.* Belmont, Calif.: Wadsworth, 1973.

[3] FOX, D.J. *Fundamentals of Research in Nursing,* 3rd ed. Englewood Cliffs, N.J.: Prentice-Hall, Inc., 1976.

[4] KERLINGER, F.N. *Foundations of Behavioral Research,* 2nd ed. New York: Holt, Rinehart & Winston, 1973.

[5] PHILLIPS, J.L. *Statistical Thinking.* San Francisco: W. H. Freeman & Co., 1973.

[6] POLIT, D., and HUNGLER, B. *Nursing Research: Principles and Methods.* Philadelphia: Lippincott, 1978.

[7] SELLTIZ, C.; WRIGHTSMAN, L.S.; and COOK, S.W. *Research Methods in Social Relations,* 3rd ed. New York: Holt, Rinehart & Winston, 1976.

[8] TREECE, E.W., and TREECE, J.W. *Elements of Research in Nursing.* St. Louis: C. V. Mosby, 1973.

[9] WANDELT, M. *Guide for the Beginning Researcher.* Englewood Cliffs, N.J.: Prentice-Hall, Inc., 1970.

[10] NIE, N.H.; HULL, C.H.; JENKINS, J.; STEINBRENNER, K.; and BENT, D.H. Organization and Coding of Data for Input into the SPSS System. In *SPSS Statistical Package for the Social Sciences,* 2nd ed., pp. 21-28. New York: McGraw-Hill Book Co., 1975.

chapter thirteen

ANAYIS DERDIARIAN, R.N., M.N.
Assistant Clinical Professor
Teaching in Graduate Nursing
Oncology Program
School of Nursing, UCLA

Nursing conceptual frameworks: Implications for education, practice, and research

INTRODUCTION

Disciplines are identified according to their methods and their underlying concepts. Such identification has not been accorded to nursing, essentially because—as this author sees it—nursing's method is not visible to the nurse, nor is it visible to the client or the professional colleague. This lack of method, and therefore of systematized practice, seems to underlie most of the ill fate experienced by the nursing profession as it attempts to maintain good balance in the practice scene of the health professions. One of the logical and practical ways to overcome this lack is to adopt "good" nursing models and utilize them as instruments for systematization of practice, development of curriculae consistent with that practice, and generation of research from such practice to improve future practice. The implied intent of the chapter is to think about the future of cancer nursing introspectively and prospectively, in the hope that cancer nursing will develop as a specialty and benefit from past mistakes of the nursing profession. Specializations have greater potential than general practice to develop their science and professional identity, because practice in a population of patients with similar health problems, age, sex, and in similar settings can be more controlled and thus more suitable for research. The development of science in cancer nursing will be dependent on the identification of the professional goal, theory development, and research—all of which begin with a consistent view of the patient and of nursing.

Within the last three decades, several conceptual frameworks for nursing practice have been developed in an attempt to answer the inevitable question raised by society and nurses with respect to the nature of nursing and its particular contribution to human welfare. Although such frameworks are still embryonic in development, elements of a few are presently undergoing empirical testing. However, the full value of those frameworks for nursing practice, research, and education remains to be realized. The realization of this value will be dependent on systematic and consistent use of such frameworks in practice, thus making possible: (1) the evaluation and improvement of practice; and (2) the generation of researchable questions related to nursing practice.

THE NEED FOR CONCEPTUAL FRAMEWORKS FOR PROFESSIONAL PRACTICE

Professional practice implies two complex and interrelated concepts— *professional* and *practice*. An understanding of these concepts is essential for understanding the matrix of interrelationships of the various professions involved in the health care system. This understanding not only sheds light on interprofessional gaps, overlaps, and conflicts—all of which are likely to affect society and the patients, the recipients of health care—but it sheds light also on the nature, scope, and method of practice of each profession in that matrix. One of the ways of developing such understanding is through developing an ability to conceptualize the goal and the method of a particular profession; that is, through developing conceptual clarity about the particular ills of the society with which the profession is concerned and about which it possesses the knowledge necessary to understand them and the method necessary to deal with them. Research in the established professions has flourished, in great part, due to the conceptual clarity of the professionals with regard to their profession's goal and its mission to human welfare. In better-established professions, such as medicine, the neophyte is socialized into the profession during generic training with: (1) conceptual clarity about the profession's goal—to cure the ills or the disease(s) of the human body; and (2) tools available to achieve this goal—through a wealth of medical technology respective to medical problems and interventions. Such conceptual clarity about professional goals has become crucial to the development of medical technology and therefore it has been directly responsible for the profession's success in acquiring society's sanction for its professional power, especially in respect to its capability to alleviate the physical ills of the society which it has accepted as its professional charge.

Professionalism and Practice

The term *professional* is defined in the dictionary as ". . . a vocation or occupation requiring advanced training in some liberal art or science, and usually involving mental rather than manual work. . . ." The term *practice* is defined as ". . . to do, exercise, or perform frequently or usually; make a habit or custom of. . . ." [6]. Thus the relationship of the term *professional* to the term *practice* is that a particular knowledge or skill is put into action in order to achieve a goal. Freidson contends that professionalism is a symbol to persuade others that: (1) one's occupational outcome is important, needed, and good; and (2) that this "good" is the function of one's particular knowledge and training of which others are deprived [4].

The formal criteria of a profession, according to Goode, are derived from two core characteristics. The first is a prolonged specialized training in a body of abstract knowledge; the second is collectivity or service orientation. Out of those core characteristics emerge the characteristics of autonomy of a profession [5]. Freidson, in addition to concurring with Goode, defines this autonomy in operational terms as: (1) a basic systematic theory that leads to a profession's skills; (2) authority that is recognized by clients; (3) authority that is recognized by the community through licensure; (4) a code of ethics; and (5) a professional culture [4].

Implicit in those authors' contentions are the notions that the profession: (1) determines the parameters of the area of its practice—thus it declares the nature of the ills of the humankind with which it is primarily concerned; (2) possesses the know-how enabling it to identify *normalcy* from *deviancy* and the tools with which to distinguish those; (3) determines the nature and the scope of the educational training of its neophytes; (4) controls the efficacy of professional practice through explicating its expectations of uniform and acceptable practice through means of licensure, peer review, research publication, and the like; and (5) assumes responsibility to maintain congruence of professional goals with societal need for the outcome of the profession's practice.

CONCEPTUAL FRAMEWORK AND PROFESSIONALISM

One of the academic reasons basic to medicine's success in establishing itself as a profession is believed, by this author, to be the fact that the medical profession possesses a conceptual framework in the biological model that undergirds its professional education, practice, development of research, and accumulation of knowledge. It is not within the scope of this chapter to discuss the morality or the "goodness" and the "badness" of using models in developing knowledge; rather, the intent here is to discuss the advantages of using models as tools in the systematization of practice, in the observation of outcome of practice, and thus in the development of professional knowledge. It was to this end that conceptual frameworks for nursing practice were created.

Characteristics of Models

Although several nursing models have been in existence, not all meet the criteria of being useful, good, or complete models. Consequently, not only are they of limited usefulness, they also cause precautious rejection of the idea of models for practice. Therefore, it is important to know the basic characteristics of good models in examining a particular model for professional education, practice, and research.

A good conceptual model must reflect the major components of a profession's practice. Those components are: (1) the goal or outcome of professional practice; (2) the nature of the problem—the potential target of the profession's action; (3) the sources of difficulty—the nature of potentially etiologic factors of the problems; (4) the actor's role—the role definition of the professional; and (5) the nature and the methods of professional interventions. Furthermore, such a model must reflect, implicitly or explicitly, the value system of the profession—the minimum acceptable outcome of professional action, the expected desired outcome of professional action and, therefore, standards of professional practice [1].

Functions of Models

As a general attribute, models provide meaningful contexts within which specific findings can be located as significant details [6].

Although this is true and important, it is not an attribute distinctive of models. Theories in general guide data collection and their subsequent analysis by indicating beforehand where data are to be fitted and what is to be done with them when they are obtained. Without theory, observations are a loose variety of incidences having no significance either in themselves or in the context or situation from which they have been arbitrarily or accidentally selected. Besides data organization, some of the more salient functions of models include theory explication, theory stabilization, establishment of communication, and theory validation.

Data Organization. Although theories guide observations, thus moving observations further away from intuitive, subjective data, they do not guide the observer in gathering discrete, useful data. If the theory is ill defined in the mind of the observer, the resulting observations are vague, untidy, and flighty. Theories are remote and illusive inventions of the mind until they are explicated. Models, on the other hand, make the theory conscious, explicit, tangible, and more definite. Thus, models not only crystallize theory in the mind that invents it, but in so doing, they also render the theory tangible to the minds of others [6].

Theory Explication. In making theory more explicit and tangible, the model makes the major concepts of the theory more clearly visible in terms of their nature, relations, and the underlying scheme which orders the relationship. Each such component becomes available for individual treatment in terms of understanding of its functional contribution to the theory.

Theory Stabilization. Explication of theory renders it more stable in the minds of the inventor and others alike. This not only allows the holding of an idea in an "as if" fashion until data supports its validity, totally or partially, but it also forms a basis for reference for future reenvisionment of the theory [6].

Establishment of Communication. Models, as described, generate communication about the idea among those who have the theory as the subject matter. This not only renders communication more effective and efficient but also allows input of many who discuss it, use it, or evaluate it, in relation to its validity and usefulness in describing or testing the congruence of theory with the piece of reality it represents [6].

Generation of Theory Validation. In making theory explicable, tangible, and mediatory for communication, models not only provide enhancement of evaluation of the theory as valid or complete, but they also potentiate the validation of the theory through testing in multiplicative efforts.

Shortcomings of Models

Models, like other human inventions, are not exempt from imperfections. Those, however, are not reasons for discarding the idea of models. If better-established disciplines such as chemistry, physics, mathematics, biology, sociology, or psychology had done this, these disciplines would have deprived humankind of knowledge and progress. By taking into account the shortcomings, and thus using their respective models skillfully, the scientists in those fields have: (1) generated knowledge; and (2) modified the models they used to obtain more knowledge. Since the usefulness of models depends on the skill and sophistication of the one using them, the following shortcomings may not inhibit the potential benefits of models, except when they are used by unskilled hands.

Overemphasis on Models. Models are symbolic representations of theories and not of the truth temporarily represented in the theory. A pictorial or written representation of an individual, an object, a place, or a concept is not the actual individual, object, place, or concept [6]. Thus placing more emphasis on models, as if they were the reflection of truth or the representation of reality, impedes scientific inquiry. Therefore, models need to be referred to as temporary symbols.

Overemphasis on Structure. Models, as representations of theories invented by the mind, hold an isomorphic resemblance to those theories. As such, their explications represent particular structures. Often, it is assumed that there is a certain logic or rationality about that structure in representing the theory—which, scientifically speaking, may represent imperfect truth. Thus, utilization and testing of models, in time, would yield knowledge about the congruence of the structure with the truth represented in the theory [6].

Oversimplification of Form. Although models reduce theories to understandable form, thus simplifying them, they may simplify them to the extent that they no longer represent details essential to enhancing the understanding of the theory they represent. Thus, those who create and use models need to take into account this potential problem [6].

Nursing is ill defined as a field of practice or inquiry at the present. Although the generally agreed upon statement, that nursing is concerned first with the person who is ill rather than the illness, implies a strong commitment to a goal of health for the members of society, the fact is that there is no identifiable professional goal commonly recognized and accepted by all nurses [2]. Furthermore, there is no common, specific, identifiable description of nursing practice. More tragically, while nurses think that they have a common goal for patient welfare, they are unable to distinguish this goal from those of other health professionals such as the physician, the psychiatrist, or the social worker. Consequently, each nurse practices according to the individual conception she or he holds as to the proper focus of nursing's concern and, thus, nursing's goal in patient care. This state of affairs, in turn, only exacerbates the confusion about professional goals, modes of practice, outcomes of practice, and objects of research.

This confusion also explains the lack of certain elements common to the practice of nurses. For example, the outcome of nursing is not visible, in measurable terms, to the nurse; neither is it so visible to the collaborating professions or to the recipient of nursing care. In general, nursing's role is seen as supplementary rather than complementary to the practices of other professionals in physical or mental health care. However, defining the role of nursing as primarily *complementary* is more useful in explicating the goal of nursing as it relates to the goals of other health professionals. When the goals of the various professions are clearly distinguished: (1) the goal of each individual profession is envisioned in relation to the goals of other professions within the context of the entire health care delivery system; and (2) the overlaps and the gaps among those professions' practices are more accessible for proper treatment. More importantly, defining a truly complementary role for nursing is necessary for discerning the direction for inquiry into the scientific bases of its practice consistent with this role. This complementary role must be defined in terms of: (1) the primary mission of nursing to meet the specific needs of society it claims to be its aim; and (2) the parameters of the *care,* the *cure,* and the *coordination* it claims as the core elements of its practice.

More specifically, the nature and the extent of the *care,* the *cure,* and the *coordination* aspects of nursing practice need to be defined with respect to nursing's role as it complements those of other health professions. Only then will nursing be able to distinguish its supplementary role from its complementary role and to answer the questions: Does nursing merely extend the role(s) of other health professionals or does it do this in concert with its own role? How much of extending of others' roles does nursing do in proportion to extending of its own role in delivery of care, cure, and coordination?

IMPLICATIONS FOR NURSING EDUCATION

As mentioned earlier, one of the characteristics of a profession is its ability to determine the parameters of professional education. It does this by deriving direction from the profession's goal, and for the sake of keeping the profession's goal consistent with the practice goal of the individual professional. Ideally, it does this in accordance with the society's needs for the profession's contributions [1].

Because nursing is not very well-defined as a profession at the present, the content and the methodology for training nursing professionals at various levels is largely determined by the institutions employing the products of nursing programs. Thus, the parameters for professional training are, for the most part, determined by the job descriptions formulated by the employing agencies according to their particular needs. The nature of those needs in turn are determined, for the most part, by medical and technological changes [2]. This situation, coupled with the variety of philosophies about the goal and function of nursing held by individual schools of nursing, gives rise to the diversities of content and method of curriculae among those schools. Although common ground exists, emphasis in curriculum content and practicum varies according to the goal of nursing subscribed to by a particular school. Thus, each school may justify its program in reference to its own vision of nursing rather than in reference to a vision accepted by the profession as a whole. As a result, the frame of reference for practice and the professional behavior of the neophyte professional reflect the philosophy and the ideology of the particular school. This, when viewed in the context of the multiplicity of schools of nursing, explains the confusion of the nurses—as well as that of other health-related disciplines, and of the society at large—about the goal of nursing practice.

It has been proposed, therefore, that adaptation of a nursing model would provide schools of nursing with a philosophy about nursing and a goal for nursing practice that would direct selection of content and method in curriculum development. Conceptualizing nursing in a way consistent with the school's training would provide systematic and consistent practice behavior in the practitioners individually and collectively. This, in turn, is essential for the systematization of observations *about* the practice—an essential behavior of professional practice and the basis for the development of knowledge in nursing. The use of a particular model implies that the delineation of content and method of curriculum development ought to be based on the particular goal provided by that model. A clear conceptualization of nursing's goal on the part of a school will undoubtedly help its neophytes to a clear conceptualization of the professional goal. Such clarity about the professional role of nursing will thus prevent confusion—on the part of the nurse, the other professionals, the recipient of health care, and the society—about nursing's role and function in the health care system. With conceptual clarity about nursing's professional goal the neophyte will be able to develop professional identity and maintain discretion in rendering nursing care without encroaching upon the practice domain of the physician, the clinical psychologist, the psychiatrist, the social worker, or the pharmacist. With this conceptual clarity, moreover, nursing can aid other colleagues to view and understand nursing, and thus align their practices with nursing in more efficient and economical collaboration.

Conceptual clarity and consistency derived from a model of nursing can and should provide the framework for curriculum development at all levels, including generic, graduate, postgraduate, and continuing educational programs.

IMPLICATIONS FOR NURSING PRACTICE

Although nurses generally agree on a goal of nursing, disagreement arises in the operational definition of this goal. Therefore, the operational definition of the outcomes, the methods, and the standards of nursing practice vary according to the goal viewed by the particular practitioner. It is reasonable to assume that there is a lack of consistency about the goals of nursing not only among various professionals but also within the individual nurse across various clinical situations [2].

Consistency of practice is essential for accumulation of knowledge to improve future practice. Lack of appropriate consideration and action is believed to hinder systematization of individual as well as collective practice. Systematization of practice is essential to the understanding of the elements of professional practice and thus to the derivation of the scientific bases of that practice. Systematized practice is a basic requirement for the identification and description of the nature of that practice. Furthermore, systematized practice is indispensable for the generation of knowledge about nursing practice and for the improvement of this practice over time. Systematization of practice is possible only if practice is viewed in a consistent way across clinical situations and across individual and/or collective practice. Consistency of viewing practice is in turn dependent upon the goal of nursing practice as perceived by the practitioner at a point in time. Thus, a common frame of reference for nursing practice would provide a common goal for nursing practice to all practitioners, irrespective of the changes in the clinical situations.

Although it may be argued that any goal provided by a model for nursing practice may not be acceptable, encompassing, or useful to all clinicians, the important point is to adopt a goal and model for nursing practice, at least temporarily, in order to systematize practice. In time, as the model is used, data concerning the usefulness of the model as well as indicating needed modifications of the model will be available. It must be borne in mind, as mentioned earlier, that not all models for nursing practice are "good" models; that is, not all models have the essential characteristics and scientific merits of a good model. Nurses need to discriminate against such models basing their judgments upon the characteristics basic to good models [2].

However temporarily it is used, a good nursing model would provide the clinician with a philosophy and goal of nursing and, thus, a direction for nursing practice. A goal for practice is necessary as a basis for envisioning outcomes of practice and evaluating those outcomes as "good" or "not as good." Temporary as models may be, they render practice tangible to the individual practitioner and others for examination and analysis. They engender a common reference for communication about nursing practice among practitioners using a particular nursing model. They indicate needed changes in the practice and thus make possible the improvement of practice. Therefore, data about nursing practice as well as the particular model would be available for improving both. Temporary yet practical treatment of some good models for nursing practice would, in time, help identify the elements common to those models and common to nursing. It is the belief of this author that models share commonalities more than diversities.

In essence, nursing models are instruments through which systematization of practice, observation, and analysis of practice outcomes are made possible. Their greatest potential is in their common property of being instrumental in representing nursing goals—and, therefore, nursing practice and outcomes—in a specific, defined, and identifiable way.

IMPLICATIONS FOR RESEARCH

Even though nursing has contributed abundant knowledge to the field of health, this contribution has not directly and specifically affected nursing practice. Information retrievable from empirical as well as basic research has not been consistently or systematically used to improve practice or increase the wealth of knowledge. One major reason for this failure is that generation of research or hypotheses has not taken place in a systematic way. Although information is used to expand the knowledge base of the individual practitioner and thus may have an indirect influence on practice, research findings used in a deliberate and controlled manner are not yet being used to improve practice. Generation of research has followed academic interest rather than clinical necessity. Generation of research following clinical interest can be expected to increase only if the practice is consistent and systematic. Thus the points made with respect to clinical practice are also pertinent in thinking about models as they relate to nursing research [2].

The systematization of practice which is a necessary condition for generating hypotheses related to nursing practice has been and continues to be lacking. Nursing practice has been and continues to be what the individual nurse or the employer defines it to be. Thus a definition of the field of nursing—that is, of the nature of nursing practice—is necessary. Research is necessary to identify and describe the *ingredients* of nursing practice, specifically: (1) the problems and their descriptions; and (2) the interventions and their descriptions. Research is necessary to identify and describe the *method* of nursing practice. In essence, it is necessary to identify areas of research priority related to the practice of nursing, that is, a rationale for researching what nursing must research.

Clearly, the ingredient necessary for grappling with the research objectives implied above is systematization of nursing practice, the feasibility of which is dependent upon the conceptualization of the goal of nursing in a specific way. Models, it is proposed, can serve as bases for systematization of nursing practice. Models, as inventions of the minds of nurse theorists, exemplify nursing in some organized way. Research to test the comprehensiveness and usefulness of those models is needed. Research to test the usefulness of outcomes or methods of nursing practice indicated by nursing models is necessary to the understanding of the field of nursing. Utilization of nursing models consistently and systematically would lead to hypotheses relating to nursing problems and nursing interventions.

APPLICATION OF MODELS TO CANCER NURSING

The application of models to nursing as a whole is difficult and often seemingly impractical. However, while such attempts have frequently resulted in notable failures, they have also contributed valuable understanding of some of the difficulties, and provided insight into refining future attempts. The application of models to specialties in nursing is simpler and more manageable. Specializations have a greater potential than general practice to contribute to the development of nursing theory, of nursing science, and thus to the identification of the field of nursing inquiry and practice. They address themselves to populations of patients with similar health problems, sex, age, or in similar settings; thus, they enable better identification and control of common variables. Those variables, by and large, determine and affect practice and therefore the content of education, as well as influence the development of research [2]. The application of models to various specializations, in time, would yield data for the comparison and extraction of common areas and discernment of the ingredients for building a model of nursing [2].

Cancer nursing as a specialty of the nursing profession, can create a prototype—a model—in exemplifying the methods of operationally defining models for practice, curriculum development, and research development. Such an attempt has been in effect at the UCLA School of Nursing since 1975, where the Johnson Behavioral Systems Model has been used as the conceptual base for the Cancer Nursing Specialization program. This model, along with—to a lesser extent—the Peplau, Roy, and Orem models, is used for the development of assessment tools for the nursing process. The Johnson model is favored for its comprehensiveness and sophistication of conceptualization, characteristics that have rendered possible the task of developing the theoretical constructs respective to the model's components. Also, it has proven particularly useful, in this sense, in clinical use. Research in this area is currently ongoing.

A general discussion of the application of the Johnson model to curriculum development, practice, and research development is presented here. Evaluation of outcomes with respect to the usefulness of the model to any of those areas of exploration is not possible, as data related to such outcomes is not yet available. The curriculum design and components and a synopsis of the Johnson model are given in their respective models in the following sections.

Application of the Johnson Model to Cancer Nursing Education

As discussed earlier, the goal for professional practice is the point of venture for curriculum design. Because there is currently no declared concensus about a definition of nursing, and therefore no identifiable professional goal, the goal of the Johnson model is adopted temporarily. The goal of this model is expressed in its philosophy regarding: (1) man as a biopsychosocial being striving to maintain a balance in adaptation to the influences of his or her environment; and (2) nursing's role in relation to such attempts by man. Intrinsic to this philosophy are the elements of the view of man as an open system in constant interaction with his or her environment. Eight subsystems and their respective goals and parts are identified. The function of the subsystem is to contribute to the overall system balance through maintaining: (1) intact function in the subsystems; (2) appropriate interaction; and (3) functional interdependence. The system, as influenced by internal and external forces of man's environment, sustains imbalances as man strives to bring it back to his or her usual level of equilibrium. Depending on the magnitude of the imbalance, man may need supplementary and complementary assistance from the environment to regain equilibrium. Illness is viewed as a noxious stimulus affecting the intra- and/or intersubsystem equilibrium. Nursing's role is envisioned as an external force necessary in assisting man to regain the harmony in the subsystem(s), and thus in the overall system.

This philosophy guides not only the selection and the sequencing of the content in the curriculum development, but also its implementation. Exposure to the concept of models in general and the understanding of one model in particular and its application to nursing practice come early in the education of the learner. Research and advanced research courses are taught concurrently with the nursing theory courses. Those enable the student to relate to the theoretical aspects of the model and its function in the systematization of practice and observation. The content from basic and medical sciences is taught concurrently and/or in direct sequence to the theory and research courses. This content is necessary to understand and assess comprehensively the clinical aspects of the disease and/or the treatment of cancer. The content is taught in the context of the model's application. The clinical courses follow in which the learner is expected to observe, analyze, interpret, and evaluate data relevant to the description and definition of: (1) patient problems; (2) nursing interventions; and (3) patient outcomes. The format of documentation is the Problem-Oriented Recording method. The common ultimate goal for the clinical courses is the generation of hypotheses with respect to practice of cancer nursing.

Such use of the model in curriculum design and implementation, over time, allows the learners to develop theses from their observations or from observations made previously in the areas of nursing problems in various clinical settings where care of the cancer patient takes place. Observations with respect to nursing interventions also yield similar fruitful arenas for research. Such a deliberate approach to the education of nurses specializing in cancer nursing culminates in two important and interrelated outcomes. The first is the retrieval of data relevant to understanding the patient in "nursing" terms. Presently, the most critical consideration in graduate nursing education is to provide the student with the theoretical content and skill to: (1) delineate and identify the nursing problems and nursing interventions from those of other disciplines; and (2) describe and document these for further exploration and refinement. Thus, a critical and analytical approach to and practice of nursing practice is believed to benefit not only the profession, but more importantly the cancer patient. The second outcome is the retrieval of data relevant to evaluating the useful or the unintended outcomes of utilizing the conceptual framework approach in the education of clinicians [2].

Application of the Johnson Model
to Cancer Nursing Service

There are two main elements of practice: (1) the ability of the clinician to identify, and therefore to diagnose, problems specific to his or her professional goal; and (2) the ability to intervene and obtain intended outcomes. The usefulness, and thus the compatibility of the professional goal with the need of the society the profession serves, is measured in terms of the extent of the ability of the practitioners to render cure of particular ailments of society [2]. The thrust of the model, in this respect, is in its instrumentality in rendering the practice of the practitioner systematic, analytic, deliberate, and accountable. All these characteristics can be achieved, presently, based on theoretical support through the theoretical underpinnings of the model. Thus, practice in which the model is used is not the result of intuitive, haphazard dependency on recall of observations of the past or of the others, but it is current, tangible, measurable, and modifiable.

The model, its goal, assumptions, and theoretical underpinnings come to bear on the method of the implementation of the nursing process. Since the model is the instrument consistently used in assessing patients and intervening in their processes, with the view of man and the view of the nurse's role held as constant as possible, the individual differences of patients' experiences are better identified from one cancer patient to another. Furthermore, gross differences across populations of cancer patients defined by particular descriptions of medical diagnosis, treatment, age, or sex can be identified, described, and explored in terms of prevalence of particular nursing problems. Similarly, particular nursing interventions can be so studied in terms of their specificity and effectiveness with respect to those populations.

Such deliberate practice, based on clear theoretical bases, not only renders practice accountable but also makes it more immediately beneficial to the recipients of care. Economies of time, effort, and coordination afford the patient with intended and needed care more quickly. Comprehensive and deliberate nursing assessment and intervention not only enable nursing's unique and particular contribution to the overall care that the patient and the family receive from the health care team, but they also assist the other professionals in envisioning the patient in the same consistent way the nurse does. This allows the proper orientation of the input of the other professionals into the overall care of the patient. Therefore, not only the caring and curing aspects of the nursing roles, but also the coordinating aspects are orchestrated in a systematic and therefore effective and efficient way.

Application of the Johnson Model to Cancer Nursing Research

Since Chapters 11 and 12 are devoted to the comprehensive coverage of the topic of research as it relates to cancer nursing, only the research aspects that specifically relate to the model and its implementation will be presented here. The basic philosophy underlying this section is that in order for nursing research to affect improvement of nursing care, such research must emerge from nursing practice. Hypotheses for cancer nursing research must be formulated by practitioners of cancer nursing. Furthermore, research findings need to be implemented and evaluated by practitioners of cancer nursing. The practical difficulties here are: (1) lack of a definition of nursing problems, interventions, and outcomes; (2) lack of a systematized method of assessment and intervention; and (3) lack of support for systematized nursing practice and research on the part of the health care facilities. However, graduate students training for cancer nursing specialization on the master's level, primarily, and those training on the doctoral level, would be the force facilitating the exchange of the hypotheses and research findings between the clinician and the researcher. Both will be inhibited, or toil less fruitfully, unless there is systematized practice. The model can be taught at all levels of cancer nursing education employing a degree of sophistication for its utility appropriate to the goals of education at each level.

The use of the model in practice leads to the development of concerted, coordinated effort in research. Moving toward and building on related hypotheses would render research stronger, more economical, and more immediate in its benefit to the patient [10]. In the wake of the development of cancer nursing as a specialization, research generated from systematic observations would be descriptive of the nursing problems and their associated relationships to their determinants in given populations. Explored over clinical stages of the disease and its treatment, morphological variations may be described also. Multiplied by the variety of possible population descriptions, such research would yield invaluable data relevant to defining nursing problems. Nursing interventions also can be subjected to such descriptive research. Thus, knowledge relevant to the nursing problems and intervention would increase [2].

Finally, use of the model over time would allow evaluation of its usefulness in practice, education, and research. Data generated in using the model in nursing care plans could be compared with data generated through conventional practice of nursing. Data generated through exploration of the impact of model-based education on the behavior of the practitioner may enable a comparison with the behavior of the practitioner trained through conventional programs. Evaluative research can explore the difference in the sense of professional goal and identity on the part of the nurses trained through model-based programs compared with the sense of goal and identity of those trained through conventional programs. Explorations may also be conducted to determine whether there are differences in the cancer patients', their families', and other professionals' perceptions of the nurse in relating to nurses using a model and to those not using models.

CONCLUSION

The usefulness of the conceptual frameworks for nursing is intrinsic to their nature of being instruments. They themselves are not nursing theories, but they are instrumental constructs to help develop nursing theory. Such theory building necessarily begins with systematizing practice and observation in relation to nursing education and nursing practice. The relationship of frameworks or models to actual practice, education, or research is analogous to the relationship of *potential* energy to *kinetic* energy. Their contribution to all aspects of nursing is currently *potential* and as such not too utilitarian to either the profession or the society. It is in the transformation of this *potential* to *kinetic* utility of the models, in the hands of the clinician, educator, and the researcher, that they will consume themselves in fruitful meaning for nursing and the patient. In essence, they are means to define the content and the method of nursing as a discipline.

REFERENCES

[1] DERDIARIAN. A. Education: A Way of Theory Construction in Nursing. *Journal of Nursing Education*, 18:36–45, 1979.

[2] DERDIARIAN, A. Roles and Directions in Cancer Nursing Education. *Proceedings of the Second National Conference on Cancer*, St. Louis, May 1977, pp. 17–22.

[3] JOHNSON, D. A Philosophy of Nursing. *Nursing Outlook*, 7:198–200, 1959.

[4] FREIDSON, E. *Profession of Medicine*. New York: Dodd, Mead, 1970.

[5] GOODE, W. Psychology, Medicine, and Sociology. *American Sociology Review*, 25 D60:902–914, 1960.

[6] KAPLAN, A. *The Conduct of Inquiry*. San Francisco: Chandler, 1964.

[7] NEWLIN, N. Development of Methodology and Examination of Characteristics of Oncology Patient Utilizing Johnson's Nursing Model. Unpublished thesis, UCLA School of Nursing.

[8] *Webster's New World Dictionary—College Edition*. New York: Collins and World, 1962.

[9] DERDIARIAN, A. Summation Notes. *First Conference on Cancer Nursing Research*, Los Angeles, California, May 1979.

ADDITIONAL READINGS

AUGER, J. *Behavioral Systems and Nursing.* Englewood Cliffs, N.J.: Prentice-Hall, Inc., 1976.

BRODBECK, M. Models, Meaning, and Theories. In *Symposium on Sociological Theory*, pp. 373–403. Evanston, Ill.: Row, Peterson, 1959.

CHIN, R. The Utility of System Models and Developmental Models for Practitioners. In *The Planning of Change*, pp. 201-214. New York: Holt, Rinehart, and Winston, 1961.

DILWORTH, A. Goals for Nursing. *Nursing Outlook*, 11(5):336-340, 1963.

DRISCOLL, V. Liberating Nursing Practice. *Nursing Outlook*, 20(1):24-28, 1972.

GUNTER, L. Notes on a Theoretical Framework for Nursing Research. *Nursing Research*, 11(4):219-222, 1962.

LEONARD, R. Developing Research in a Practice-Oriented Discipline. *American Journal of Nursing*, 67(7):1472-1475, 1967.

LYNAUGH, J.E., and BATES, B. The Two Languages of Nursing and Medicine. *American Journal of Nursing*, 73(1):66-69, 1973.

MOORE, M.A. The Professional Practice of Nursing. *Nursing Forum*, VIII(4): 361-373, 1969.

NEWMAN, M. Nursing's Theoretical Evolution. *Nursing Outlook*, 20(7):449-453, 1972.

ROGERS, M. Nursing: To Be or Not to Be. *Nursing Outlook*, 20(1):42-46, 1972.

ROY, SISTER CALLISTA. Adaptation: Implications for Curriculum Change. *Nursing Outlook*, 21:163-168, 1973.

ROY, C. *Conceptual Models for Nursing*, 2nd ed. Englewood Cliffs, N.J.: Prentice-Hall, Inc., in press.

ROY, SISTER CALLISTA. *Introduction to Nursing*. Englewood Cliffs, N.J.: Prentice-Hall, Inc., 1976.

WIEDENBACH, E. Nurses' Wisdom in Nursing Theory. *American Journal of Nursing*, 70(5):1057-1062, 1970.

Index